Physician Assistant
Board Review
Certification and
Recertification

Physician Assistant Board Review
Certification and Recertification

Edited by

James Van Rhee, M.S., PA-C
Chair, Physician Assistant Department
Wake Forest University
Winston-Salem, North Carolina

SAUNDERS
ELSEVIER

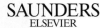

SAUNDERS
ELSEVIER

The 1600 Jhon F. Kennedy Blvd.
Suite 1800
Philadelphia, PA 19103-2899

Physician Assistant Board Review: Certification and Recertification

ISBN-13: 978-1-4160-2598-6
ISBN-10: 1-4160-2598-7

Notice

Knowledge and best practice in this field are constantly changing. As new research and experience broaden our knowledge, changes in practice, treatment and drug therapy may become necessary or appropriate. Readers are advised to check the most current information provided (i) on procedures featured or (ii) by the manufacturer of each product to be administered, to verify the recommended dose or formula, the method and duration of administration, and contraindications. It is the responsibility of the practitioner, relying on their own experience and knowledge of the patient, to make diagnoses, to determine dosages and the best treatment for each individual patient, and to take all appropriate safety precautions. To the fullest extent of the law, neither the Publisher nor the Author assumes any liability for any injury and/or damage to property arising out or related to any use of the material contained in this book.

The Publisher

Library of Congress Cataloging in Publication Data
Physician assistant board review certification and recertification / edited by James Van Rhee.
    p. cm.
  ISBN 1-4160-2598-7
  1. Physicians' assistants–Examinations, questions, etc. I. Van Rhee, James.

R697.P45P482 2006
610.76–dc22

2006045027

Acquisitions Editor: Rolla Couchman
Developmental Editor: Dylan Parker
Project Manager: David Saltzberg
Marketing Manager: Kimberly Hamm
Design Direction: Louis Forgione

Printed in the United States of America

Last digit is the print number: 9 8 7 6 5 4 3 2 1

This book is dedicated to my family, who had to put up with me during all the hours spent writing and reviewing this manuscript.

Thanks to all the physician assistant students I have had contact with over the years and to all the physician assistants who have attended my board review courses, without all of you this book would not have been possible. Thanks also to CW and EV for reviewing parts of the book, your input was most helpful.

Preface

The PANCE or PANRE are examinations that all physician assistants are familiar with. Many view the examinations with fear and trepidation. This book is here to help.

Many board review books offer a review of the examination content with sample questions and explanations. This provides the test taker with the opportunity to review material and to highlight the areas where additional review is needed. This book also provides sample tests and a review of examination content. However, this book differs in a number of ways:

- Sample questions are provided throughout the text to assist the reader in assessing their retention of knowledge.

- Numerous photos, tables, charts, and graphs are provided to enhance the learning and provide another avenue of review.
- A color plate of photos is included to provide the reader with more than just a written description o selected disease states.
- An on-line examination is also available to you after purchasing this book. This examination will provide you with a "real-life" experience taking the exam.

I think you will find this book easy to use and very helpful as you prepare for the PANCE or PANRE examination.

James Van Rhee, M.S., PA-C

Contents

Color Plate section follows Chapter 8.

Cardiovascular System

EXAM BLUEPRINT TOPICS

Cardiomyopathy
Dilated
Hypertrophic
Restrictive
Conduction Disorders
Atrial fibrillation/flutter
Atrioventricular block
Bundle branch block
Paroxysmal supraventricular tachycardia
Premature beats
Ventricular tachycardia
Ventricular fibrillation/flutter
Congenital Heart Disease
Atrial septal defect
Coarctation of aorta
Patent ductus arteriosus
Tetralogy of Fallot
Ventricular septal defect
Congestive Heart Failure
Hypertension
Essential
Secondary
Malignant
Hypotension
Cardiogenic shock
Orthostatic/postural
Ischemic Heart Disease
Acute myocardial infarction
Angina pectoris

- Stable
- Unstable
- Prinzmetal's variant

Vascular Disease
Acute rheumatic fever

Aortic aneurysm
Aortic dissection
Arterial embolism/thrombosis
Chronic/acute arterial occlusion
Giant cell arteritis
Phlebitis/thrombophlebitis
Venous thrombosis
Varicose veins
Valvular Disease
Aortic stenosis
Aortic insufficiency
Mitral stenosis
Mitral insufficiency
Mitral valve prolapse
Tricuspid insufficiency
Pulmonary stenosis
Other Forms of Heart Disease
Acute/subacute bacterial endocarditis
Acute pericarditis
Cardiac tamponade
Pericardial effusion

CARDIOMYOPATHY

I. Dilated
   a. General
      i. Caused by malfunction of the myocardium.
      ii. Most common cause is alcohol abuse.
         1. Etiology may also be idiopathic, infectious, or drugs.
      iii. Cardiac dilatation leads to right and left systolic dysfunction and then congestive heart failure.
   b. Clinical manifestations
      i. Most common first symptom is exertional intolerance.

NOTES

ii. Other signs and symptoms are same as congestive heart failure.
1. Include dyspnea, orthopnea, and edema in the lower extremities.
2. Chest pain may also be noted.
iii. Physical examination reveals an S_3 on cardiac exam, and crackles are noted on examination of the lungs.
1. Mitral regurgitation may also be noted.

c. Diagnosis
i. On electrocardiogram (EKG), nonspecific ST and T wave changes may be noted along with left bundle branch block (LBBB).
ii. Chest X-ray reveals cardiomegaly and pulmonary vascular congestion.
iii. Echocardiogram reveals dilated chambers, thin left ventricular wall, and poor wall movement.
1. Ejection fraction is decreased, typically less than 30%.

d. Treatment
i. Withdraw offending agents, such as alcohol.
ii. Treatment of the congestive heart failure includes diuretics, possible use of digoxin, and sodium restriction.
1. Angiotensin-converting enzyme (ACE) inhibitors are helpful unless contraindicated.
2. Beta-blockers are indicated in patients with stable heart failure.
iii. Cardiac transplantation may be needed.

II. Hypertrophic
a. General
i. Most common cause of sudden death in young athletes.
1. Due to ventricular tachyarrhythmias.
ii. An autosomal dominant genetic cause seen in most cases.
iii. Pathogenesis
1. Hypertrophy of cardiac septum leads to left ventricular outflow obstruction and impaired diastolic filling.
2. Impaired diastolic filling leads to pulmonary congestion.
b. Clinical manifestations
i. Most patients are asymptomatic.

ii. Most common presenting symptom is dyspnea on exertion.
1. May also note angina and syncope.
iii. Physical examination reveals mitral regurgitation, S_4, and prominent left ventricular impulse.
1. Murmur of mitral regurgitation increases with Valsalva maneuver and decreases with handgrip and leg elevation.

c. Diagnosis
i. Echocardiogram makes diagnosis.
1. Note septal wall thickness and ejection fraction are typically greater than 60%.
ii. EKG reveals left ventricular hypertrophy (LVH).

d. Treatment
i. With presence of symptoms, treatment includes beta-blockers (propranolol) and calcium channel blockers (verapamil).
1. Beta-blockers slow the heart rate and allow increased diastolic filling time.
2. Calcium channel blockers improve ventricular compliance.
ii. Diuretics are used for fluid overload.

III. Restrictive
a. General
i. Often caused by an infiltrative process.
1. Such as amyloidosis, sarcoidosis, and hemochromatosis.
ii. Pathogenesis
1. Myocardium changes lead to diastolic noncompliance with elevated filling pressures.
2. Elevated filling pressures lead to pulmonary congestion.
b. Clinical manifestations
i. Most common first symptom is exertion intolerance and fluid retention.
1. Signs of right side heart failure.
(a) Elevated jugular venous distention (JVD).
ii. On physical examination, a pronounced S_4 is noted along with mitral and tricuspid regurgitation.
c. Diagnosis
i. Echocardiogram reveals an ejection fraction between 25% and 50%; normal left ventricular wall thickness, and increased atrial size.

NOTES

ii. EKG reveals low-voltage QRS complexes and nonspecific ST-T wave changes.

iii. Specific diagnosis made by tissue biopsy.

d. Treatment

i. Treat the underlying cause if possible.

ii. Diuretics used to treat congestive heart failure.

CONDUCTION DISORDERS

I. Atrial fibrillation/flutter

a. Atrial fibrillation

i. General

1. Most common sustained arrhythmia in adults.

2. Increase risk with increasing age.

3. Increased risk of intra-atrial clot formation.

ii. EKG findings

1. Rapid, irregular atrial rate of over 400 beats/minute.

2. Ventricular response is irregularly irregular.

3. Atrial fibrillation waves may be coarse, fine, and difficult to discern.

4. R-R interval is irregular.

5. Ventricular rate varies from 100 to 200 beats/minute.

iii. Treatment

1. Rate control is very important.

(a) Rate control with beta-blockers (esmolol, metoprolol), calcium channel blockers (verapamil, diltiazem), or digoxin.

2. Anticoagulation is vital.

(a) Long-term anticoagulation is needed.

QUESTION

Which of the following is a common cause of dilated cardiomyopathy?

A. Iron

B. Alcohol

C. Sarcoidosis

D. Amyloidosis

(b) Heparin is used acutely, and warfarin sodium (Coumadin) long-term.

3. Rhythm control

(a) Amiodarone is most effective, but side effects are common.

(b) Cardioversion can be attempted if no sign of atrial clots.

b. Atrial flutter

i. General

1. Causes regular atrial rates from 250 to 400 beats/minute.

2. Symptoms include dizziness, palpitations, chest pain, and dyspnea.

ii. EKG findings

1. Present with a sawtooth pattern of P waves in leads II, III, and aVF.

2. Ventricular response is 2:1 to 4:1.

(a) Ventricular rates are then 75 to 150 beats/minute.

iii. Treatment

1. Cardioversion should be attempted if no contraindications.

2. Acute treatment with beta-blockers (esmolol, metoprolol) and calcium channel blockers (verapamil, diltiazem) to control rate.

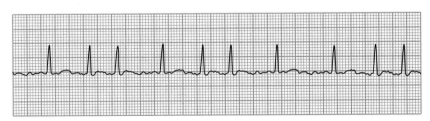

Figure 1-1   Atrial fibrillation.

NOTES

ANSWER B EXPLANATION: *Alcohol is the most common cause of dilated cardiomyopathy. The other options are all causes of restrictive cardiomyopathy.*

correct ☐   incorrect ☐

(a) Long-term treatment with amiodarone, sotalol, quinidine, or procainamide.
3. If site of reentrant is known, catheter ablation can be attempted.
c. Multifocal atrial tachycardia
   i. General
      1. Noted in patients with chronic obstruction pulmonary disease or severe systemic illness.
   ii. EKG findings
      1. Presence of multiple shaped P waves.
      2. Differing PR intervals.
   iii. Treatment
      1. Treat underlying cause.

2. Calcium channel blockers are agents of choice.
II. Atrioventricular (AV) block
   a. General
      i. AV block is defined as when some impulses are delayed or do not reach the ventricle.
      ii. Syncope may be noted.
   b. EKG findings
      i. First-degree block
         1. Prolonged PR interval
            (a) Greater than 0.2 second
      ii. Second-degree block
         1. General
            (a) Some P waves fail to produce a QRS complex.
         2. Mobitz type I (Wenckebach)
            (a) Have a progressive increase in PR interval, until a P wave is blocked, and the cycle is repeated.
            (b) The PR interval after the block is typically the longest.

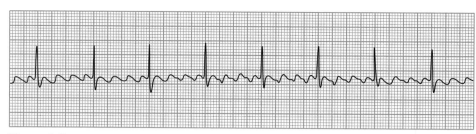

Figure 1-2   Atrial flutter.

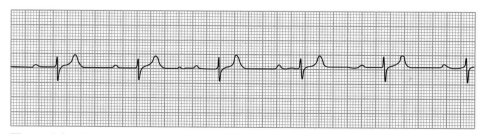

Figure 1-3   First-degree atrioventricular block.

NOTES

3. Mobitz type II
   (a) Have a sudden block of a P wave with no change in PR interval.
iii. Third-degree block
   1. Occurs when atria and ventricle are controlled by different pacemakers.
   2. The atrial and ventricular rhythms are independent of each other.
iv. See Table 1-1 for summary of EKG findings.

c. Treatment
   i. Asymptomatic patients do not require treatment.
   ii. Correct any reversible causes.
   iii. Symptomatic patients may need to be treated with atropine or isoproterenol.
   iv. Permanent pacing may be needed.
III. Bundle branch block
   a. General
      i. May develop after acute myocardial infarction (MI), cardiomyopathy, massive

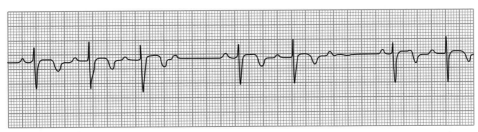

Figure 1-4   Second-degree atrioventricular block: Wenckebach type.

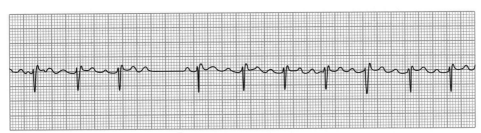

Figure 1-5   Second-degree atrioventricular block: Mobitz type II.

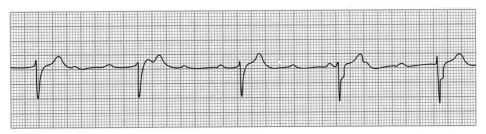

Figure 1-6   Third-degree atrioventricular block.

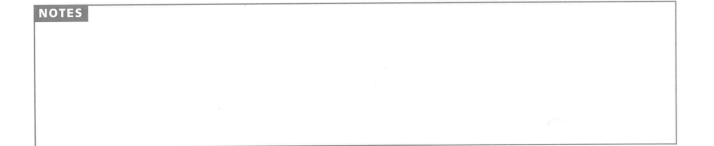

NOTES

Table 1-1 • Comparison of Heart Blocks

	First Degree	Second Degree I	Second Degree II	Third Degree (Complete)
P waves	Yes	Yes	Yes	Yes
1:1	Yes	No	No	No
PR interval	Long	Progressively longer	Long or constant	No association noted
PR constant	Yes	No	Yes, but more P waves not conducted through	No

pulmonary embolism, or aortic stenosis, or may be normal.
   ii. Due to conduction delay in the right or left bundles.
     1. Represented by changes in the QRS complex.
   iii. Conduction across an accessory pathway can occur and leads to Wolff-Parkinson-White (WPW) syndrome.
     1. Patients with WPW are at greater risk for developing other cardiac arrhythmias.
  b. EKG findings
   i. Right bundle branch block (RBBB)
     1. QRS complex is wide.
       (a) QRS complex greater than or equal to 0.11 second.
     2. An rSR in lead V_1.

3. Wide terminal S wave in leads I and V_6.
4. May note ST-T wave changes.
   (a) ST depression in V_1 and elevation in leads I and V_6.
  ii. LBBB
    1. QRS complex is wide.
     (a) QRS complex at least 0.12 second.
    2. Upright and notched QRS complex in leads I and V_6.
    3. Mostly negative QRS in lead V_1.
    4. May note ST-T wave changes.
     (a) ST elevation in V_1 and depression in leads I and V_6.
  iii. Intraventricular conduction delay
    1. QRS complex is wide.
    2. Lacks either RBBB or LBBB signs on EKG.

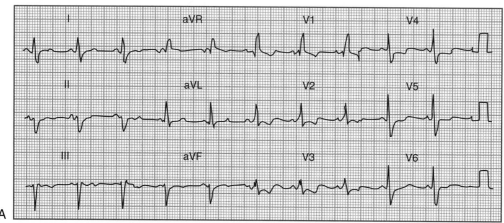

Figure 1-7 **A.** Right bundle branch block.

NOTES

iv. WPW
   1. QRS is wide.
   2. A delta wave is present at the start of the QRS complex.
   3. PR interval is short.
   c. Treatment
      i. Treat underlying cause.
      ii. In WPW, medications such as digoxin or calcium channel blockers, which slow down the heart rate, are contraindicated.

QUESTION

On an EKG, P-waves are noted to have a saw-tooth pattern in lead II and the ventricular rate is 150 beats/minute. Which of the following is the most likely diagnosis?

A. Atrial fibrillation
B. Atrial flutter
C. Ventricular tachycardia
D. Ventricular fibrillation

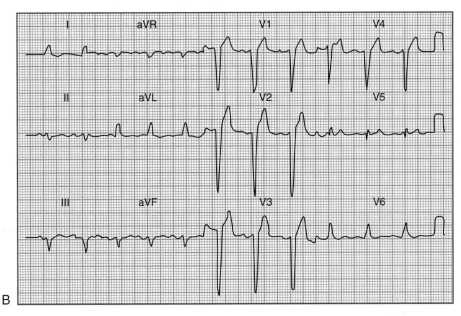

B

Figure 1-7—Cont'd **B.** Left bundle branch block. (From Goldman L, Ausiello D [eds]: Cecil Textbook of Medicine, 22nd ed. Philadelphia: WB Saunders, 2004:272, Fig. 50-4B.)

IV. Paroxysmal supraventricular tachycardia
   a. General
      i. A reentry tachycardia.
      ii. Also called AV nodal reentry tachycardia.
      iii. Commonly noted in elderly patients with underlying heart disease.
      iv. Patients may present with palpitations or anxiety.

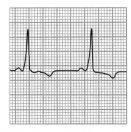

Figure 1-8 Wolff-Parkinson-White syndrome. Note delta wave and short PR interval.

ANSWER **B** EXPLANATION: *With atrial flutter note a sawtooth pattern in leads II, AVF, and aVF with a ventricular response of 2:1 to 4:1. Ventricular rates are typically 75–150 beats/minute.*

correct ☐   incorrect ☐

b. EKG findings
   i. Rate is between 150 and 250 beats/minute, and rhythm is regular.
   ii. Atrial activity is typically not seen.
c. Treatment
   i. A vagal maneuver or antianxiety medication may be helpful.
   ii. Drug of choice is adenosine.
      1. Other rate-slowing medications (e.g., calcium channel blockers, beta-blockers, or digoxin) may be helpful.
V. Premature beats
   a. Premature atrial contractions
      i. General
         1. Underlying rhythm interrupted by an early beat originating from the atria other than the sinoatrial node.
      ii. EKG findings
         1. Impulse is conducted with a narrow QRS complex, similar in appearance to normal sinus conducted beat.
      iii. Treatment
         1. Treat underlying cause.
         2. Antiarrhythmic drugs may be needed.
            (a) Side effects are common.

   b. Premature ventricular contractions (PVCs)
      i. General
         1. Underlying rhythm interrupted by an early beat originating from the ventricles.
      ii. EKG findings
         1. Impulse conducted with a wide QRS complex, different from normal sinus conducted beat.
      iii. Treatment
         1. Treat underlying cause.
         2. If noted in presence of acute ischemic heart disease, PVCs may lead to life-threatening ventricular arrhythmia.
         3. Antiarrhythmic drugs may be needed. See Table 1-2 for list of antiarrhythmic drugs.
            (a) Use of beta-blockers is common.
            (b) Side effects are common.
VI. Ventricular tachycardia (VT)
   a. General
      i. Originates from below the bundle of His at a rate greater than 100 beats/minute.
      ii. Precipitating causes include electrolyte imbalance, acid–base abnormalities, hypoxemia, MI, or drugs.
      iii. Patients typically remain alert and stable with short runs of VT.
         1. If prolonged, patient may become hypotensive and develop myocardial ischemia.
      iv. VT may present with the patient unstable.
         1. Syncope, chest pain, and dyspnea may be noted.
         2. Can cause sudden cardiac death.
      v. Torsades de pointes
         1. Polymorphic VT in which the QRS complexes change amplitude around an isoelectric axis.

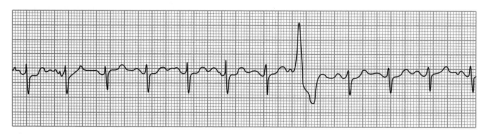

Figure 1-9   Premature ventricular contractions.

2. Long QT interval noted on EKG.
3. Treatment includes removing any offending agents and use of antiarrhythmics.
  b. EKG findings
    i. Rate greater than 100 beats/minute.
    ii. QRS complex is wide.
  c. Treatment
    i. If VT lasts longer than 30 seconds, treatment is needed.
    ii. Antiarrhythmic drugs, such as amiodarone, lidocaine, or procainamide, may be needed if patient is unstable.
    iii. If patient remains unstable, cardioversion is required.
VII. Ventricular fibrillation/flutter
  a. Ventricular fibrillation
    i. General
      1. Malignant arrhythmia with disorganized electrical activity leading to failure of cardiac contraction and failure to maintain cardiac output.

2. Typically occurs in patients with ischemic heart disease and left ventricular dysfunction.
  ii. EKG findings
    1. Irregular rhythm with an undulating low-amplitude baseline with no organized QRS complexes or T waves.
  iii. Treatment
    1. Electrical defibrillation is required.
  b. Ventricular flutter
    i. General
      1. Very rapid, unstable form of VT.
      2. Typically progresses to ventricular fibrillation.
    ii. EKG findings
      1. Sinus QRS complexes without distinct ST segment or T wave.
      2. Rate is 240 to 280 beats/minute.
    iii. Treatment
      1. Treat underlying cause.
      2. Electrical defibrillation is required.

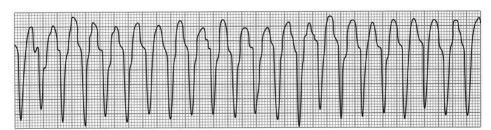

Figure 1-10   Ventricular tachycardia.

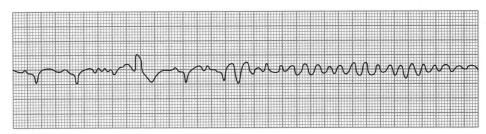

Figure 1-11   Ventricular fibrillation.

NOTES

Table 1-2 • Antiarrhythmic Drugs

Class	Mechanism of Action	Drugs
Ia	Sodium channel blocker	Quinidine, procainamide, disopyramide
Ib	Shorten repolarization	Mexiletine, lidocaine
Ic	Decrease phase 0 repolarization	Flecainide, propafenone
II	Beta-blocker	Beta-blockers
III	Prolong action potential	Amiodarone, sotalol
IV	Slow calcium channel blockers	Calcium channel blockers

CONGENITAL HEART DISEASE

I. Atrial septal defect
  a. General
    i. Defect in the atrial septum allowing shunting of blood between the atria.
    ii. Most common type is the ostium secundum defect noted in the mid-portion of the atrial septum.
  b. Clinical manifestations
    i. Are not typically associated with symptoms.
      1. May have a history of slow weight gain and recurrent lower respiratory tract infections.
    ii. On physical examination, there is a right ventricular heave, wide and constantly split S_2, and a systolic ejection murmur in the pulmonic area and a mid-diastolic rumble in the lower right sternal border.
      1. Murmurs and rumble are due to increased blood flow across the pulmonic and tricuspid valves.
    iii. Chest X-ray reveals cardiomegaly and increased pulmonary vascularity.
    iv. EKG reveals right ventricular hypertrophy and right ventricular conduction delay.
  c. Diagnosis
    i. Echocardiogram reveals an enlarged right ventricle and flow across the defect.
  d. Treatment
    i. Spontaneous closure is likely to occur in most cases in the first year of life.
    ii. If symptomatic, the defect should be closed as soon as possible.
    iii. If asymptomatic, most patients undergo closure between ages 2 and 4 years.
II. Coarctation of aorta
  a. General
    i. Male-to-female ratio is 2:1.
      1. When occurs in a female, must consider presence of Turner's syndrome.
    ii. Obstruction is located in the descending aorta, at the insertion site of the ductus arterious.
  b. Clinical manifestations
    i. May present with or without cardiovascular symptoms.
      1. Congestive heart failure may develop.
    ii. On physical examination, note weak or absent femoral pulses and delayed when compared with upper extremities.
    iii. Upper extremity hypertension.
    iv. A systolic ejection murmur may be heard at the apex.
    v. Chest X-ray reveals an enlarged aortic knob.
      1. Notching of the ribs may be noted.
    vi. EKG shows right ventricular hypertrophy in the neonate and LVH in older children.

NOTES

c. Diagnosis
  i. Based on echocardiogram findings of the coarctation.
    1. If the ductus arteriosus is still patent, the coarctation may not be seen.
d. Treatment
  i. Signs of heart failure must be treated aggressively.
  ii. Prostaglandin E_1 can be used to dilate the patent ductus arteriosus (PDA).
  iii. Repair via balloon angioplasty or surgical anastomosis.
III. Patent ductus arteriosus
  a. General
    i. Higher incidence in premature neonates with a female-to-male ratio of 2:1.
    ii. Function of the ductus arteriosus is to connect the aorta and the left pulmonary artery.
      1. If pulmonary resistance is above systemic resistance, a right-to-left shunt develops.
      2. Typically closes spontaneously by 4 days of age.
  b. Clinical manifestations
    i. Symptoms vary with degree of shunting.
      1. Small defect causes no symptoms.
      2. Large defect may present with signs of congestive heart failure, slow growth, and recurrent lower respiratory tract infections.
        (a) Symptoms include shortness of breath, dyspnea on exertion, and cyanosis.
    ii. Physical exam in the patient with a large shunt reveals bounding pulses and a machine-like murmur.
      1. Murmur starts after S_1, peaks at S_2, and softens during diastole.
    iii. Chest X-ray
      1. In a small PDA, it is often normal.
      2. In a large PDA, cardiomegaly, left atrial and ventricular enlargement, and increased pulmonary congestion are noted.
    iv. EKG
      1. Normal EKG in patients with a small PDA.

QUESTION

Which of the following heart blocks presents with a prolonged and constant PR interval and a P wave to QRS complex ratio of 1:1?

A. First degree AV block
B. Mobitz type I
C. Mobitz type II
D. Complete AV block

      2. Left or biventricular hypertrophy may be noted with a large PDA.
  c. Diagnosis
    i. Echocardiogram confirms presence of PDA.
  d. Treatment
    i. Indomethacin is often effective in closing a PDA.
      1. Works by decreasing prostaglandin E_1 levels.
    ii. Surgical ligation may be needed.
IV. Tetralogy of Fallot
  a. General
    i. A cause of cyanotic congenital heart disease.
    ii. Cyanosis is due to right-to-left shunting and decreased pulmonary flow.
    iii. Are four defects:
      1. Ventricular septal defect (VSD)
      2. Right ventricular outflow obstruction lesion
      3. Right ventricular hypertrophy
      4. Overriding large ascending aorta
  b. Clinical manifestations
    i. Degree of cyanosis is related to severity of right ventricular outflow obstruction.
    ii. Neonates present with cyanosis and agitation.
      1. Episodes of cyanosis are called "tet spells."
        (a) May last minutes to hours.
    iii. On cardiac examination, a right ventricular heave is noted with a loud systolic ejection murmur at the left sternal border.
    iv. EKG reveals right atrial enlargement.
    v. Chest X-ray shows normal heart size and decreased pulmonary vascularity.

NOTES

ANSWER A EXPLANATION: *First-degree AV block presents with a prolonged PR internal and P to QRS ratio of 1:1. Mobitz type I, type II, and complete heart block do not have a 1:1 ratio of P waves to QRS complexes.*

correct ☐   incorrect ☐

   c. Diagnosis
      i. Based on clinical findings and cardiac echocardiogram results.
         1. Echocardiogram reveals thick right ventricular wall, overriding of the aorta, and a VSD.
   d. Treatment
      i. Must decrease right-to-left shunting by increasing systemic vascular resistance and decreasing pulmonary vascular resistance.
         1. Acute treatment options include vagal maneuvers, oxygen, vasoconstrictors, beta-blockers, morphine, and fluid administration.
      ii. Surgical repair is performed during the first 3 to 6 months of life.
V. Ventricular septal defect
   a. General
      i. Most common congenital heart defect.

      ii. Have presence of a communication between the right and left ventricles.
      iii. Have increased pulmonary blood flow that may lead to pulmonary hypertension.
   b. Clinical manifestations
      i. Symptoms vary with size of defect and range from being asymptomatic to presenting with signs of congestive heart failure.
         1. Signs include tachypnea, tachycardia, poor weight gain, trouble feeding, and edema.
      ii. Physical examination reveals a holosystolic murmur heard best at the middle to lower left sternal border.
         1. The smaller the defect, the louder the murmur.
      iii. Chest X-ray may be normal in small defects and reveal cardiomegaly and increased pulmonary vascularity in large defects.
      iv. EKG is normal in small defects and reveals left atrial, left ventricular, or biventricular hypertrophy.
   c. Diagnosis
      i. Echocardiogram confirms the presence of the defect.
   d. Treatment
      i. Most small VSDs close without intervention by age 10 years.
      ii. Large VSDs will require surgical closure.

Table 1-3 • Summary of Common Congenital Heart Defects

Defect	Cyanosis	Cardiovascular Findings
Ventricular septal defect	No	Pansystolic murmur
Tetralogy of Fallot	Yes	Rough, systolic ejection murmur
Aortic stenosis	No	Systolic ejection murmur at right upper sternal border and a systolic click at the apex
Atrial septal defect	No	Fixed split S_2 Systolic ejection murmur at left sternal border Mid-diastolic murmur at left sternal border, 4th intercostal space
Patent ductus arteriosus	No	Continuous machine-like murmur
Coarctation of aorta	No	Decreased femoral pulses
Transposition of great vessels	Yes	Vary depending on presence of ventricular septal defect

NOTES

CONGESTIVE HEART FAILURE

I. General
   a. Abnormal cardiac function leads to a decreased cardiac output that is not able to meet metabolic demands of the body.
   b. Valvular heart disease, coronary artery disease, arrhythmias, hypothyroidism, high-cardiac output syndromes, and hypertension can lead to heart failure.
      i. Disease may be precipitated by reduction or discontinuing medications, increased sodium intake, anemia, infection, or pulmonary embolism.
II. Clinical manifestations
   a. Presenting symptoms include dyspnea, orthopnea, paroxysmal nocturnal dyspnea, fatigue, exercise intolerance, and edema.
   b. Physical examination reveals a restless, dyspneic patient.
      i. Neck exam reveals JVD.
      ii. Pulmonary exam reveals rales (crackles).
      iii. Cardiac exam reveals tachycardia, a displaced point of maximal impulse (PMI), and presence of an S_3 and S_4.
      iv. Abdominal and extremity exam reveals right upper quadrant tenderness, ascites, and peripheral edema.
      v. Laboratory tests show a prerenal azotemia, elevated liver function tests, and elevated B-natriuretic peptide.
         1. Complete blood count (CBC) and thyroid-stimulating hormone should be checked to rule out anemia and thyroid disease as possible causes of failure.
      vi. Chest X-ray may reveal cardiomegaly and increase in pulmonary vasculature.
         1. Pleural effusions may also be present.
         2. Kerley B lines may be noted.
            (a) Due to fluid accumulation in the subpleural interlobular septa.
      vii. EKG reveals LVH.
         1. Acute MI may also be noted.
III. Diagnosis
   a. Echocardiogram will reveal signs of systolic or diastolic dysfunction and decreased ejection fraction.
IV. Treatment
   a. Must treat the underlying cause, discontinue smoking, and control diet.
      i. Diet is low sodium, 1 to 2 g daily.
   b. Pharmacologic therapy
      i. Goals are to control fluid retention, control neurohormonal activation, and control symptoms.

QUESTION

Which of the following tests is best used to diagnose congenital heart disease?

   A. Chest x-ray

   B. Electrocardiogram

   C. Echocardiogram

   D. CT scan

Table 1-4 • Functional Classification of Heart Failure	
Class	**Definition**
I	No cardiac symptoms with ordinary activity
II	Cardiac symptoms with marked activity but asymptomatic at rest
III	Cardiac symptoms with mild activity but asymptomatic at rest
IV	Cardiac symptoms at rest

NOTES

ANSWER C EXPLANATION: *Congenital heart disease are typically structural abnormalities that are best evaluated with an echocardiogram.*

correct ☐   incorrect ☐

ii. Diuretics are used to control fluid retention.
iii. ACE inhibitors, which interfere with the renin–angiotensin system, are required of all patients with cardiac failure unless contraindicated.

iv. Vasodilators, including hydralazine and nitrates, are used when use of ACE inhibitors is not possible.
v. Beta-blockers should be used in patients with left ventricular dysfunction, unless contraindicated.
vi. Digitalis can improve symptoms and exercise tolerance by increasing cardiac contractility.
vii. Other medications include oxygen and morphine.
viii. Aspirin, nonsteroidal anti-inflammatory drugs (NSAIDs), and calcium channel blockers should be avoided.

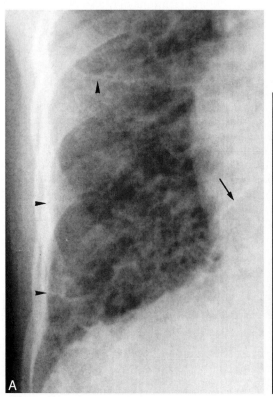
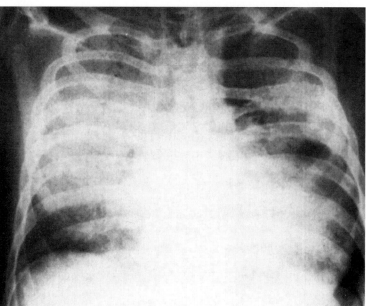

Figure 1-12 Chest X-ray in a patient with severe congestive heart failure.(From Grainger RG, Allison D, Adam A, Dixon AK [eds]: Diagnostic Radiology: A Textbook of Medical Imaging, 4th ed. London: Harcourt, 2001:874, Fig. 39.3A, B.)

NOTES

HYPERTENSION

I. Essential
   a. General
      i. Definition based in The Seventh Report of the Joint National Commission on Prevention, Detection, Evaluation, and Treatment of High Blood Pressure (JNC VII) guidelines.
      ii. Incidence in the adult population is 10% to 15%.
      iii. End-organ damage may occur to the brain, kidney, and heart.
   b. Clinical manifestations
      i. Physical examination may be completely normal, except for elevated blood pressure.
         1. Physical examination should include evaluation of possible end-organ damage secondary to hypertension.
   c. Diagnosis
      i. Based on two or more elevated blood pressure readings.
      ii. EKG may show LVH.
   d. Treatment
      i. Lifestyle modifications
         1. Weight loss
         2. Limit alcohol intake
         3. Regular aerobic exercise
         4. Discontinue smoking
         5. Reduce sodium intake
         6. Reduce saturated fat and cholesterol intake
      ii. Pharmacologic therapy
         1. Therapy should be started in patients with stage 1 hypertension.
            (a) Initial therapy is thiazide diuretics or beta-blockers.
            (b) Other options include ACE inhibitors, calcium channel blockers, and alpha-blockers.
         2. Stage 2 typically requires two-drug combination.
         3. Therapy options may vary with presence of comorbid conditions.
II. Secondary
   a. General
      i. Defined as hypertension due to an identifiable cause.

Table 1-6 • Target-Organ Damage
Left ventricular hypertrophy
Angina
Heart failure
Stroke
Chronic kidney disease
Peripheral artery disease
Retinopathy

Table 1-5 • Classification of Hypertension	
Classification	**Blood Pressure Levels**
Normal	<120 mm Hg systolic and <80 mm Hg diastolic
Prehypertension	Systolic 120–139 mm Hg or diastolic 80–89 mm Hg
Stage 1 hypertension	Systolic 140–159 mm Hg or diastolic 90–99 mm Hg
Stage 2 hypertension	Systolic ≥ 160 mm Hg or diastolic ≥ 100 mm Hg

NOTES

Table 1-7 • Treatment of Hypertension in Patients with Concomitant Disease

Concomitant Disease	Primary Choice	Secondary Choice	Avoid
Angina	Beta-blockers	Diuretics	
	Calcium channel blockers	Angiotensin-converting enzyme (ACE) inhibitors	
Diabetes	ACE inhibitors Ca⁺⁺ channel blockers		Diuretics
Hyperlipidemia	ACE inhibitors Ca⁺⁺ channel blockers		Diuretics Beta-blockers
Congestive heart failure	Diuretics ACE inhibitors		Beta-blockers Ca⁺⁺ channel blockers (verapamil)
Previous myocardial infarction	Beta blockers ACE inhibitors	Diuretics Ca⁺⁺ channel blockers	
Chronic renal failure	Diuretics Ca⁺⁺ channel blockers	Beta-blockers ACE inhibitors	
Asthma, chronic obstructive pulmonary disease	Diuretics Ca⁺⁺ channel blockers	ACE inhibitors	Beta-blockers

    ii. Major etiologies include:
      1. Renovascular disease
      2. Coarctation of the aorta
      3. Primary aldosteronism
      4. Cushing's syndrome
      5. Pheochromocytoma
      6. Obstructive sleep apnea
      7. Renal parenchymal hypertension
  b. Clinical manifestations
    i. Symptoms and laboratory results vary with etiology.
    ii. See Table 1-8 for clinical signs and symptoms.
  c. Diagnosis
    i. Based on finding of hypertension.
    ii. See Table 1-8 for evaluation testing.
  d. Treatment
    i. Treat underlying cause.

    ii. Renovascular cause
      1. Beta-blockers used in patients with elevated renin.
      2. ACE inhibitors should be avoided in patients with bilateral renal artery stenosis.
      3. Diuretics used in combination with ACE inhibitors.
      4. Surgical revascularization
III. Malignant
  a. General
    i. Potentially life-threatening situation.
    ii. Hypertension plus retinopathy, cardiovascular or renal compromise, or encephalopathy.
    iii. Etiologies
      1. Acute aortic dissection
      2. Post coronary artery bypass graft
      3. Acute MI

NOTES

Table 1-8 • Symptoms and Laboratory Findings in Secondary Hypertension

Etiology	Clinical	Evaluation
Renovascular disease	Elevated serum creatinine	Captopril renogram Magnetic resonance angiography of renal arteries
Coarctation of the aorta	Unequal pulses Rib notching Claudication	Magnetic resonance imaging
Primary aldosteronism	Hypokalemia	Plasma renin and aldosterone
Cushing's syndrome	Truncal obesity	Plasma cortisol Dexamethasone suppression test
Pheochromocytoma	Tachycardia Polyuria Headache Diaphoresis	Plasma metanephrine and normetanephrine
Obstructive sleep apnea	Snoring Obesity	Sleep study
Renal parenchymal	Elevated serum creatinine Abnormal urinalysis	24-hour urine for creatinine and protein Renal ultrasound

     4. Unstable angina

     5. Eclampsia

     6. Head trauma

     7. Severe burns

  b. Clinical manifestations

    i. Hypertension with end-organ disease.

  c. Diagnosis

    i. Based on severely elevated blood pressure, greater than 220/140 mm Hg, and presence of headache, confusion, blurred vision, nausea and vomiting, seizures, grade II or IV hypertensive retinopathy, heart failure, and oliguria.

  d. Treatment

    i. Requires immediate blood pressure reduction.

     1. Gradual decrease in blood pressure by 10% in the first hour of treatment and then 15% over the next 3 to 12 hours, to a target blood pressure of 170/110 mm Hg.

     2. Further decrease to a normal value over the next 48 hours.

    ii. Choice of agent varies with the cause.

     1. Nitroprusside for patients with hypertensive encephalopathy, intracranial bleeding, and heart failure.

      (a) Used in combination with propranolol for dissecting aneurysm.

     2. Oral clonidine can also be used for hypertensive urgency.

      (a) Sedation is common.

HYPOTENSION

I. Cardiogenic shock

  a. General

    i. Tissue hypoperfusion due to acute MI or end-stage heart failure.

NOTES

ii. Overall prognosis in cardiogenic shock is poor.
1. Accounts for most deaths after acute MI.
iii. Etiologies
1. Acute MI
(a) Pump failure
(b) VSD
(c) Ventricular rupture
2. Tachyarrhythmia
3. Valvular heart disease
(a) Acute mitral regurgitation
(b) Acute aortic regurgitation
(c) Aortic or mitral stenosis
4. Traumatic cardiac injury
5. Myocarditis
b. Clinical manifestations
i. Hypotension is defined as a systolic blood pressure less than 90 mm Hg or a decrease from baseline by more than 30 mm Hg.
ii. Symptoms include altered mental status, cyanosis, oliguria, and cool, clammy extremities.
iii. Physical examination reveals signs of hypoperfusion and hypovolemia.
iv. Acute MI may be noted on EKG.
c. Diagnosis
i. Echocardiogram is very helpful in diagnosing cardiogenic shock.
1. May note left ventricular wall motion abnormalities and decreased left ventricular function.
d. Treatment
i. Adequate oxygenation and treatment of arrhythmias are very important.
ii. Improving blood pressure is critical.
1. Intravenous (IV) fluids

(a) Trial of volume expansion is warranted.
2. Vasopressor agents
(a) Dopamine can increase systemic pressure and cardiac output.
(b) Dobutamine can increase cardiac output, but does not increase systemic blood pressure.
(c) Risks of vasopressor drugs include aggravation of arrhythmias and increase in myocardial oxygen demand.
3. Intra-aortic balloon pump
(a) Will increase diastolic coronary artery perfusion, decrease left ventricular afterload, improve cardiac output, and decrease myocardial oxygen demand.
II. Orthostatic/postural
a. General
i. May result in syncope that could be recurrent.
ii. Defined as a fall in systolic blood pressure of 30 mm Hg or more or diastolic blood pressure fall of 10 mm Hg or more between recumbent and upright posture.
iii. Etiologies include:
1. Drugs
(a) Antipsychotic agents
(b) Diuretics
(c) Alpha-adrenergic blockers
(d) ACE inhibitors
(e) Alcohol
(f) Tranquilizers
(g) Vasodilators
(h) Methyldopa

Table 1-9 • Categories of Shock			
Hypovolemic	**Cardiogenic**	**Obstructive Noncardiogenic**	**Distributive**
Hemorrhage	Myocardial dysfunction	Pericardial tamponade	Septic shock
Volume depletion	Valvular heart defects	Tension pneumothorax	Neurogenic
Extravascular spacing		Severe pulmonary embolism	Anaphylactic
		Left ventricular outflow obstruction	Drug induced

NOTES

2. Polyneuropathies
3. Parkinson's disease
b. Clinical manifestations
    i. Symptoms include change in mental status (confusion), secondary to cerebral hypoperfusion, weak pulse, cool extremities, tachypnea, and reduced urine output.
    ii. Physical examination reveals hypotension, tachycardia, and tachypnea.
c. Diagnosis
    i. Based on clinical findings.
d. Treatment
    i. Treat underlying cause, remove offending medications if possible, and support blood pressure.

ISCHEMIC HEART DISEASE

I. Acute myocardial infarction
    a. General
        i. Myocardial necrosis brought on by ischemia.
        ii. Most deaths occur within 1 hour of onset of symptoms.
            1. Most deaths caused by ventricular fibrillation.
            2. Rapid defibrillation can reverse ventricular fibrillation.
        iii. See Table 1-10 for list of risk factors for coronary atherosclerosis.
    b. Clinical manifestations
        i. Pain is retrosternal and described as heavy, pressure-like, squeezing, or bandlike.
            1. Pain may radiate to the neck, jaw, or left arm.

Table 1-10 • Risk Factors for Coronary Atherosclerosis

Increasing age	Male gender
Positive family history	Smoking
Hypertension	Diabetes
Hyperlipidemia	Stress
Obesity	Sedentary lifestyle

2. Pain typically lasts longer, 20 minutes to several hours, than angina.
3. Elderly patients or patients with diabetes may have acute MI that is painless.
4. Watch for atypical presentation of pain.
    ii. Associated symptoms include nausea, vomiting, diaphoresis, dyspnea, and weakness.
    iii. Physical examination reveals no findings that are diagnostic for acute MI.
        1. Blood pressure may be elevated, an S_4 may be noted, and signs of heart failure may be evident.
    iv. Laboratory studies
        1. Myoglobin
            (a) Detectable within 1 to 2 hours after acute MI.
            (b) Found in skeletal and cardiac muscle.
        2. Creatine phosphokinase (CPK)
            (a) Total CPK correlates with infarct size.
            (b) CPK-MB is specific for cardiac muscle.
        3. Troponin
            (a) Not normally present in blood.
            (b) Elevated in acute MI.
        4. See Table 1-11 for comparison of cardiac enzyme markers.
        5. Other tests
            (a) Leukocytosis is noted on CBC.
            (b) Lipid profile should be obtained to determine if lipid-lowering therapy is indicated.
            (c) C-reactive protein is elevated.
    v. EKG reveals ST elevation.
        1. See Table 1-12 for acute MI patterns.

NOTES

ANSWER C EXPLANATION: *Class I congestive heart failure is defined as no cardiac symptoms with activity, class II symptoms with marked activity, class III symptoms with mild activity, and class IV symptoms at rest.*

correct ☐   incorrect ☐

c. Diagnosis
  i. Based on clinical and laboratory findings.
  ii. Echocardiogram is obtained to evaluate global and regional cardiac function.
  iii. Coronary angiography confirms location of injury and coronary vessel involved.

Table 1-11 • Cardiac Enzyme Markers in Acute Myocardial Infarction

Marker	Time to Appearance	Duration of Elevation	Note
Troponin I	2–6 hr	5–10 days	Test of choice
Creatine kinase Mb	3–6 hr	2–4 days	
Myoglobin	1–2 hr	<1 day	Low specificity

Table 1-12 • Locating Myocardial Damage

Affected Wall	EKG Leads	Artery Involved	EKG Leads Reciprocal Changes
Inferior	II, III, aVF	RCA	I, aVL
Lateral	I, aVL, V_5, V_6	Circumflex	V_1, V_2
Anterior	V_1–V_4, I, aVL	LCA	II, III, aVF
Posterior	V_1, V_2	RCA Circumflex	
Apical	V_3–V_6	LAD RCA	None
Anterolateral	I, aVL, V_4–V_6	LAD Circumflex	II, III, aVF
Anteroseptal	V_1–V_3	LAD	None

LAD, left anterior descending; LCA, left coronary artery; RCA, right coronary artery.

NOTES

d. Treatment
  i. Aspirin should be given to all patients, unless contraindicated.
  ii. Initial therapy
    1. Oxygen
      (a) Given to avoid hypoxia.
    2. Beta-blockers
      (a) Control blood pressure and decrease probability of sudden cardiac death.
    3. Nitroglycerin
      (a) Used for coronary artery dilatation.
    4. Morphine
      (a) Pain and blood pressure control.
    5. Continuous EKG monitoring.
  iii. Specific therapy
    1. Recanalization therapy
      (a) Thrombolytic therapy
        (i) Includes streptokinase and tissue plasminogen activator.
          (1) Major risk factor is bleeding, intracerebral hemorrhage.
          (2) Candidates for therapy include patients with ST elevation or new LBBB presenting within 12 hours of onset of symptoms and without contraindications.
          (3) See Table 1-13 for contraindications to thrombolytic therapy.

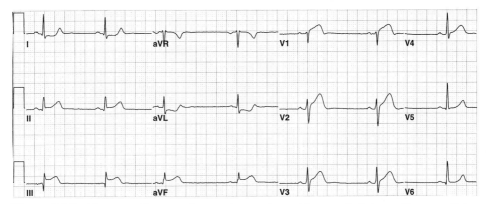

Figure 1-13 Electrocardiogram changes in a patient with acute inferior wall myocardial infarction. (From Goldberger AL: Clinical Electrocardiography: A Simplified Approach, 6th ed. St. Louis: Mosby–Year Book, 1999:89, Fig. 8-12.)

Table 1-13 • **Contraindications to Thrombolytic Therapy**	
Absolute	**Relative**
Active bleeding/bleeding disorders	Severe/uncontrolled hypertension
Prior hemorrhagic stroke/other stroke within 1 year	Anticoagulation: therapeutic or elevated INR
Intracranial or spinal cord cancer	Old ischemic stroke
Suspected/known aortic dissection	Recent major surgery/trauma Pregnancy

NOTES

(b) Primary percutaneous coronary intervention.
- (i) Mechanical recanalization by inflation of catheter-based balloon.

2. Antiplatelet therapy
- (a) Aspirin
  - (i) Inhibits platelet aggregation and development of coronary thrombi.
- (b) Clopidogrel
  - (i) Antiplatelet effects and used in aspirin allergic patients.
- (c) Glycoprotein IIb/IIIa receptor inhibitor
  - (i) Inhibits fibrinogen receptor and benefits high-risk patients by improving coronary artery patency.

3. Antithrombin therapy
- (a) Heparin inactivates thrombin and factor X.
- (b) Used in combination with thrombolytic therapy.

4. Other
- (a) Nitrates
  - (i) Induce vascular smooth muscle relaxation and reduce cardiac preload and afterload.
- (b) Beta-blockers
  - (i) Reduce heart rate, blood pressure, and myocardial contractility, and stabilize the heart electrically.
    - (1) Limit myocardial oxygen consumption.
- (c) ACE inhibitors
  - (i) Improves remodeling after acute MI.
  - (ii) Avoid in presence of hypotension.

iv. Complications
1. Arrhythmias
- (a) Ventricular
- (b) Atrial fibrillation
2. Heart failure
- (a) Left ventricular dysfunction
- (b) Cardiogenic shock
3. Mechanical
- (a) Papillary muscle rupture
- (b) Left ventricular wall rupture
- (c) Left ventricular aneurysm
4. Thromboembolic

II. Angina pectoris
a. Stable
- i. General
  1. A symptom, pain that builds up rapidly in 30 seconds and disappears within 5 to 15 minutes.
  - (a) Disappears more promptly if nitroglycerin is used.
  2. Is precipitated by activity and relieved by rest.
  3. Related to a fixed stenosis of one or more coronary arteries.
- ii. Clinical manifestations
  1. Pain presents as a tightness, squeezing and is described as aching or dull discomfort.
  - (a) Pain is midsternal with radiation to neck, left shoulder, or left arm.
  2. Risk factors should be sought.
  3. Physical examination may be totally normal.
  - (a) A transient S_4 or S_3 gallop may be noted.
  4. EKG, when patient is pain-free, may reveal arrhythmia, prior MI, or LVH.
  - (a) EKG obtained during episode of pain, or shortly after, may reveal ST segment depression and T wave inversion.
- iii. Diagnosis
  1. Exercise testing used to detect myocardial ischemia.
  - (a) Ischemia indicated when ST segment depression of greater than 1 mV, during early stages of exercise.
  2. Perfusion scintigraphy testing
  - (a) Performed with exercise, adenosine, or dipyridamole injection.
  - (b) Can localize site of active ischemia.
  3. Coronary angiography
  - (a) Required to exclude coronary artery disease with certainty.

NOTES

iv. Treatment
  1. General
    (a) Smoking cessation
    (b) Control hypertension
    (c) Control diabetes
    (d) Exercise plan
  2. Reduce progression
    (a) Manage lipids
    (b) Antiplatelet medications
      (i) Includes aspirin, clopidogrel, or warfarin.
    (c) Beta-blockers
    (d) ACE inhibitors
  3. Control symptoms
    (a) Beta-blockers
    (b) Nitrates
      (i) Excellent response to nitrates.
    (c) Calcium channel blockers
  4. Revascularization
    (a) Includes percutaneous coronary interventions or coronary artery bypass graft.
b. Unstable
 i. General
  1. Diagnosed clinically when:
    (a) Patient has new-onset angina.
    (b) Increasing angina.
    (c) Angina occurring at rest.
  2. An acute, nonocclusive thrombus is found in most cases.
    (a) Plaque rupture or erosion with overlying thrombus is the initiating mechanism.
 ii. Clinical manifestations
  1. Patient presents with dyspnea, palpitations, and fatigue.
  2. Pain is located retrosternal or epigastric.
    (a) Described as a pressure, burning, or squeezing pain.
    (b) May have associated nausea, shortness of breath, and diaphoresis.
      (i) These may be the only symptoms in elderly or diabetic patients.

  3. Physical examination may be normal or reveal an S_4 gallop, mitral regurgitation murmur, and rales on lung exam.
  4. EKG may be normal.
    (a) Nonspecific signs, such as transient ST changes and inverted T waves, may be noted.
  5. Laboratory testing reveals normal cardiac enzymes.
 iii. Diagnosis
  1. Based on clinical findings.
  2. Must rule out acute myocardial infarction.
 iv. Treatment
  1. Reduce progression to or size of MI.
    (a) Antiplatelet medications
      (i) Includes aspirin, clopidogrel, platelet glycoprotein IIb/IIIa receptor inhibitors, or heparin.
    (b) Beta-blockers
    (c) ACE inhibitors
  2. Treatment of ischemic signs and symptoms
    (a) Beta-blockers
    (b) Nitrates
      (i) Responds poorly to nitrates.
    (c) Calcium channel blockers
  3. Revascularization
    (a) Includes coronary angioplasty or coronary artery bypass graft.
c. Prinzmetal's variant
 i. General
  1. Pain occurs mainly at rest, but may occur during exercise.
  2. Pain may awaken patient in the morning.

QUESTION

Which of the following is the drug of choice for life threatening hypertensive crisis?

A. IV Nitroprusside (Nipride)
B. IV Propranolol (Inderal)
C. PO Nifedipine (Procardia)
D. PO Diltiazem (Cardizem)

NOTES

ANSWER **A** EXPLANATION: *Malignant hypertension is acute hypertension with end-organ disease. Nitroprusside is the drug of choice, with clonidine used for hypertensive urgency.*

correct ☐   incorrect ☐

(a) Due to increased sympathetic activity.
3. Caused by occlusive spasm superimposed on a nonsevere coronary artery stenosis.
4. Syndrome X is myocardial ischemia that occurs in patients with normal coronary arteries.

(a) Due to disease of coronary microcirculation.
ii. Clinical manifestations
1. Pain is noted as above.
(a) May be associated with Raynaud's phenomenon and migraine headache.
iii. Diagnosis
1. Diagnosed when transient ST segment elevation is documented during an episode of chest pain.
2. Coronary angiography, with injection of ergonovine or acetylcholine, can cause focal vasospasm.
iv. Treatment
1. Episodes respond well to nitrates and calcium channel blockers.

Table 1-14 • Etiologies of Chest Pain

| Ischemic | | Nonischemic | |
Cardiac	Noncardiac	Cardiac	Noncardiac
Coronary atherosclerosis	Anemia	Pericarditis	Gastrointestinal Esophagitis Gastroesophageal reflux disease Cholecystitis Peptic ulcer disease Pancreatitis
Coronary spasm	Sickle cell disease	Aortic dissection	Psychogenic Anxiety Panic Somatization
Cocaine induced	Hyperviscosity		Pulmonary Pulmonary embolism Pneumothorax Pneumonia
Aortic stenosis	Hyperthyroidism		Neuromuscular Costochondritis Herpes zoster
Hypertrophic cardiomyopathy	Adrenergic stimulation Hypoxia		

NOTES

(a) Beta-blockers may exacerbate vasospasm.

VASCULAR DISEASE

I. Acute rheumatic fever
  a. General
    i. Inflammatory disease that occurs as a response to an upper respiratory tract infection due to group A streptococci.
      1. Have exudative and proliferative inflammatory lesions on connective tissue, mainly of the heart, joints, and subcutaneous tissue.
    ii. Range of time from infection to onset of symptoms is 1 to 5 weeks.
    iii. Mechanism is unknown.
    iv. Peak incidence in the 5- to 15-year age group.
      1. Rare in children younger than 4 years.
  b. Clinical manifestations
    i. Major manifestations (Jones criteria)
      1. Carditis
        (a) Can involve the endocardium, myocardium, or pericardium.
        (b) Present with cardiac murmur, cardiomegaly, pericarditis, and congestive heart failure.
        (c) Cardiac murmur is an apical systolic murmur, blowing and high pitched in nature.
      2. Polyarthritis
        (a) A migratory arthritis, typically involves larger joints, knees, and ankles.
        (b) Synovial fluid reveals increase in neutrophils, but no bacteria.
      3. Chorea
        (a) Rapid, purposeless, involuntary movements, involving the face and extremities.
        (b) Speech is slurred and the tongue, when protruded, retracts involuntarily.
      4. Erythema marginatum
        (a) Erythematosus macule or papule that extends over the skin with central clearing.

      5. Subcutaneous nodules
        (a) Firm, painless subcutaneous nodules that vary in size from a few millimeters to 2 cm.
        (b) Occur over bony surfaces and tendons, of the elbows, knees, and wrists.
    ii. Earliest manifestations include fever and joint involvement.
      1. See Table 1-15 for Jones criteria.
  c. Diagnosis
    i. No laboratory tests are diagnostic for rheumatic fever.
      1. CBC reveals a leukocytosis and anemia of chronic disease.
      2. Sedimentation rate and C-reactive protein are elevated.
    ii. Documentation of a recent streptococcal infection is noted.
      1. Includes ASO titer, anti-DNase, or antihyaluronidase.
    iii. Diagnosis is based on the Jones criteria.
      1. Two major or one major and two minor manifestations indicate a high probability of acute rheumatic fever.
  d. Treatment
    i. Antibiotics do not modify the course of the disease.
    ii. Anti-inflammatory drugs suppress the signs and symptoms but are not curative.

NOTES

ANSWER B EXPLANATION: *Acute inferior wall myocardial infarction presents with ST elevation in leads II, III, and aVF. See table 1-12 for summary.*

correct ☐   incorrect ☐

1. Major drugs include aspirin and corticosteroids.
iii. Decrease risk for disease by prevention with appropriate and timely treatment of streptococcal throat infections.
iv. Secondary prevention of rheumatic fever, prevention of recurrent attacks, includes penicillin G or V, or sulfadiazine.
1. Erythromycin is used in the penicillin-allergic person.

II. Aortic aneurysm
a. General
i. Pathologic dilatation of the aorta.
ii. May involve any portion of the aorta, but abdominal aorta is the most common location.
1. Abdominal aorta aneurysms are more common in men.
iii. Atherosclerosis is the major underlying cause.

b. Clinical manifestations
i. Most are asymptomatic.
ii. When symptoms are noted, include hypogastric or low back pain.
1. Pain is a steady gnawing pain.
iii. With rupture, the pain worsens, and blood pressure drops.
iv. On physical examination, a pulsatile abdominal mass may be noted.
c. Diagnosis
i. Ultrasound or computed tomography (CT) scan makes diagnosis.
1. Ultrasound is an excellent screening test.
2. Monitor change in aneurysm by CT scan.
d. Treatment
i. Goal is to reduce the risk for expansion and rupture.
ii. Serial imaging should be obtained to monitor size, and beta-blockers should be used to reduce aortic pressure.
1. Imaging should be done every 6 months for abdominal aortic aneurysm greater than 4 cm in size.
iii. Abdominal aortic aneurysm greater than 5 cm in size should be surgically repaired.

Table 1-15 • Jones Criteria for Diagnosis of Acute Rheumatic Fever

Major	Minor	Supporting
Carditis	Arthralgia	Positive strep screen or throat culture
Polyarthritis	Fever	Elevated or increasing ASO titer
Chorea	Prolonged PR interval	
Erythema marginatum	Laboratory findings: Increased erythrocyte sedimentation rate Increased C-reactive protein Increased acute-phase reactants	
Subcutaneous nodules		

NOTES

III. Aortic dissection
   a. General
      i. Begins with a tear in the aorta intima, blood enters the media, cleaving it into two layers.
      ii. Increased risk in patients with Marfan syndrome.
      iii. Peak incidence, in patients without Marfan syndrome, is age 60 to 80 years.
      iv. Typically, patients have a history of hypertension.
   b. Clinical manifestations
      i. Present with severe retrosternal pain, described as a tearing or sharp pain.
      ii. Elevated blood pressure is common.
      iii. Pulse deficits are common.
      iv. Chest X-ray may reveal an enlarged mediastinum.
   c. Diagnosis
      i. Diagnosis can be made via CT scan, aortograph, magnetic resonance imaging (MRI), or transesophageal echocardiogram.
   d. Treatment
      i. Primary goal is to halt further progression of the dissection and reduce chance of rupture.
      ii. Blood pressure control with a beta-blocker, nitroprusside, or calcium channel blockers.
      iii. Surgical repair is the definitive treatment.
IV. Arterial embolism/thrombosis
   a. General
      i. Cause of acute arterial insufficiency.
      ii. Arterial embolism secondary to atrial fibrillation/flutter, mitral stenosis, transmural infarct, trauma, hypercoagulable states, and postarterial procedures.
   b. Clinical manifestations
      i. Present with acute onset of severe pain, diminished pulses, cold limbs, and cyanosis.
      ii. Typically presents unilaterally.
      iii. Physical examination reveals the five P's:
         1. Pain
            (a) Constant and worse with any movement.

QUESTION

In which of the following disorders is an S4 typically noted?

   A. Congestive heart failure
   B. Abdominal aortic aneurysm
   C. Myocardial infraction
   D. Mitral valve prolapse

---

         2. Pallor
            (a) Occurs first, followed by cyanosis.
         3. Pulseless
            (a) Associated with a cold limb.
         4. Paresthesias
            (a) Caused by damage to peripheral nerves.
         5. Paralysis
            (a) Due to damage to muscle and motor nerves.
   c. Diagnosis
      i. Echocardiogram obtained to evaluate for source of thrombus.
      ii. Arteriogram to identify location.
   d. Treatment
      i. Heparin should be started immediately.
      ii. Emergent embolectomy-thrombectomy is needed to restore blood flow.
      iii. Complications include limb loss and compartment syndrome.
V. Chronic/acute arterial occlusion
   a. General
      i. Decrease in 50% of arterial lumen will produce clinical symptoms, ischemia, and necrosis.
      ii. Risk factors include smoking, hypercholesterolemia, diabetes, and hypertension.
      iii. Most common cause is atherosclerosis.
      iv. Lower extremities are most common location.
   b. Clinical manifestations
      i. Patients may be asymptomatic due to collateral circulation.
      ii. Major symptom is pain, followed by claudication.

NOTES

ANSWER C EXPLANATION: *A S4 gallop may be heard in acute myocardial infarction and angina pectoris. An S3 is noted in congestive heart failure.*

correct ☐   incorrect ☐

 1. Primary area involved is the calf.
 2. Area of occlusion is distal to the site of claudication.
 iii. Occlusion of certain vessels brings about certain conditions.
   1. Carotid artery—transient ischemic attack
   2. Ophthalmic artery—amaurosis fugax
 iv. Physical examination reveals decreased peripheral pulses, bruits, ischemic skin changes, and painful ischemic ulcers.
 c. Diagnosis
   i. Ankle/brachial index can provide information regarding severity of disease.
     1. See Table 1-16 for interpretation of ankle/brachial index.
   ii. Doppler with ultrasound can be used to evaluate blood flow.
   iii. Arteriography is used to determine location of occlusion.
 d. Treatment
   i. Pharmacologic therapies include:
     1. Pentoxifylline
       (a) Decrease blood viscosity and increase flexibility of red blood cells.

 2. Aspirin
   (a) Inhibits platelet aggregation.
 3. Ticlopidine
   (a) Inhibits platelet aggregation.
 4. Heparin and warfarin have no therapeutic use.
 ii. Thromboendarterectomy can be used to repair diseased arteries.
 iii. Patient should be educated to stop smoking.
VI. Giant cell arteritis
 a. General
   i. A granulomatous vasculitis that affects the temporal artery.
   ii. Typically affects patients older than 50 years.
   iii. Etiology is unknown.
   iv. May coexist with polymyalgia rheumatica.
 b. Clinical manifestations
   i. Most common symptom is new onset of headache, located in the temporal region.
   ii. Jaw claudication and visual disturbances are also noted.
     1. Transient vision loss or complete blindness may be noted.
   iii. On physical examination, enlargement, tenderness, and erythema may be noted of the artery.
     1. Bruit may also be present.
   iv. Laboratory testing reveals an elevated erythrocyte sedimentation rate (ESR), anemia, and leukocytosis.
 c. Diagnosis
   i. Diagnosis is made by biopsy.

Table 1-16 • Interpretation of Ankle/Brachial Index	
Ankle/Brachial Index Result	Interpretation
>1.0	Normal
0.5–0.9	Arterial claudication
<0.4	Severe arterial stenosis

NOTES

d. Treatment
  i. Corticosteroids should be started as soon as possible.

VII. Phlebitis/thrombophlebitis
  a. General
    i. Inflammatory thrombosis involving the superficial veins of the lower extremity.
    ii. Associated with varicose veins, pregnancy, and catheter placement.
    iii. Septic thrombophlebitis is more common in IV drug abusers.
  b. Clinical manifestations
    i. Vein is palpable and tender.
    ii. Induration, redness, and tenderness are localized along the course of the vein.
      1. A palpable cord is present.
    iii. There is no swelling of the extremity.
  c. Diagnosis
    i. Must rule out deep venous thrombosis (DVT).
    ii. Diagnosis based on clinical findings.
  d. Treatment
    i. Warm, moist compresses to the area.
      1. No restriction of activity is needed.
    ii. NSAIDs to relieve pain.
    iii. If septic thrombophlebitis, antibiotics are needed.
      1. Antibiotics should cover staphylococci.

VIII. Venous thrombosis
  a. General
    i. DVT is development of clot in the deep veins of the extremities or pelvis.
    ii. Predisposing factors include venous stasis, activation of coagulation system, and vascular damage.
    iii. Risk factors for DVT.
      1. Prolonged immobilization
      2. Postoperative
      3. Pelvic or extremity trauma
      4. Birth control pills
      5. Cancer
      6. Hypercoagulable state
      7. Pregnancy
      8. Obesity
      9. Smoking
  b. Clinical manifestations
    i. Present with pain and swelling at the site and distal from the clot.

QUESTION

Which of the following tests is best used for screening of possible abdominal aortic aneurysm?

A. Electrocardiogram
B. Echocardiogram
C. Ultrasound
D. Angiography

    ii. Physical examination may be normal.
      1. Homans' sign, pain with dorsiflexion of the foot, may be positive.
  c. Diagnosis
    i. Compression ultrasound and venogram are diagnostic.
      1. Serial ultrasounds may be needed to confirm diagnosis.
    ii. D-Dimer may be useful in ruling out thrombosis in patients with low probability for DVT.
  d. Treatment
    i. Complications include pulmonary embolism.
    ii. Prophylaxis is required for all high-risk patients and includes:
      1. Low molecular weight heparin
      2. Elastic stockings
      3. Intermittent pneumatic leg compression
    iii. Anticoagulation therapy is required.
      1. IV unfractionated heparin or low molecular weight heparin is required acutely until warfarin levels are therapeutic.
        (a) Heparin is continued for at least 5 days and until warfarin levels are therapeutic.
          (i) Heparin-associated thrombocytopenia may occur within 5 to 10 days of starting heparin.
            (1) Platelet count should be monitored.

NOTES

ANSWER C EXPLANATION: *Due to non-invasive nature, ultrasound is an excellent screening test for abdominal aortic aneurysm. Serial measurements are used to monitor size.*

correct ❏   incorrect ❏

      (b) With warfarin therapy, the INR should be greater than 2 to be therapeutic.

      (c) Warfarin therapy is typically continued for 3 to 6 months in patients with reversible risk factors.

         (i) Indefinite therapy may be needed in high-risk patients.

    2. An inferior vena cava filter may be needed to prevent pulmonary embolism in patients with contraindications to anticoagulation.

IX. Varicose veins

  a. General

    i. Caused by incompetence of the saphenous vein.

      1. Due to increased intravascular pressure or defective valves.

    ii. Occurs primarily in the superficial veins of the medial and anterior thigh, calf, and ankle.

    iii. Contributing factors include prolonged standing, pregnancy, and obesity.

      1. More common in females.

  b. Clinical manifestations

    i. Typically asymptomatic, but may have local aching and fatigue.

    ii. Physical examination will reveal tortuous veins that are easily compressed.

  c. Diagnosis

    i. Based on clinical findings.

  d. Treatment

    i. Conservative management with elastic support stockings.

    ii. Surgical therapy consists of vein stripping or vein ligation.

    iii. Small varicose veins can be treated with a sclerosing agent.

VALVULAR DISEASE

I. Aortic stenosis

  a. General

    i. Symptoms due to left ventricular outflow obstruction leading to increased left ventricular pressure, muscle hypertrophy, and decreased ejection fraction.

    ii. More common in men than women.

    iii. Etiology

      1. Rheumatic inflammation

      2. Congenital

  b. Clinical manifestations

    i. Symptoms include angina, syncope, and congestive heart failure.

    ii. Physical examination

      1. Delayed carotid upstroke.

      2. Strong apical impulse

      3. Narrowing pulse pressure

      4. Loud, rough, systolic, diamond-shaped murmur

        (a) Heard best at the base of the heart with radiation to the neck.

        (b) Associated with an ejection click.

  c. Diagnosis

    i. Chest X-ray reveals dilatation of the ascending aorta and pulmonary congestion.

      1. Heart is boot shaped.

    ii. EKG reveals LVH and ST-T wave changes.

    iii. Doppler echocardiogram shows thickening of the left ventricular wall and valvular calcifications.

    iv. Diagnosis confirmed by cardiac catheterization.

  d. Treatment

    i. Strenuous activity should be avoided.

    ii. Treatment of congestive heart failure, if present, with diuretics and sodium restriction.

      1. ACE inhibitors are contraindicated.

    iii. Valve replacement is the treatment of choice in symptomatic patients.

    iv. Subacute bacterial endocarditis (SBE) antibiotic prophylaxis is required.

NOTES

II. Aortic insufficiency
  a. General
    i. Aortic insufficiency results in increased end-diastolic volume, ventricular dilatation, leading to regurgitation.
    ii. Etiology
      1. Rheumatic fever
      2. Infectious endocarditis
      3. Hypertension
      4. Syphilis
      5. Collagen vascular disease
      6. Marfan syndrome
  b. Clinical manifestations
    i. Symptoms include dyspnea on exertion, syncope, chest pain, and congestive heart failure.
    ii. Physical examination reveals the following:
      1. Wide pulse pressure
      2. Bounding "water hammer" pulses
      3. Presence of an S_3
      4. Displaced cardiac impulse, downward and to the left.
      5. Decrescendo, blowing diastolic murmur heard along left sternal border
        (a) Low-pitched, apical diastolic murmur (Austin-Flint murmur)
  c. Diagnosis
    i. Chest X-ray reveals LVH with or without signs of congestive heart failure.
    ii. Echocardiogram reveals left ventricular enlargement.
    iii. Cardiac catheterization confirms wide pulse pressure and evaluates left ventricular dysfunction.
  d. Treatment
    i. SBE antibiotic prophylaxis is required.
    ii. Congestive heart failure is treated with digoxin, diuretics, ACE inhibitors, and salt restriction.
      1. Long-term treatment with nifedipine and/or ACE inhibitors delays need for valve replacement.
    iii. Surgical valve replacement is required when signs of decompensation occur.
      1. Surgery should be performed before ejection fraction is less than 55%.
III. Mitral stenosis

QUESTION

A 75-year-old patient presents with headache, sudden loss of vision in the right eye, and tenderness in the right temporal area. Which of the following tests would most likely be increased or elevated?

  A. Erythrocyte sedimentation rate
  B. White blood cell count
  C. Lactic dehydrogenase
  D. Haptoglobin

  a. General
    i. Stenosis leads to increased atrial pressure and atrial enlargement, pulmonary congestion, pulmonary hypertension, and right side heart failure.
    ii. More common in women, between ages 25 and 45 years.
    iii. Etiology
      1. Rheumatic fever
      2. Congenital defect
  b. Clinical manifestations
    i. Symptoms include exertional dyspnea, orthopnea, and paroxysmal nocturnal dyspnea.
      1. Hemoptysis may occur secondary to vessel rupture.
    ii. Physical examination
      1. Prominent jugular A wave
      2. Opening snap in early diastole
      3. Soft, low-pitched, diastolic rumble heard best at the apex in the left decubitus position.
      4. A palpable right ventricular heave may be noted at the left sternal border.
  c. Diagnosis
    i. Echocardiogram and cardiac catheterization are diagnostic.
    ii. Chest X-ray reveals left atrial enlargement and prominent pulmonary arteries.
    iii. EKG reveals left atrial enlargement or atrial fibrillation.
  d. Treatment

NOTES

ANSWER **A** EXPLANATION: *Giant cell arteritis (Temporal arteritis) is most common in the elderly and presents with sudden loss of vision and a headache in the temporal region. The sedimentation rate will be elevated.*

correct ❑   incorrect ❑

    i. Control atrial fibrillation and congestive heart failure.
    ii. SBE antibiotic prophylaxis is required.
    iii. Valve replacement or percutaneous transvenous mitral valvotomy is required in patients who respond poorly to medical treatment.
IV. Mitral insufficiency
  a. General
    i. Increased volume in left atrium from left ventricular leads to ineffective cardiac output.
    ii. Etiology
      1. Rheumatic fever
      2. Papillary muscle rupture
      3. Chordae tendineae rupture
      4. Calcification
      5. Mitral valve prolapse
      6. Systemic lupus erythematosus (SLE)
  b. Clinical manifestations
    i. Symptoms include fatigue, dyspnea, orthopnea, and congestive heart failure.
      1. Hemoptysis may be noted.
    ii. Physical examination
      1. Left ventricular lift or apical thrill
      2. Holosystolic murmur at apex with radiation to the base or left axilla.
      3. S_3 may be present.
  c. Diagnosis
    i. Echocardiogram is diagnostic.
    ii. EKG reveals LVH.
  d. Treatment
    i. SBE antibiotic prophylaxis is required.
    ii. Treat congestive heart failure with salt restrictions, digoxin, ACE inhibitors, and diuretics.
    iii. Valve replacement must be performed early and is the only definite treatment.
V. Mitral valve prolapse

Table 1-17 • Summary of Major Valvular Disease

	Aortic Stenosis	Mitral Stenosis	Aortic Regurgitation	Mitral Regurgitation
Etiology	Rheumatic	Rheumatic	Endocarditis Marfan syndrome	Mitral prolapse Endocarditis Papillary muscle dysfunction
Symptoms	Angina Syncope	Dyspnea Orthopnea PND	Dyspnea Orthopnea Angina	Dyspnea Orthopnea PND
Cardiac signs	Systolic ejection murmur Delayed carotid upstroke	Diastolic rumble Opening snap	Diastolic blowing murmur	Holosystolic apical murmur
EKG	LVH	RVH	LVH	LVH
Chest X-ray	Boot-shaped heart	Straight left heart border	Cardiac enlargement	Cardiac enlargement

LVH, left ventricular hypertrophy; PND, paroxysmal nocturnal dyspnea; RVH, right ventricular hypertrophy.

NOTES

    a. General
      i. More common in young females.
        1. Typically have a narrow anteroposterior chest diameter, low body weight, and hypotension.
    b. Clinical manifestations
      i. Symptoms include chest pain and palpitations.
      ii. Physical examination findings include mid to late click, heard best at the apex, and a crescendo mid to late systolic murmur.
    c. Diagnosis
      i. Echocardiogram is diagnostic and reveals valve leaflets bulging posteriorly in systole.
    d. Treatment
      i. Avoid stimulates.
      ii. Beta-blockers may be tried in symptomatic patients.
      iii. SBE prophylaxis is required only if significant regurgitation is noted.
VI. Tricuspid insufficiency
    a. General
      i. Typically due to hemodynamic load in the right ventricle and not structural.
        1. Increases right atrial pressure, which leads to venous hypertension.
      ii. Etiology
        1. Pulmonary hypertension
        2. Endocarditis
          (a) Suspect in drug addicts.
    b. Clinical manifestations
      i. Symptoms are those of right side heart failure.
        1. Includes ascites, edema, and right upper quadrant pain.
      ii. Physical examination reveals hepatic enlargement, JVD, and a parasternal lift.
        1. Holosystolic murmur noted along left sternal border.
    c. Diagnosis
      i. Diagnosis made by echocardiogram.
    d. Treatment
      i. Treat underlying cause.
      ii. Surgery is rarely needed.
VII. Pulmonary stenosis

QUESTION

Which of the following produces a loud, snapping S1, an opening snap and a diastolic rumble?

    A. Mitral stenosis
    B. Mitral regurgitation
    C. Aortic stenosis
    D. Aortic regurgitation

    a. General
      i. A congenital disease due to fusion of the valve cusps.
    b. Clinical manifestations
      i. Symptoms include angina and syncope.
      ii. Physical examination reveals an early systolic opening ejection click followed by a systolic ejection murmur, which radiates to the base.
    c. Diagnosis
      i. Diagnosis made by echocardiogram.
    d. Treatment
      i. If asymptomatic, no treatment is needed.
      ii. If symptoms are present, commissurotomy is needed.

OTHER FORMS OF HEART DISEASE

I. Acute/subacute bacterial endocarditis
    a. General
      i. Infection of the endothelial surface of the heart.
      ii. More common in elderly people and males.
      iii. Predisposing conditions that increase risk for endocarditis
        1. Mitral valve prolapse
        2. Degenerative valvular disease
        3. IV drug abuse
        4. Prosthetic valve
        5. Congenital abnormalities
      iv. Microorganisms that cause endocarditis vary with setting.
        1. Community acquired
          (a) *Staphylococcus aureus*
          (b) Viridans streptococci

NOTES

          (c) Enterococci
      2. Nosocomial
          (a) *S. aureus*
          (b) *Staphylococcus epidermidis*
          (c) Enterococci
          (d) Fungal
      3. Prosthetic valve
          (a) *S. epidermidis*
          (b) *S. aureus*
          (c) Enterococci
  b. Clinical manifestations
      i. Symptoms include fever, fatigue, malaise, weight loss, arthritis, and myalgias.
      ii. Physical examination reveals the following:
          1. Petechiae
          2. Osler's nodes
              (a) Small, painful nodules on the palmar surface of the fingers and toes.
          3. Janeway's lesions
              (a) Hemorrhagic, nonpainful macules on palms and soles.
          4. Splinter hemorrhages
              (a) Nonblanching, linear brownish-red lesions in the nail beds perpendicular to the growth of the nails.
          5. Roth's spots on funduscopic exam.
              (a) Retinal hemorrhages with pale centers.
          6. Cardiac murmur
              (a) May be diastolic or systolic depending on valve involved.
          7. Splenomegaly
      iii. Laboratory tests reveal leukocytosis, elevated ESR, and hematuria.
  c. Diagnosis
      i. Based on Duke criteria.
          1. Major
              (a) Positive blood cultures

              (b) Endocardial involvement on echocardiogram or new murmur.
          2. Minor
              (a) Predisposing condition: cardiac or IV drug abuse.
              (b) Fever
              (c) Vascular phenomena
              (d) Immunologic phenomena
      ii. Definitive diagnosis with two major criteria or one major and three minor criteria.
  d. Treatment
      i. Antibiotics are selected based on culture results, but may need empirical treatment.
          1. Empiric treatment
              (a) Native valve, community acquired, methicillin-resistant *S. aureus* (MRSA) unlikely.
                  (i) Nafcillin plus penicillin plus gentamicin
              (b) Hospital acquired, hemodialysis, suspect MRSA, or penicillin allergic
                  (i) Vancomycin plus gentamicin
              (c) Prosthetic valve
                  (i) Vancomycin plus gentamicin plus rifampin
                  (ii) Valve may need to be replaced.
      ii. Antibiotics should be bactericidal, and therapy is prolonged, lasting 4 to 6 weeks.
      iii. See Table 1-18 for treatment options for infectious endocarditis.
      iv. Prevention
          1. Required for select high- and moderate-risk patients and for certain invasive procedures.
              (a) Antibiotics typically given before the procedure so that peak level is at the time of the procedure.
          2. Needed for high-risk and moderate-risk patients
              (a) High-risk
                  (i) History of prosthetic valves
                  (ii) Past history of endocarditis
                  (iii) Complex cyanotic congenital heart disease
              (b) Moderate-risk
                  (i) Rheumatic or acquired valvular dysfunction
                  (ii) Hypertrophic cardiomyopathy

NOTES

(iii) Mitral valve prolapse with regurgitation
3. Invasive procedures include:
(a) Dental procedures
(b) Tonsillectomy and adenoidectomy
(c) Surgery involving intestinal or respiratory mucosa
(d) Sclerotherapy of esophageal varices
(e) Endoscopic retrograde cholangiography
(f) Gallbladder surgery in high-risk patients
(g) Cystoscopy, urethral dilatation, or prostate surgery
4. Antibiotic selection
(a) Dental, oral, and upper respiratory procedures
(i) Amoxicillin or penicillin V before the procedure.
(ii) If penicillin allergic can use clindamycin, azithromycin, or clarithromycin before the procedure.
(b) Genitourinary or gastrointestinal procedures
(i) High risk
(1) Ampicillin plus gentamicin before the procedure followed by ampicillin or amoxicillin after the procedure.

(ii) High risk, penicillin allergic
(1) Vancomycin plus gentamicin
(iii) Moderate risk
(1) Amoxicillin or ampicillin
(iv) Moderate risk, penicillin allergic
(1) Vancomycin
II. Acute pericarditis
a. General
i. Inflammation of the pericardium.
ii. Etiologies include:
1. Viral: Coxsackie virus B, hepatitis B, and cytomegalovirus
2. Bacterial: *Staphylococcus, Streptococcus,* and tuberculosis.
3. Post-MI
4. Drugs: procainamide
5. Malignancy: lung or breast metastases
6. Collagen vascular disease: SLE

Table 1-18 • Treatment Options for Infectious Endocarditis	
Organism	**Treatment**
Viridans streptococci	Penicillin G or ampicillin plus gentamicin, *or* Ceftriaxone plus gentamicin, *or* Vancomycin
Enterococci	Ampicillin or penicillin G plus gentamicin
Staphylococcus aureus	Nafcillin or oxacillin plus gentamicin
Methicillin-resistant *S. aureus*	Vancomycin
Staphylococcus epidermidis	Vancomycin plus gentamicin plus rifampin

NOTES

ANSWER **D** EXPLANATION: *Physical examination findings in endocarditis include Osler's nodes, Janeway's lesions, splinter hemorrhages, Roth's spots, and cardiac murmur.*

correct ☐   incorrect ☐

  iii. Constrictive pericarditis is thickening and fibrosis of the pericardium after an episode of acute pericarditis.
 b. Clinical manifestations
  i. Present with chest pain that worsens with deep breathing, cough, or lying down.
   1. Pain improved with sitting and leaning forward.
  ii. Physical examination reveals a pericardial friction rub.
   1. Friction rub is diagnostic for pericarditis.
 c. Diagnosis
  i. EKG reveals ST elevation in all precordial leads without reciprocal ST depression.
  ii. Cardiac enzymes are normal.
  iii. Echocardiogram reveals a pericardial effusion.
 d. Treatment
  i. Treat underlying cause.
  ii. NSAIDs are used to treat the pain and inflammation.
  iii. Steroids may be needed.
  iv. Constrictive pericarditis is treated with pericardiectomy.
III. Cardiac tamponade
 a. General
  i. Accumulation of fluid that results in an increase in pericardial pressure and impairs ventricular filling.
  ii. Typically a complication of pericardial effusion.
 b. Clinical manifestations
  i. Symptoms include hypotension, tachycardia, and dyspnea on exertion.
  ii. Physical examination reveals distended neck veins, indistinct heart sounds, narrow pulse pressure, and pulsus paradoxus.
 c. Diagnosis
  i. Echocardiogram is diagnostic for tamponade.
 d. Treatment
  i. Pericardiocentesis by echocardiogram guidance.
  ii. Treat underlying cause.
IV. Pericardial effusion
 a. General
  i. Prolonged and severe inflammation leads to fluid accumulation around the heart.
 b. Clinical manifestations
  i. Small effusion causes no symptoms, whereas large effusions lead to cardiac tamponade.
  ii. Physical examination reveals diminished heart sounds.
   1. Friction rub may be noted if effusion secondary to pericarditis.
  iii. See Table 1-19 for comparison of cardiac tamponade and pericarditis.
 c. Diagnosis
  i. EKG reveals low-voltage QRS complexes and ST changes due to pericarditis.
  ii. Chest X-ray reveals an enlarged water-bottle–shaped heart.
  iii. Echocardiogram shows fluid between the layers of the pericardium.
   1. This is diagnostic for pericardial effusion.
  iv. Pericardiocentesis confirms the diagnosis.
 d. Treatment
  i. If symptoms are severe, pericardiocentesis is required to remove the fluid.

NOTES

Table 1-19 • Comparison of Tamponade and Pericarditis

	Cardiac Tamponade	Constrictive Pericarditis	Restrictive Cardiomyopathy
Pulsus paradoxus	Positive	Negative	Negative
S_3	Negative	Positive	Positive
S_4	Negative	Negative	Positive
Cardiomegaly	Positive	Negative	Negative
Pericardial effusion	Positive	Negative	Negative

Cardiology Drugs

Name	Mechanism	Therapeutic Use	Side Effects	Notes
Captopril	ACE inhibitor	CHF Hypertension	Postural hypotension Cough Hyperkalemia Altered taste	Should not be used in pregnancy.
Enalapril	ACE inhibitor	CHF Hypertension	Postural hypotension Cough Hyperkalemia Altered taste	Should not be used in pregnancy.
Lisinopril	ACE inhibitor	CHF Hypertension	Postural hypotension Cough Hyperkalemia Altered taste	Should not be used in pregnancy.
Hydralazine	Direct smooth muscle relaxant	CHF Hypertension	Headache Nausea Sweating Lupus-like syndrome	
Isosorbide	Direct smooth muscle relaxant	CHF Angina	Headache	
Minoxidil	Vasodilator (arterioles)	CHF Hypertension	Reflex tachycardia Edema Hypertrichosis	
Sodium nitroprusside	Vasodilation	CHF Hypertension emergency	Hypotension	Given IV only

(continued)

NOTES

Cardiology Drugs—cont'd

Name	Mechanism	Therapeutic Use	Side Effects	Notes
Bumetanide	Inhibit Na/K/Cl transport in the ascending Loop of Henle	CHF Hypertension	Ototoxicity Hyperuricemia Hypovolemia Hypokalemia	Rapid onset of action
Furosemide	Inhibit Na/K/Cl transport in the ascending Loop of Henle	CHF Hypertension	Ototoxicity Hyperuricemia Hypovolemia Hypokalemia	Rapid onset of action
Hydrochloro-thiazide	Increase sodium and water excretion	CHF Hypertension	Hypokalemia Hyperglycemia	
Digoxin	Enhances cardiac muscle contractility	CHF Antiarrhythmic (Atrial flutter, SVT)	Dysrhythmia Nausea and vomiting Headache Confusion Altered color perception	Not indicated in right-sided heart failure
Dobutamine	Direct-acting catecholamine that is a beta-receptor agonist.	CHF	Anxiety Headache Pulmonary edema	Use with caution in patients with A. fib.
Amrinone	Phosphodiesterase inhibitor	CHF		
Disopyramide	Sodium channel blocker	Antiarrhythmic	Dry mouth Urinary retention Blurry vision Constipation	
Flecainide	Sodium channel blocker	Antiarrhythmic	Dizziness Blurred vision Headache Nausea	
Lidocaine	Sodium channel blocker	Antiarrhythmic (VT or V fib)	Drowsiness Slurred speech Paresthesia Confusion Convulsions	
Mexiletine	Sodium channel blocker	Antiarrhythmic		

NOTES

Cardiology Drugs—cont'd

Name	Mechanism	Therapeutic Use	Side Effects	Notes
Procainamide	Sodium channel blocker	Antiarrhythmic	SLE Depression Hallucination Psychosis	
Quinidine	Sodium channel blocker	Antiarrhythmic (Atrial flutter or fibrillation)	SA/AV blocks Asystole Nausea/vomiting Diarrhea	
Esmolol	Beta-blocker	Antiarrhythmic	Fatigue Lethargy Insomnia Impotence Hypotension	Rebound hypotension
Metoprolol	Beta-blocker	Antiarrhythmic Hypertension	Fatigue Lethargy Insomnia Impotence Hypotension	Rebound hypotension
Propranolol	Beta-blocker	Antiarrhythmic (Atrial flutter or fibrillation, SVT) Angina Hypertension	Fatigue Lethargy Insomnia Impotence Hypotension	Rebound hypotension
Amiodarone	Potassium channel blocker	Antiarrhythmic (A fib, SVT, or VF)	Pulmonary fibrosis Hyper or hypothyroidism Liver toxic Photosensitivity Blue skin discoloration	Full effects may take 6 weeks.
Bretylium	Potassium channel blocker	Antiarrhythmic (VF or VT)	Postural hypotension	
Sotalol	Potassium channel blocker	Antiarrhythmic (VT)	Torsade de pointes	
Diltiazem	Calcium channel blocker	Antiarrhythmic Angina Hypertension	Hypotension Constipation	Avoid in patients with depressed cardiac function

(*continued*)

NOTES

Cardiology Drugs—cont'd

Name	Mechanism	Therapeutic Use	Side Effects	Notes
Verapamil	Calcium channel blocker	Antiarrhythmic (Atrial flutter, SVT) Angina Hypertension Migraine headache	Hypotension Constipation	Avoid in patients with depressed cardiac function
Adenosine	Decreases conduction velocity	Antiarrhythmic (SVT)	Flushing Chest pain Hypotension	Very short duration of action
Nitroglycerin	Smooth muscle relaxant	Angina	Headache Hypotension	
Nifedipine	Calcium channel blocker	Hypertension Angina Hypertension	Flushing Headache Hypotension Edema Constipation	
Spironolactone	Inhibit sodium reabsorption and potassium secretion	Hypertension	Gynecomastia Hyperkalemia Nausea	
Triamterene	Block Na-K exchange	Hypertension	Leg cramps Increased BUN and uric acid	
Atenolol	Beta blocker	Hypertension	Fatigue Lethargy Insomnia Impotence Hypotension	Rebound hypotension
Labetalol	Beta blocker	Hypertension	Fatigue Lethargy Insomnia Impotence Hypotension	Rebound hypotension
Timolol	Beta blocker	Hypertension	Fatigue Lethargy Insomnia Impotence Hypotension	Rebound hypotension

NOTES

Cardiology Drugs—cont'd

Name	Mechanism	Therapeutic Use	Side Effects	Notes
Ramipril	ACE inhibitor	Hypertension	Postural hypotension Cough Hyperkalemia Altered taste	
Losartan	Angiotensin II antagonist	Hypertension	Hypotension Hyperkalemia	Fetotoxic
Prazosin	Alpha blocker	Hypertension	First dose syncope Reflex tachycardia	
Clonidine	Alpha-2 agonist	Hypertension	Sedation Dry nose	Does not worsen renal function

Question 1

Which of the following describes the murmur of patent ductus arteriosus?

 A. Rough, systolic murmur
 B. Systolic ejection murmur
 C. Continuous, machine-like murmur
 D. Mid-diastolic murmur

Question 2

A 55-year-old presents with orthopnea and paroxysmal nocturnal dyspnea. On physical examination jugular venous distension and pulmonary rales are noted. Which of the following laboratory tests would most likely be elevated in this patient?

 A. Thyroid stimulating hormone
 B. Brain natriuretic peptide
 C. Myoglobin
 D. Renin

NOTES

Question 3

A 35-year-old presents with chest pain that worsens with lying down. Electrocardiogram reveals diffuse ST elevation in all the precordial leads. Which of the following is the most likely diagnosis?

A. Dilated cardiomyopathy
B. Subacute bacterial endocarditis
C. Acute inferior wall infarct
D. Acute pericarditis

Question 4

A large ventricular septal defect is noted on echocardiogram of an 8-month old male. Which of the following is the most appropriate intervention?

A. Beta-blocker
B. Indomethacin
C. Surgical repair
D. Balloon angioplasty

Question 5

A 65-year-old male with a history of benign prostatic hypertrophy develops hypertension. Which of the following would be the best treatment option for this patient's hypertension?

A. Alpha blocker
B. Beta blocker
C. ACE inhibitor
D. Diuretic

Question 6

Control of which of the following conduction disorders will decrease the risk of intra-atrial clot formation?

A. Ventricular tachycardia
B. Atrial fibrillation
C. Premature atrial contractions
D. Wolff-Parkinson White Syndrome

Question 7

Which of the following coronary arteries is typically involved in a lateral wall myocardial infarction?

A. Right coronary artery
B. Circumflex artery
C. Left anterior descending artery
D. Left coronary artery

Answer 1

ANSWER D EXPLANATION: *In cases of patent ductus arterious with a large shunt the patient will have bounding pulses and a machine like murmur starting after S1, peaking at S2, and softening during diastole.*

Topic: Patent ductus arterious

correct ☐   incorrect ☐

NOTES

Answer 2

ANSWER **B** EXPLANATION: *The patient with congestive heart failure typically presents with dyspnea, orthopnea, paroxysmal nocturnal dyspnea, fatigue, and edema. On physical examination jugular venous distention and pulmonary rales are noted. Laboratory evaluation will reveal prerenal azotemia, elevated liver function tests, and elevated B-natriuretic peptide.*

Topic: Congestive heart failure

correct ☐   **incorrect** ☐

Answer 3

ANSWER **D** EXPLANATION: *In pericarditis chest pain is worsens with deep breathing, coughing, or lying down. EKG reveals ST elevation in all precordial leads without reciprocal ST depression.*

Topic: Acute pericarditis

correct ☐   **incorrect** ☐

Answer 4

ANSWER **C** EXPLANATION: *Large ventricular septal defects will not close spontaneously but require surgical repair.*

Topic: Ventricular septal defects

correct ☐   **incorrect** ☐

Answer 5

ANSWER **A** EXPLANATION: *The use of a single medication to treat two disorders is encouraged to decrease the risk of side effects. Alpha blockers treat both hypertension and benign prostatic hypertrophy.*

Topic: Hypertension

correct ☐   **incorrect** ☐

Answer 6

ANSWER **B** EXPLANATION: *Atrial fibrillation presents with an irregular, irregular rate with no visible p wave activity. Atrial fibrillation increases the risk of intra-atrial clot formation and requires long-term anticoagulation.*

Topic: Atrial fibrillation.

correct ☐   **incorrect** ☐

Answer 7

ANSWER **B** EXPLANATION: *Lateral wall myocardial infarction presents with EKG changes in leads I, AVL, V5, and V6. These changes correspond to occlusion of the circumflex artery.*

Topic: Myocardial infarction

correct ☐   **incorrect** ☐

NOTES

Pulmonary System

EXAM BLUEPRINT TOPICS

Infectious Disorders
Acute bronchitis
Acute bronchiolitis
Acute epiglottitis
Croup
Influenza
Pertussis
Pneumonia
Respiratory syncytial virus infection
Tuberculosis
Neoplastic Disease
Bronchogenic carcinoma
Carcinoid tumors
Metastatic tumors
Pulmonary nodules
Obstructive Pulmonary Disease
Asthma
Status asthmaticus
Bronchiectasis
Chronic bronchitis
Cystic fibrosis
Emphysema
Pleural Diseases
Pleural effusion
Pneumothorax

- Primary
- Secondary
- Traumatic
- Tension

Pulmonary Circulation
Pulmonary embolism
Pulmonary hypertension
Cor pulmonale
Restrictive Pulmonary Disease
Idiopathic pulmonary fibrosis
Pneumoconiosis

Sarcoidosis
Other Pulmonary Disease
Acute respiratory distress syndrome
Hyaline membrane disease
Foreign body aspiration

INFECTIOUS DISORDERS

I. Acute bronchitis
  a. General
    i. Inflammation of the large airways of the tracheobronchial tree.
    ii. Caused by infectious agents.
      1. Most frequently due to viruses.
        (a) Adenovirus
        (b) Influenza A and B
        (c) Coronavirus
        (d) Rhinovirus
        (e) Respiratory syncytial virus (RSV)
      2. Bacterial causes include:
        (a) *Haemophilus influenzae*
        (b) *Mycoplasma pneumoniae*
        (c) *Moraxella catarrhalis*
        (d) *Chlamydia pneumoniae*
        (e) *Streptococcus pneumoniae*
    iii. Most prevalent during the winter and early spring.
  b. Clinical manifestations
    i. Major complaint is cough preceded by nasal congestion, sore throat, malaise, headache, and sneezing.
    ii. Physical examination reveals findings of upper respiratory tract infection.
      1. Lung exam may reveal rhonchi, crackles, or wheezing.
    iii. Chest X-ray is normal.
  c. Diagnosis
    i. Based on clinical findings.

NOTES

   d. Treatment
      i. Supportive measures, including rest, cough suppressants, oral hydration, and rest.
      ii. Decongestants and inhaled bronchodilators may be helpful.
II. Acute bronchiolitis
   a. General
      i. Infection and inflammation of the smaller airways.
      ii. Most common cause is RSV.
   b. Clinical manifestations
      i. Present with diffuse wheezing, variable fever, cough, tachypnea, difficulty feeding, and cyanosis.
      ii. Physical examination reveals hyperinflation, crackles, and prolonged expiration, and wheezing.
   c. Diagnosis
      i. Based on clinical findings and isolation of offending organism.
   d. Treatment
      i. Bronchodilator can be used for wheezing.
      ii. Antiviral, ribavirin, is given by aerosolization for RSV.
      iii. Some patients may develop wheezing later in life.
III. Acute epiglottitis
   a. General
      i. Rare condition, medical emergency.
      ii. Noted more frequently in adolescents and adults.
         1. Decreased frequency in children with development and use of the *H. influenzae* type b vaccine.
      iii. Etiologies include:
         1. *H. influenzae* type b
         2. *S. pneumoniae*
         3. *Staphylococcus aureus*
         4. *Candida albicans*
         5. Herpes simplex virus
   b. Clinical manifestations
      i. On presentation, patient appears anxious and toxic.
      ii. Fever, muffled voice, and cyanosis may be noted.
      iii. Patients prefer the sitting position; children have the classic "sniffing" or "tripod" position.
         1. Sitting up with chin forward and neck slightly extended.
      iv. Late symptoms include stridor, drooling, and trouble handling secretions.
      v. Examination of the upper airway should be avoided.
         1. If patient is examined, the epiglottis is cherry red and swollen.
   c. Diagnosis
      i. Based on clinical findings.
      ii. Lateral soft tissue neck X-rays reveal an enlarged epiglottis and surrounding structures.
         1. Thumbprint sign noted on lateral X-ray.

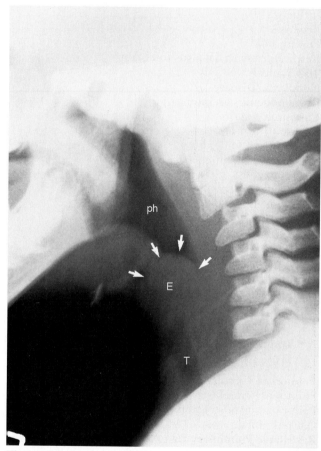

Figure 2-1   Lateral soft tissue neck X-ray in a patient with epiglottitis.

d. Treatment
    i. Airway management is key to treatment.
    ii. Humidified oxygen and intravenous (IV) fluids.
    iii. Antibiotic options include:
       1. Cefuroxime
       2. Chloramphenicol
       3. Cefotaxime
       4. Ceftriaxone
       5. Cefazolin
       6. Ampicillin-sulbactam

IV. Croup
  a. General
    i. Acute inflammatory disease of the larynx.
       1. Involves mainly the subglottic area.
    ii. Affects younger children in the fall and early winter.
    iii. Etiologies:
       1. RSV
       2. Influenza
       3. Adenovirus
       4. *Mycoplasma pneumoniae*
  b. Clinical manifestations
    i. Prodrome of upper respiratory tract symptoms followed by a barking cough and stridor.
    ii. Fever is typically absent.
  c. Diagnosis
    i. Based on clinical findings.
    ii. Lateral neck X-ray reveals narrowing of the subglottic area and normal epiglottis.
  d. Treatment
    i. Supportive care, oral hydration, mist therapy, and minimal handling, for mild croup.
    ii. Patients with stridor are treated with active intervention.
       1. Oxygen
       2. Racemic epinephrine
       3. Glucocorticoids
    iii. Artifical airway may be needed in severe cases.

V. Influenza
  a. General
    i. Common respiratory infection caused by influenza A or B.
    ii. Spread by respiratory droplets.
    iii. Incubation period is 1 to 3 days.
    iv. Outbreaks occur every winter.

  b. Clinical manifestations
    i. Present with abrupt onset of fever, chills, myalgias, headache, and a nonproductive cough.
       1. Coryza and sore throat are also common.
    ii. Physical examination is normal or reveals mild pharyngeal erythema, cervical adenopathy, and clear nasal drainage.
  c. Diagnosis
    i. Viral culture from throat and nasal specimens or immunofluorescence and enzyme immunoassays can be used for rapid detection.
  d. Treatment
    i. Rimantadine and amantadine can be used to shorten the course of influenzae A.
       1. Both medications can lead to central nervous system side effects.
    ii. Zanamivir and oseltamivir are active against both influenza A and B.
       1. Are neuraminidase inhibitors.
       2. Side effects include bronchospasms with zanamivir and nausea and vomiting with oseltamivir.
    iii. Prevention
       1. Mainstay of prevention is inactivated influenzae vaccine.
       2. High-risk groups in need of vaccine include:
         (a) Elderly people
         (b) Nursing home residents
         (c) History of chronic obstructive pulmonary disease (COPD) and cardiac disease
         (d) Chronic disease, such as diabetes, renal disease, or hemoglobinopathies.
         (e) Pregnant women, second or third trimester
         (f) Children, ages 6 to 24 months
         (g) Groups in contact with high-risk patients
    iv. Complications include bacterial pneumonia.

VI. Pertussis
  a. General
    i. Whooping cough is a highly communicable respiratory illness.
    ii. More common in young children and infants.

NOTES

iii. Etiology is *Bordetella pertussis.*
iv. Incubation period is 6 to 14 days.
  b. Clinical manifestations
    i. Three stages
      1. Catarrhal stage
        (a) Present with sneezing, injected conjunctivae, and nocturnal cough.
      2. Paroxysmal stage
        (a) Paroxysmal cough with a whooping sound.
        (b) Mucous plug may be expelled, followed by vomiting.
        (c) Physical examination may reveal scattered rhonchi.
      3. Convalescent stage
        (a) Cough disappears.
  c. Diagnosis
    i. Diagnosis based on clinical findings and whooping cough.
    ii. Lymphocytosis may be noted.
    iii. Nasal swab culture for *B. pertussis* is diagnostic.
  d. Treatment
    i. Antibiotic options include erythromycin (drug of choice), trimethoprim-sulfamethoxazole, azithromycin, or clarithromycin.
    ii. Prevention
      1. Exposed susceptible individuals can be treated with erythromycin.
      2. Active immunization
        (a) DTaP is given every 8 weeks, starting at 2 months, for a total of three injections.
        (b) A fourth dose is given at 15 to 18 months, booster at age 5 years.
        (c) Does not confer lifelong immunity.
VII. Pneumonia
  a. Bacterial
    i. General
      1. Due to microaspiration of oral contents, inhalation of small droplets, or hematogenous spread.
      2. Etiologies: see Table 2-1 for common bacterial, viral, fungal, rickettsial, and other causes of pneumonia.
    ii. Clinical manifestations
      1. Symptoms include productive cough, dyspnea, pleuritic chest pain, and fever.
      2. Nonspecific symptoms such as confusion, dehydration, loss of appetite, or failure to thrive may be noted.
      3. Aspiration pneumonia presents with foul-smelling sputum.
      4. Physical examination
        (a) Increased respiratory rate
        (b) Pulmonary exam
          (i) Bronchial breath sounds and egophony
          (ii) Dullness to percussion
          (iii) Decreased breath sounds
      5. Exposure history or underlying disease states may provide clue to etiology.
    iii. Diagnosis
      1. Laboratory testing reveals leukocytosis and positive sputum Gram stain and culture.
      2. In patients with pneumonia, sputum Gram stain will contain less than 10 epithelial cells per low-power field and more than 25 white blood cells per low-power field.
      3. Urine testing for legionella may be positive.
      4. Chest X-ray reveals five classic patterns. See Figure 2-2.
        (a) Lobar pneumonia
          (i) Density that involves a distinct segment of the lung.
          (ii) Noted in infection due to *S. pneumoniae, H. influenzae,* and *Legionella* species.
        (b) Bronchopneumonia
          (i) Patchy infiltrates involving multiple areas of the lung.
          (ii) Noted in infection due to *S. aureus,* Gram-negative bacilli, mycoplasma, chlamydia, and viruses.
        (c) Interstitial pneumonia
          (i) Present with fine, diffuse, granular infiltrates.
          (ii) Noted in infection due to influenza, cytomegalovirus, and *Pneumocystis carinii.*
        (d) Lung abscess
          (i) Present with loss of lung tissue and cavity formation.

NOTES

(ii) Noted in infection due to anaerobes.
(e) Nodular lesions
(i) Multiple or single nodular lesions.
(ii) Noted in infection due to histoplasmosis, coccidioidomycosis, and cryptococcosis.
iv. Treatment
1. Empiric therapy based on most likely organism and clinical setting.

QUESTION

An 18-month old presents with a 2-week history of cough, coryza, and decreased appetite. Today the child developed coughing spells that end in a deep high-pitched inspiration or whooping sound. Which of the following is the most likely diagnosis?

A. Croup
B. Pertussis
C. Influenzae
D. Epiglottitis

Table 2-1 • Etiologies of Pneumonia

Bacterial	Viral	Fungal
Streptococcus pneumoniae	Adenovirus	*Aspergillus* species
Staphylococcus aureus	Respiratory syncytial virus	*Candida albicans*
Haemophilus influenzae	Parainfluenza virus	*Cryptococcus neoformans*
Anaerobes	Influenza A and B	*Histoplasma capsulatum*
Bacteroides species	Rhinovirus	*Coccidioides immitis*
Peptostreptococcus species	Hantavirus	
Fusobacterium species	Varicella-zoster virus	
Enterobacteriaceae		**Rickettsia species**
Escherichia coli		*Coxiella burnetii*
Klebsiella pneumoniae		*Rickettsia rickettsiae*
Enterobacter species		
Pseudomonas aeruginosa		
Legionella pneumophila		**Other**
Actinomyces species		*Mycoplasma pneumoniae*
Nocardia species		*Chlamydia pneumoniae*
Moraxella catarrhalis		*Chlamydia psittaci*
		Mycobacterium tuberculosis

NOTES

ANSWER **B** EXPLANATION: *Pertussis, whooping cough, is a highly communicable respiratory disease in young children. A paroxysmal cough with a whooping sound is noted.*

correct ☐   incorrect ☐

b. Viral
  i. General
    1. Etiologies include:
      (a) *M. pneumoniae*
        (i) Typically seen in patients younger than 40 years.
        (ii) Higher incidence in late summer and early fall.

Table 2-2 • Factors Related to Specific Etiologies

Factor	Etiology
Smoking, chronic obstructive pulmonary disease	*Streptococcus pneumoniae* *Haemophilus influenzae*
Nursing home residence	*Streptococcus pneumoniae* Gram-negative bacilli *Haemophilus influenzae* Tuberculosis
Alcoholism	*Streptococcus pneumoniae* Gram-negative bacilli, such as *Klebsiella pneumoniae* Anaerobes
Exposure to bats	*Histoplasma capsulatum*
Exposure to birds	*Cryptococcus neoformans* *Chlamydia psittaci*
Recent history of influenza	*Staphylococcus aureus* *Streptococcus pneumoniae* *Haemophilus influenzae*
Cystic fibrosis	*Pseudomonas aeruginosa* *Pseudomonas cepacia*
Intravenous drug abuse	*Staphylococcus aureus* Anaerobes Tuberculosis
Aspiration	Anaerobes
HIV/AIDS	*Pneumocystis carinii*

NOTES

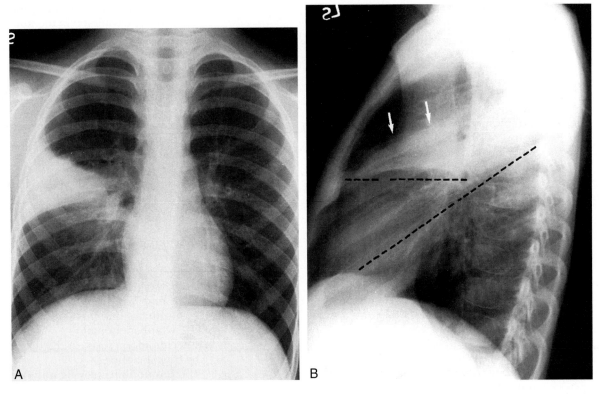

Figure 2-2 Chest X-ray in a patient with pneumonia. (From Mettler FA. Essentials of Radiology, 2nd ed. Philadelphia: Elsevier Saunders, 2005:80, Fig. 3-44.)

Table 2-3 • Empiric Treatment of Pneumonia			
Community-Acquired Pneumonia, Inpatient	Community-Acquired Pneumonia, Outpatient	Aspiration (Community)	Aspiration (Hospital)
Clarithromycin	Ceftriaxone or cefotaxime plus a macrolide	Penicillin G	Ceftriaxone plus metronidazole
Azithromycin	Fluoroquinolone	Clindamycin	Fluoroquinolone plus metronidazole
Erythromycin			Piperacillin-tazobactam
Doxycycline			Ticarcillin-clavulanate
Amoxicillin-clavulanate			
Second-generation cephalosporins			

NOTES

(b) *C. pneumoniae*
(c) Viruses including adenovirus, parainfluenzae, influenza A and B, and RSV.

ii. Clinical manifestations
1. Subacute disease with patients typically having symptoms for 7 to 10 days before seeking medical attention.
2. Symptoms are less severe than other forms of pneumonia.
   (a) Cough is nonproductive.
   (b) Also present with fever, malaise, and headache.
       (i) Headache and sore throat are common in mycoplasma and chlamydia infections.
3. Viral infection presents with nonproductive cough, malaise, and fever.

iii. Diagnosis
1. Chest X-ray in mycoplasma and chlamydia infections reveals unilateral or bilateral patchy lower lobe infiltrates.
2. Rapid viral screens are available for detection of influenza.

iv. Treatment
1. Treat mycoplasma and chlamydia with tetracycline and macrolides.
2. Influenzae A can be treated with amantadine and rimantadine.
   (a) Neuraminidase inhibitors can be used for treatment of influenza A and B.
   (b) Prevention can be obtained with influenza vaccine.

c. Fungal
i. General
1. Includes *Histoplasma capsulatum* and *Coccidioides immitis*.
2. Histoplasmosis
   (a) More common in Midwestern (Ohio and Mississippi river valleys) and southeastern United States.
   (b) A dimorphic fungus that is found in the soil.
   (c) Infection is noted in cave explorers, due to exposure to bat guano.
3. Coccidioidomycosis
   (a) More common in central California, Arizona, New Mexico, and Texas.
   (b) A dimorphic fungus found in the soil and more common in the summer.

ii. Clinical manifestations
1. Histoplasmosis presents as a flulike illness.
   (a) Two weeks after exposure, patients develop high fever, headache, nonproductive cough, and dull chest pain.
   (b) May disseminate to other parts of the body.
2. Coccidioidomycosis patients may be asymptomatic or present with fever, pleuritic chest pain, dry cough, and shortness of breath.
   (a) Disease may disseminate to other parts of the body, such as the central nervous system.

iii. Diagnosis
1. Fungal culture or antigen testing can diagnose histoplasmosis.
   (a) Chest X-ray reveals a patchy infiltrate and mediastinal lymphadenopathy.
2. Coccidioidomycosis can be diagnosed by fungal culture.
   (a) Eosinophilia may be noted.
   (b) Sputum sample may reveal spherules.
   (c) Organism can be noted on silver stain.
   (d) Multiple serologic tests are available.

iv. Treatment
1. Histoplasmosis
   (a) Itraconazole or amphotericin B can be used to treat.
2. Coccidioidomycosis
   (a) Most cases resolve spontaneously.
   (b) Disseminated disease should be treated with amphotericin B.

d. HIV related
i. General
1. Due to *P. carinii*.
2. Patients typically have a CD4 count less than $200/\mu L$.

ii. Clinical manifestations
1. Present with fever, dry cough, dyspnea, weight loss, fatigue, and tachypnea.
2. Physical examination is typically normal for pulmonary complaints.

NOTES

iii. Diagnosis
1. Lactate dehydrogenase (LDH) is elevated.
2. Gallium scan is positive, reveals increased uptake in the infected areas.
3. Gram stain is negative for bacteria.
4. Chest X-ray may be normal or reveals diffuse interstitial infiltrates.
    (a) A butterfly pattern may be noted.
iv. Treatment
1. Treatment of choice is trimethoprim-sulfamethoxazole or pentamidine.
2. Steroids can be given if presence of severe respiratory compromise.

VIII. RSV infection
a. General
i. Cause of lower respiratory tract infection in young.
ii. Increase risk for severe disease in children with congenital heart disease, chronic lung disease, or premature infants.
b. Clinical manifestations
i. First symptoms are those of an upper respiratory tract infection.
ii. Low-grade fever may be present.
iii. Physical examination reveals wheezing, retractions, crackles, and hyperinflation.
c. Diagnosis
i. Rapid detection of RSV antigen, via enzyme-linked immunosorbent assay or fluorescent antibody staining, in nasal or pulmonary secretion is very sensitive.
d. Treatment
i. Supportive care with humidified oxygen and IV fluids.
ii. Bronchodilators may be used for wheezing.
iii. Antiviral, ribavirin can be given by continuous aerosolization.
1. Antibiotics, decongestants, expectorants, and steroids are not helpful.
iv. RSV monoclonal antibodies can be given monthly to high-risk patients, during peak periods.
v. Complications include secondary bacterial infection of the lungs or middle ear.
1. May cause exacerbation of asthma.

IX. Tuberculosis
a. General
i. Caused by *Mycobacterium tuberculosis*.

QUESTION

Which of the following is a common infectious cause of nodular lesions on chest x-ray?

A. Pneumocystis carinii
B. Legionella species
C. Histoplasmosis
D. Mycoplasma

ii. Spread by aerosolization of contaminated respiratory secretions.
1. Organism reaches the alveolar surface, macrophages fail to control infection and infection spreads via the pulmonary lymphatics to the hilar lymph nodes (Ghon complex).
2. From there may spread via the systemic circulation to other parts of the body or become latent.
    (a) Reactivation occurs when macrophages can no longer contain the infection.
3. Only 10% of people infected will have clinical disease at some point in their lifetime.
iii. HIV and AIDS have contributed to the rise in tuberculosis infections.
b. Clinical manifestations
i. Pulmonary disease symptoms include cough, fever, and night sweats.
1. Cough starts dry, then becomes productive with hemoptysis.
ii. Extrapulmonary disease symptoms depend on site involved.
1. See Table 2-4 for summary.
c. Diagnosis
i. Chest X-ray is very important in making the diagnosis.
1. Apices show fibronodular scarring that develops into fluffy and then cavitary lesions.
ii. Sputum smears and culture are specific for making the diagnosis.
1. Acid-fast smears identify mycobacteria, but are not species specific.

NOTES

ANSWER **C** EXPLANATION: *Nodular lesions on chest x-ray are noted in infection due to histoplasmosis, coccidioidomycosis, and cryptococcus. See table 13-2 for summary of systemic fungal organisms.*

correct ☐   incorrect ☐

   2. Cultures are the gold standard, but require 3 to 6 weeks to make the identification of the organism.
iii. Tuberculin skin test used to identify latent disease.
   1. Interdermal injection given and read 48 to 72 hours later.
      (a) Read induration only, not erythema.
      (b) See Table 2-5 for interpretation of tuberculin skin test.
   2. Becomes positive 4 to 5 weeks after infection.
   3. Use of bacille Calmette-Guérin (BCG) vaccine is not a contraindication to a tuberculin skin test.
      (a) In high-risk patients, the history of prior BCG vaccine should not alter the interpretation of the tuberculin skin test.
d. Treatment
   i. Treatment should be based on a patient-centered case management system with direct observation of therapy.

   ii. Multiple agents are needed to improve bacteria clearance and decrease the development of drug resistance.
   iii. A four-drug regimen is recommended, with two of the drugs being isoniazid and rifampin.
      1. Other drugs include rifabutin, pyrazinamide, ethambutol, and streptomycin.
   iv. Preventive therapy for latent infection
      1. Before treatment begins must rule out active tuberculosis.
      2. First-line drugs include isoniazid, rifampin, rifabutin, pyrazinamide, ethambutol, or pyrotomycin.
         (a) Drugs can be given daily, two times per week, or three times per week.
      3. Patients should be monitored for signs of hepatitis.

NEOPLASTIC DISEASE

I. Bronchogenic carcinoma
   a. General
      i. Lung cancer is the leading cause of cancer deaths in both men and women in the United States.
         1. Overall 5-year survival rate is 14%.
      ii. Arise from the respiratory epithelium cells.
      iii. Two subtypes.

Table 2-4 • Clinical Manifestations of Extrapulmonary Tuberculosis	
Organ System	**Clinical Manifestations**
Lymphatic	Painless, unilateral cervical adenopathy
Genitourinary	Hematuria, pyuria, routine culture negative
Bone	Lumbar spine pain in older patient with high dorsal pain in the young
Disseminated	Fever, night sweats
Central nervous system	Fever, headache, vomiting, focal neurologic deficits
Pericardial	Substernal pain, signs of heart failure

NOTES

1. Non–small cell lung cancer
   (a) Adenocarcinoma
       (i) Noted in the periphery of the lung or central airway.
       (ii) Tumor cells contain mucins.
       (iii) Bronchoalveolar carcinoma is a subtype of adeno-carcinoma.
            (1) Arise in the periphery of the lung.
   (b) Squamous cell carcinoma
       (i) Originate in the central airways.
   (c) Large cell carcinoma
2. Small cell lung cancer
iv. Risk factors
   1. Smoking
   2. Passive smoke exposure
   3. Asbestos exposure
      (a) Also linked to mesothelioma.
   4. Ionizing radiation
   5. Radon
   6. COPD

b. Clinical manifestations
   i. Clinically silent for most of the course of the disease, with symptoms only appearing late in the disease.
   ii. Symptoms include new cough, change in chronic cough, hemoptysis, chest pain, dyspnea, weight loss, and hoarseness.

QUESTION

A 50-year-old alcoholic and IV drug abuser presents with the complaint of weight loss, night sweats, and hemoptysis. A chest x-ray reveals a cavitary lesion in the right upper lobe. Which of the following is the most likely diagnosis?

A. Bacterial pneumonia
B. Lymphoma
C. Tuberculosis
D. Sarcoidosis

Table 2-5 • Interpretation of Tuberculin Skin Test

≥5 mm of induration is a positive test in the following groups:	≥10 mm induration is a positive test in the following groups:	≥15 mm induration is a positive test in the following groups:
HIV positive	Recent arrivals from high prevalence countries	No known risk factors for tuberculosis
Contact with person with clinically active tuberculosis	Intravenous drug abusers	
Findings of old healed tuberculosis (fibrotic changes on chest X-ray)	Residents and employees of high-risk settings: Prisons and jails Nursing homes Hospitals Homeless shelters	
Organ transplant recipient	Clinical condition that places patient at high risk	
Other immunosuppressed patients	Children < 4 years of age Children exposed to adults in high-risk settings	

NOTES

ANSWER **C** EXPLANATION: *Symptoms of pulmonary Tuberculosis include fever, cough, and night sweats. Hemoptysis may be noted. Chest x-ray reveals cavitary lesions in apices. Diagnosis is based on sputum culture.*

correct ☐   incorrect ☐

iii. Physical examination findings include wheezing due to airway obstruction, and findings due to various syndromes.
iv. Other syndromes may present.
  1. Superior vena cave syndrome
    (a) May be noted with local invasive disease.
    (b) Present with facial swelling due to blockage of superior vena cava by local tumor.

2. Horner's syndrome
  (a) Due to disruption of cervical sympathetic nerves.
  (b) Present with unilateral facial anhidrosis, ptosis, and miosis.
3. Pancoast's syndrome
  (a) Due to tumor invading apex and superior sulcus and invasion of brachial plexus and cervical sympathetic nerves.
  (b) Present with arm and shoulder pain and signs of Horner's syndrome.
c. Diagnosis
  i. Chest X-ray may reveal pleural effusions and lung masses or nodules.
  ii. Computed tomography (CT) scan is used to detect abnormalities in lymph nodes or metastases to surrounding structures.
  iii. Sputum cytology, biopsy of lymph nodes, and tissue from bronchoscopy determine lung cancer cell type.

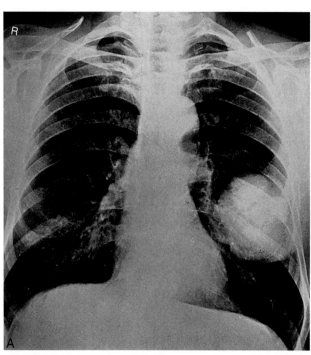 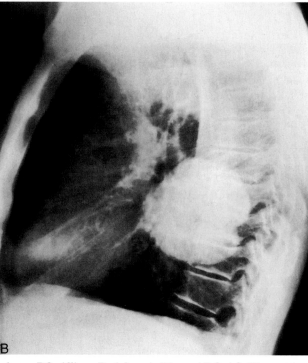

Figure 2-3 Bronchial carcinoma in left lower lobe. (From Grainger RG, Allison D, Adam A, Dixon AK [eds]: Diagnostic Radiology: A Textbook of Medical Imaging, 4th ed. London: Harcourt, 2001:464, Fig. 22.1.)

NOTES

        iv. Lung cancer tends to metastasize to brain, bone, adrenal glands, and liver.

    d. Treatment

        i. Staging is required to predict prognosis and determine appropriate therapy.

        ii. Treatment varies with subtype of lung cancer.

           1. Non–small cell lung cancer is treated with surgery, offers the best chance for survival.

              (a) Chemotherapy and radiation therapy are effective in combination with surgery.

           2. Small cell lung cancer is treated with chemotherapy and radiation therapy.

        iii. Prevention

           1. Smoking cessation is the most important strategy in the prevention of lung cancer.

II. Carcinoid tumors

    a. General

        i. Low-grade malignant neoplasms.

           1. Slow growing and rarely metastasize.

        ii. Most cases are noted in patients younger than 60 years and equally common in males and females.

        iii. Complications include bleeding and airway obstruction.

    b. Clinical manifestations

        i. Symptoms include hemoptysis, cough, wheezing, and recurrent pneumonia.

        ii. Carcinoid syndrome, with flushing, diarrhea, and hypotension, is rare.

    c. Diagnosis

        i. On chest X-ray may present with solitary pulmonary nodules.

        ii. Diagnosis is confirmed by biopsy.

        iii. Octreotide scintigraphy is used to localize tumor.

    d. Treatment

        i. Surgery is treatment of choice; chemotherapy and radiation therapy are not helpful.

III. Metastatic tumors

    a. General

        i. Due to spread of other malignant tumors to the lung, via vascular or lymphatics system, or direct extension.

        ii. Most any cancer can spread to the lung.

    b. Clinical manifestations

        i. Symptoms are uncommon, but include cough, hemoptysis, and dyspnea.

        ii. Most symptoms related to primary tumor.

    c. Diagnosis

        i. Chest X-ray and CT scan reveal multiple nodules.

        ii. Diagnosis is confirmed by percutaneous needle biopsy or transbronchial biopsy.

    d. Treatment

        i. Management consists of treatment of primary tumor and pulmonary complications.

        ii. Local resection of the tumors is available in selected cases.

IV. Pulmonary nodules

    a. General

        i. A nodule is a round or oval, sharply circumscribed lesion, up to 5 cm in diameter.

           1. If larger than 5 cm, it is termed a *mass*.

        ii. A central cavity or calcification, with or without surrounding lesions may be noted.

        iii. One fourth of bronchogenic carcinomas present with a solitary pulmonary nodule.

        iv. Benign nature of the nodule is favored if nodule is of small size (<2 cm in diameter), has smooth margins, patient is of a young age, and absence of symptoms.

    b. Clinical manifestations

        i. Are asymptomatic or present with symptoms of the underlying malignancy.

    c. Diagnosis

        i. CT scan is obtained to determine location and effect on surrounding structures.

        ii. Biopsy is used to determine whether nodule is benign or malignant, or has an infectious etiology.

    d. Treatment

        i. All nodules must be monitored closely.

        ii. All solitary nodules in patients older than 35 years should be considered potentially malignant.

           1. Resection is indicated.

NOTES

OBSTRUCTIVE PULMONARY DISEASE

I. Asthma
  a. General
    i. Respiratory disease with intermittent, reversible obstruction of the airways.
    ii. Three basic pathophysiologic changes:
      1. Airway inflammation
      2. Airway obstruction
      3. Airway hyperresponsiveness
    iii. Disease classified based on frequency of symptoms
  b. Clinical manifestations
    i. Most common symptoms include episodic wheezing, cough, chest tightness, and shortness of breath.
      1. Symptoms typically more prevalent at night and most severe in the morning.
    ii. Physical examination reveals diffuse wheezing, tachypnea, tachycardia, and prolonged expiration.
      1. In severe cases, may note accessory muscle use, intercostal retractions, and distant breath sounds.
  c. Diagnosis
    i. Laboratory testing reveals elevated white blood cell count with eosinophilia.
    ii. Sputum examination reveals eosinophils, Curschmann's spirals (mucus casts of small airways) or Charcot-Leyden crystals.
    iii. Early in an asthmatic episode, the arterial blood gases reveal respiratory alkalosis and hypoxia.
      1. A normalizing P_{CO_2} or development of respiratory acidosis indicates impending respiratory failure.
    iv. Pulmonary function testing shows an obstructive pattern.
      1. Improvement in pulmonary function tests noted after treatment with bronchodilators.
      2. See Table 2-7 for comparison of pulmonary function tests in obstructive and restrictive lung disease.
  d. Treatment
    i. Based on classification of chronic asthma with addition of agents as severity increases.
    ii. Acute exacerbations
      1. Inhaled, short-acting beta-agonist is the first agent of choice.
      2. This should be followed by oral or IV corticosteroids.
      3. Oxygen may also be required.
    iii. Exercise-induced asthma
      1. A beta-agonist or cromolyn sodium is used 15 minutes before exercise.
    iv. Prevention
      1. Decrease exposure to allergens.
      2. Avoid exposure to smoking.
      3. Annual influenza vaccine to reduce risk of influenza.
      4. Long-acting beta-agonist, salmeterol, can be used as maintenance therapy.
II. Status asthmaticus
  a. General
    i. Unremitting asthma with rapidly increasing severity.

Table 2-6 • Classification of Chronic Asthma

Step	Classification	Frequency of Symptoms	Nocturnal Symptoms
1	Mild intermittent	<2 times per week	<2 times per month
2	Mild persistent	>2 times per week	>2 times per month
3	Moderate persistent	Daily	>6 times per month
4	Severe persistent	Continuous	Frequent

NOTES

    ii. Respiratory failure develops due to two mechanisms.
      1. Diffuse bronchial obstruction leading to ventilation-perfusion mismatch and hypoxia.
      2. Respiratory muscle fatigue.
  b. Clinical manifestations
    i. Symptoms include acute onset of chest tightness, shortness of breath, and cough.
    ii. Physical examination reveals tachycardia, tachypnea, cyanosis, use of accessory muscles, intercostal retractions, pulsus paradoxus, and absence of wheezing.
  c. Diagnosis
    i. Laboratory findings include hypoxemia and hypercapnia.
    ii. Spirometry very useful in assessment of status asthmaticus.
      1. Peak flow and FEV_1 will be decreased.
      2. Monitor peak flow or FEV_1 before and after treatment.
    iii. Chest X-ray reveals hyperinflation and increased anteroposterior diameter.
  d. Treatment
    i. Treatment consists of:
      1. Oxygen
        (a) Supplemental oxygen needed to raise Po_2 to 80 to 100 mm Hg.
      2. Bronchodilators
        (a) Aerosolized beta-adrenergic agonists to open airways.
          (i) Are safe in pregnancy.

QUESTION

A 60-year-old patient presents with dyspnea, hemoptysis, and bone pain. Chest x-ray reveals a right hilar mass and widen mediastinum. Labs reveal a hyponatremia. Which of the following is the most likely diagnosis?

  A. Squamous cell carcinoma of the lung
  B. Adenocarcinoma of the lung
  C. Small cell carcinoma of the lung
  D. Non-Hodgkin's lymphoma

          (ii) Salmeterol, long-acting beta-adrenergic agonist, is not indicated in acute disease.
        (b) Subcutaneous epinephrine can be used, but side effects include tachycardia, increased myocardial oxygen requirement, and hypertension.
        (c) Intravenous magnesium is also an effective bronchodilator.
      3. Corticosteroids
        (a) IV or oral corticosteroids are recommended early in treatment.
        (b) Are safe in pregnancy and should not be withheld if needed.
        (c) Work by decreasing inflammation.

Table 2-7 • Obstructive and Restrictive Patterns on Pulmonary Function Testing		
	Obstructive	**Restrictive**
Vital capacity	Normal or decreased	Decreased
FEV_1	Decreased	Normal or decreased
$FEV_{1\%}$	<75%	Normal or increased
Residual volume (RV)	Normal or increased	Decreased
Total lung capacity (TLC)	Normal or increased	Decreased
RV/TLC	Increased	Normal or increased

NOTES

ANSWER **A** EXPLANATION: *Bronchogenic carcinoma presents with cough, hemoptysis, dyspnea, weight loss, and hoarseness. Chest x-ray reveals a mass. Hyponatremia is noted in small cell carcinoma of the lung do to secretion of anti-diuretic hormone.*

correct ☐   incorrect ☐

4. Mechanical ventilation
   (a) Indications include altered mental status, acute CO_2 retention, poor response to therapy, or impending respiratory muscle fatigue.
5. See Table 2-8 for summary of medication options in treatment of asthma.

Table 2-8 • Asthma Medications			
Drug	**Classification**	**Side Effects**	**Notes**
Albuterol	Beta-adrenergic agonist	Tachycardia Hyperglycemia Hypokalemia	
Metaproterenol	Beta-adrenergic agonist	Tachycardia Hyperglycemia Hypokalemia	
Pirbuterol	Beta-adrenergic agonist	Tachycardia Hyperglycemia Hypokalemia	
Salmeterol	Beta-adrenergic agonist	Tachycardia Hyperglycemia Hypokalemia	Long-acting agent, not used for acute therapy
Terbutaline	Beta-adrenergic agonist	Tachycardia Hyperglycemia Hypokalemia	
Ipratropium bromide	Anticholinergics	No real side effects	Very useful in chronic obstructive pulmonary disease, helps dry secretions
Theophylline	Not established	Anorexia Nausea Abdominal pain Seizures Arrhythmias	Must monitor serum drug levels
Aminophylline	Not established	Anorexia Nausea Abdominal pain Arrhythmias	Must monitor serum drug levels

NOTES

III. Bronchiectasis
    a. General
        i. Abnormal dilatation of the large conducting airways.
       ii. Due to congenital structural abnormalities or acquired process.
           1. Congenital causes include cystic fibrosis and alpha-1-antitrypsin deficiency.
           2. Acquired processes include viral and bacterial infections, foreign bodies, and tumors.
    b. Clinical manifestations
        i. Major symptom is cough, which is daily and productive with purulent sputum.

QUESTION

A patient presents with myalgias, fever, chills, dry cough, and coryza. The symptoms started last night. He states that many people in his dorm are also sick with the same symptoms. Which of the following is the most likely diagnosis?

    A. Influenzae
    B. Acute bronchitis
    C. Lobar pneumonia
    D. Asthma exacerbation

Table 2-8 • Asthma Medications—cont'd

Drug	Classification	Side Effects	Notes
Beclomethasone dipropionate	Anti-inflammatory agent	Osteoporosis Edema Increased appetite	Increased risk for oral candidiasis
Budesonide	Anti-inflammatory agent	Osteoporosis Edema Increased appetite	Increased risk for oral candidiasis
Flunisolide	Anti-inflammatory agent	Osteoporosis Edema Increased appetite	Increased risk for oral candidiasis
Fluticasone propionate	Anti-inflammatory agent	Osteoporosis Edema Increased appetite	
Methylprednisolone	Anti-inflammatory agent	Osteoporosis Edema Increased appetite	
Prednisone	Anti-inflammatory agent	Osteoporosis Edema Increased appetite	
Triamcinolone	Anti-inflammatory agent	Osteoporosis Edema Increased appetite	

(continued)

NOTES

ANSWER **A** EXPLANATION: *Influenzae is a common respiratory infection, which is spread by respiratory droplets, and presents with abrupt onset of chills, fever, myalgias, headache, and cough.*

correct ☐   incorrect ☐

       1. Hemoptysis may accompany the cough.
       2. As disease progresses, exercise intolerance and dyspnea develop.
    ii. Physical examination reveals coarse crackles with wheezing.
  c. Diagnosis
    i. Chest X-ray reveals thickened bronchial walls, "signet ring" sign on airways projecting on end.
       1. Multiple ectatic airways extending from the hila to the periphery may be noted.
          (a) Gives a finger-in-glove appearance on chest X-ray.
    ii. CT scan is the standard test for diagnosing disease.

       1. Shows failure of bronchi to taper and increased wall thickness.
    iii. Pulmonary function tests may be normal at first, later develop an obstructive, restrictive, or combined pattern.
  d. Treatment
    i. Treatment of underlying cause is crucial.
    ii. Anti-inflammatory medications may also be used.
IV. Chronic bronchitis
  a. General
    i. A clinical diagnosis of excessive sputum production with chronic or recurring cough on most days for at least 3 months of the year for at least 2 consecutive years.
    ii. Cigarette smoking is major risk factor.
       1. Increases risk by 10 to 30 times over nonsmokers.
  b. Clinical manifestations
    i. Early symptoms include cough and wheezing, later develop dyspnea on exertion.
    ii. Physical examination reveals an overweight, cyanotic patient with pedal edema.
       1. Signs of right-sided heart failure may be common.

Table 2-8 • Asthma Medications—cont'd

Drug	Classification	Side Effects	Notes
Montelukast	Leukotriene inhibitor	Elevated liver function tests Headache Dyspepsia	
Zafirlukast	Leukotriene inhibitor	Elevated liver function tests Headache Dyspepsia	Will interfere with warfarin
Cromolyn sodium	Mast cell stabilizer	Sore throat Cough Mouth dryness	Has value only when used prophylactically
Nedocromil sodium	Mast cell stabilizer	Sore throat Cough Mouth dryness	Has value only when used prophylactically

NOTES

2. Become dyspneic almost immediately when lying flat.
3. Digital clubbing is rare.
iii. See Table 2-9 for comparison of emphysema and chronic bronchitis.
c. Diagnosis
i. Pulmonary function test reveals an obstructive pattern. See Table 2-7.
ii. Arterial blood gases reveal mild to moderate hypoxemia with normal PCO_2.
iii. Electrocardiogram (EKG) will be normal early in disease and later develop right-axis deviation.
iv. Chest X-ray may reveal cardiac enlargement, congestion, increased lung markings, and bronchial wall thickening.
d. Treatment
i. Smoking cessation is the number one intervention.
ii. First-line therapy is beta-agonists.
1. Used to reverse bronchospasm.
2. Side effects include palpitations, tachycardia, nervousness, and hypertension.

3. Long-acting salmeterol is used for chronic treatment only.
iii. Theophylline is a weak bronchodilator and used as an adjunct with beta-agonists.
1. Side effects include nausea, vomiting, tachycardia, hypertension, and tremor.
iv. Corticosteroids can be helpful in reducing inflammation.
v. Mucokinetics facilitates mucociliary clearance by decreasing viscosity of mucus.
vi. Oxygen has been shown to improve survival and quality of life.
V. Cystic fibrosis
a. General
i. Autosomal recessive disease and most common lethal inherited disease in American whites.
1. Incidence is 1 in 2000 live births.
2. Most patients diagnosed in the preteen years.
3. Due to defect in cystic fibrosis transmembrane conductance regulator.

Table 2-9 • Comparison of Emphysema and Chronic Bronchitis

	Emphysema	Chronic Bronchitis
Description	"Pink puffer"	"Blue bloater"
Major complaint	Dyspnea	Chronic cough
Age at onset	After age 50 years	Late 30s and 40s
Body habitus	Thin	Overweight
Lung exam	No adventitious sounds	Rhonchi are present
Peripheral edema	Negative	Positive
Hemoglobin	Normal	Elevated
Blood gases	PO_2 normal or reduced PCO_2 normal or reduced	PO_2 reduced PCO_2 elevated
Chest X-ray	Hyperinflated with flat diaphragms	Increased interstitial markings and normal diaphragms

NOTES

ii. Symptoms are due to development of thick secretions that block the airways and ductal system in other organs.
   1. Other organ systems include pancreatic and hepatic.
   2. Many males with cystic fibrosis are infertile due to obstructive azoospermia.
iii. Airways commonly infected with *S. aureus* and *H. influenzae* as a child and *Pseudomonas aeruginosa* as adults.

b. Clinical manifestations
   i. Common symptoms include chronic cough with sputum production and dyspnea.
      1. Newborns with cystic fibrosis present with intestinal obstruction and meconium ileus.
   ii. Physical examination reveals weight loss, wheezing, and a salty taste on the skin.
   iii. Patients typically have a history of recurrent pneumonia, sinusitis, or asthma.

c. Diagnosis
   i. Most specific test result for cystic fibrosis is elevated sweat chloride.
      1. Values greater than 60 mEq/L in children are abnormal.
   ii. Pancreatic insufficiency is diagnosed by demonstrating fat malabsorption with a qualitative or quantitative fecal fat test.

d. Treatment
   i. Maintenance therapy goal is to slow the progression of lung damage by improving mucus clearance, controlling infection, and controlling inflammation.
      1. Mucus clearance is improved with percussion and postural drainage.
   ii. Pancreatic insufficiency is treated with pancreatic enzyme supplements.
   iii. Antibiotic selection should include coverage for pseudomonal with anti-pseudomonal beta-lactam agents and an aminoglycoside or ciprofloxacin.

VI. Emphysema
   a. General
      i. Defined as destructive changes to the alveoli walls and enlargement of air spaces.

1. Affects lung parenchyma distal to terminal bronchioles.
ii. Cigarette smoking is major risk factor.
   1. Increase risk by 10 to 30 times over nonsmokers.
iii. Alpha-1-antitrypsin should be suspected in patients who develop emphysema in their late 30s.
   1. Treatment consists of recombinant antiprotease replacement therapy.

b. Clinical manifestations
   i. Early symptoms include cough and wheezing, later develop dyspnea on exertion.
   ii. Physical examination reveals a thin patient with pursed-lip breathing and pink skin color.
      1. See Table 2-9.

c. Diagnosis
   i. Pulmonary function test reveals an obstructive pattern. See Table 2-7.
   ii. Arterial blood gases reveal severe hypoxemia and hypercapnia.
   iii. Chest X-ray may be normal or show overinflation, flat diaphragm, and increased retrosternal space.

d. Treatment
   i. Smoking cessation is the number one intervention.
   ii. First-line medical therapy is anticholinergic agents
      1. Agents should be given on a regular basis.
      2. Side effects include dry month, skin flushing, blurry vision, tachycardia, and urinary retention.
   iii. Theophylline is a weak bronchodilator and used as an adjunct with anticholinergic agents.
      1. Side effects include nausea, vomiting, tachycardia, hypertension, and tremor.
   iv. Oxygen has been shown to improve survival and quality of life.

PLEURAL DISEASES

I. Pleural effusion
   a. General

NOTES

i. Pleural space lies between the lung and chest wall.
ii. Effusion is present when there is excess quantity of fluid in the pleural space.
iii. Mechanisms of pleural effusion development
    1. Increased hydrostatic pressure in microcirculation
      (a) Seen in left-sided heart failure.
      (b) Most common cause of pleural effusions.
    2. Decreased oncotic pressure in microcirculation.
      (a) Seen in hypoalbuminemia.
    3. Decreased pressure in the pleural space.
      (a) Seen in collapsed lung.
    4. Increased permeability in microcirculation.
      (a) Seen in pneumonia.
    5. Impaired lymphatic drainage.
      (a) Seen in malignancy.
      (b) Most commonly noted in lung cancer, breast cancer, and lymphoma.
    6. Movement of fluid from peritoneal space.
      (a) Seen in ascites.
iv. Must determine whether fluid is a transudate or exudate.
    1. Transudates occur when systemic factors that control formation and absorption of pleural fluid are altered.
      (a) Causes include left-sided heart failure, pulmonary embolism, and cirrhosis.
    2. Exudates occur when local factors that control formation and absorption of pleural fluid are altered.
      (a) Causes include bacterial pneumonia, malignancy, viral infection, and pulmonary embolism.
b. Clinical manifestations
  i. Symptoms include dyspnea, cough, and chest pain.
  ii. Lung exam reveals decreased breath sounds, dullness to percussion, and absent tactile fremitus.
c. Diagnosis
  i. Chest X-ray reveals blunting of margins.

    1. Free pleural fluid can be demonstrated with a lateral decubitus film.
  ii. Laboratory results
    1. Exudates meet the following criteria, while transudates meet none.
      (a) Pleural fluid protein–to–serum protein ratio greater than 0.5
      (b) Pleural fluid LDH–to–serum LDH ratio greater than 0.6
      (c) Pleural fluid LDH more than two thirds the normal upper limit for serum
d. Treatment
  i. Thoracentesis can be diagnostic as well as therapeutic.
II. Pneumothorax
a. General
  i. Due to presence of gas in the pleural space.
  ii. Clinical manifestations include sudden onset of dyspnea and pleuritic chest pain.
  iii. Physical examination reveals decreased or absent breath sounds.
  iv. Chest X-ray is essential to confirm the diagnosis and reveals a collapsed lung with loss of lung markings at the periphery.
b. Types
  i. Primary spontaneous
    1. Occur in the absence of underlying lung disease.
      (a) Seen most commonly in thin males aged 30 to 40 years.
    2. Typically due to rupture of pleural blebs and occur almost exclusively in smokers.

QUESTION

A 55-year-old male presents with a long history of a productive cough. The patient states the cough has been present for 6 months each of the last three years. The patient is afebrile and chest x-ray is unremarkable. Which of the following is the most likely diagnosis?

A. Viral pneumonia
B. Chronic bronchitis
C. Emphysema
D. Asthma

NOTES

ANSWER **B** EXPLANATION: *Chronic bronchitis is defined as chronic cough with excessive sputum production for at least three months of the years for at least two consecutive years.*

correct ☐   incorrect ☐

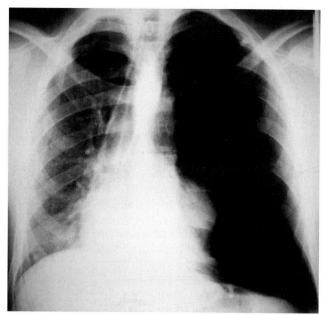

Figure 2-5 Tension pneumothorax on the left with mediastinal shift to the right. (From Grainger RG, Allison D, Adam A, Dixon AK [eds]: Diagnostic Radiology: A Textbook of Medical Imaging, 4th ed. London: Harcourt, 2001:337, Fig. 16.44.)

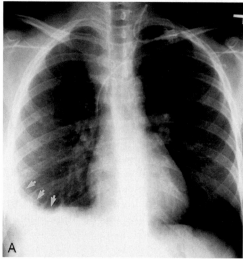

Figure 2-4 Pleural effusion. Moderate-sized right-sided pleural effusion. Note blunting of costophrenic angle. (From Mettler FA Jr. [ed]: Essentials of Radiology, 2nd ed. Philadelphia: Elsevier, Inc, 2004:107, Figure 3-79A.)

3. Recurrence is common.
4. Treatment is simple aspiration or pleural abrasion in preventing recurrences.
  ii. Secondary spontaneous
1. Occurs in the presence of underlying lung disease, such as COPD.
2. More life threatening.
3. Treatment consists of a chest tube and use of a sclerosing agent.
  iii. Traumatic
1. Results from penetrating or nonpenetrating chest injuries.

2. Treat with chest tube unless pneumothorax is very small.
  iv. Tension
1. Pneumothorax in which the pressure in the pleural space is positive throughout the respiratory cycle.
  (a) Occurs most commonly during mechanical ventilation or pulmonary resuscitation.
2. Life threatening due to positive pressure in thorax decreasing venous return and cardiac output.
3. Physical examination reveals decreased or absent breath sounds on affected side and shift of the mediastinum to the contralateral side.
4. Treatment consists of rapid placement of a large-bore needle into the pleural space through the second anterior intercostal space.

NOTES

PULMONARY CIRCULATION

I. Pulmonary embolism (PE)
  a. General
    i. Most pulmonary emboli arise from venous thrombi in the deep veins of the lower extremities, followed by right-sided heart chamber, pelvic veins, and venous catheters.
      1. Emboli are usually multiple and bilateral and typically found in the lower lobes.
    ii. Risk factors include:
      1. Hypercoagulable states
      2. Pregnancy and birth control pills
      3. Recent orthopedic, neurologic, or gynecologic surgery with general anesthesia
      4. Recent major trauma
      5. Atrial fibrillation
      6. Right ventricular myocardial infarction
      7. Immobilization
      8. History of prior PE
    iii. Pathophysiology
      1. Total stoppage of blood flow to the distal lung leads to respiratory and hemodynamic changes.
        (a) Respiratory changes
          (i) Development of an area of lung that is ventilated but not perfused.
          (ii) Pneumoconstriction leading to stoppage of pulmonary capillary flow.
          (iii) Loss of surfactant leading to alveolar collapse.
        (b) Hemodynamic changes
          (i) Increased resistance to blood flow through the lung, which leads to acute right ventricular strain and decrease in cardiac output and an increase in heart rate.
  b. Clinical manifestations
    i. Must have a high index of suspicion.
    ii. Symptoms include acute onset of dyspnea, pleuritic chest pain, cough, hemoptysis, syncope, and substernal chest pain.
    iii. Physical examination reveals tachycardia and tachypnea.
      1. In most patients, lung exam is normal.
      2. In a massive PE, an S_3 may be noted.

QUESTION

A tall, thin patient presents with shortness of breath. On examination you note the patient is breathing through "pursed" lips, his expiratory phase is prolonged and lung sounds are distant. Which of the following is the most likely diagnosis?

  A. Asthma
  B. Bronchiectasis
  C. Cystic fibrosis
  D. Emphysema

  c. Diagnosis
    i. Laboratory results
      1. Arterial blood gases reveal an acute respiratory alkalosis.
      2. EKG may show the classic $S_1Q_3T_3$ with or without a right bundle branch block.
      3. Chest X-ray
        (a) Most abnormalities are nonspecific.
        (b) May note Westermark's sign, an area of decreased pulmonary vascularity with a cutoff sign, or Hampton's hump, a shadow or density in contact with one or more pleural space corresponding to lung segment involved.
      4. Elevated D-dimer
        (a) Excellent test for ruling out pulmonary embolism in low-probability patients.
    ii. Diagnosis is made with one of the following.
      1. $\dot{V}/\dot{Q}$ scan
        (a) Scoring system
          (i) Normal: 9% PE rate
          (ii) Low probability: 14% PE rate
          (iii) Intermediate probability: 30% PE rate
          (iv) High probability: 87% PE rate
        (b) Use limited if other lung pathology is present.
      2. Spiral CT scan
        (a) Increase use with 95% sensitivity for large PE and 75% sensitivity for subsegmental PE.

NOTES

ANSWER D EXPLANATION: *The emphysema, or "pink puffer" patient is typically thin and presents with dyspnea, pursed-lip breathing and pink skin color. Arterial blood gases reveal hypoxia and hypercapnia. See table 2-9 for comparison of emphysema and chronic bronchitis.*

correct ☐   incorrect ☐

3. Pulmonary angiography
   (a) The gold standard for diagnosis.
   (b) Very invasive with increased morbidity and mortality rate.
d. Treatment
   i. Prevention
      1. Includes early ambulation after surgery or delivery, heparin therapy for high-risk patients, or compression stockings.
   ii. Anticoagulation
      1. Heparin is the gold standard for acute therapy.
         (a) Low molecular weight heparin can be used.
            (i) Less bleeding likely, and no laboratory monitoring is needed.

2. Long-term therapy includes warfarin sodium (Coumadin).
3. See Table 2-10 for comparison of heparin and Coumadin.
   iii. Pulmonary embolectomy
      1. Rarely needed except for large saddle emboli.
   iv. Vena cava filter
      1. Indications include absolute contraindication to anticoagulation, recurrence of PE or major bleeding while on anticoagulation, or septic emboli from a pelvic source.
II. Pulmonary hypertension
   a. General
      i. Occurs when resistance to flow across the pulmonary vasculature increases.
      ii. Three groups based on pathophysiology
         1. Precapillary
            (a) Abnormality that leads to elevated pressures is located in the pulmonary arteries or arterioles.
            (b) Etiologies
               (i) Pulmonary embolism
               (ii) Congenital heart disease with pulmonary vascular disease
                  (1) Left-to-right shunts
                  (2) Ventricular septal defect
                  (3) Patent ductus arteriosus

Table 2-10 • Comparison of Heparin and Coumadin		
	Heparin	**Coumadin**
Mechanism of action	Catalyzes antithrombin III inactivation allowing increased levels of activated coagulation factors in the blood	Inhibits vitamin K–dependent factors (II, VII, IX, X, and protein C and S)
Half life	1–2 hr	36 hours
Monitoring test	Partial thromboplastin time	Prothrombin time/INR
Side effects	Bleeding Overdose (treat with protamine sulfate) Heparin-associated thrombocytopenia	Fetal toxic Bleeding Overdose (treat with fresh frozen plasma or vitamin K)
Notes	Safe in pregnancy	Multiple drug interactions

NOTES

(iii) Collagen vascular disease
(iv) Sickle cell anemia
(v) Portal hypertension
(vi) COPD
(vii) Diffuse interstitial lung disease
(viii) Cystic fibrosis
2. Passive
   (a) Abnormality that leads to elevated pressure is due to diseases that increase pulmonary venous return.
   (b) Etiologies
      (i) Left ventricular failure
      (ii) Hypertension
      (iii) Ischemic heart disease
      (iv) Mitral stenosis
      (v) Obstruction of major pulmonary veins
3. Reactive
   (a) Patients have long-standing increased pulmonary venous pressure complicated by pulmonary arteriolar vasoconstriction.
   (b) Etiologies
      (i) Mitral stenosis
iii. Primary pulmonary hypertension
   1. Disease of unknown origin.
   2. Patients do not have pulmonary or cardiac disease.
   3. Present with exertional dyspnea without orthopnea, as well as syncope, chest pain, weakness, and palpitations.
   4. Physical examination
      (a) Pulmonic ejection sound and flow murmur
      (b) Hepatomegaly, peripheral edema, and ascites.
      (c) Right ventricular heave
   5. Diagnosis confirmed by cardiac catheterization or pulmonary angiography.
b. Clinical manifestations
   i. Precapillary present with dyspnea, but no orthopnea, paroxysmal nocturnal dyspnea, or pulmonary edema.
      1. Physical examination reveals tachypnea with normal lung exam.
   ii. Passive presents with dyspnea, orthopnea, and paroxysmal nocturnal dyspnea.
      1. Physical examination reveals findings consistent with underlying etiology.

QUESTION

Which disease state typically produces a pleural effusion that is transudative?

A. Congestive heart failure
B. Rheumatoid arthritis
C. Lung cancer
D. Pancreatitis

iii. Reactive presents with severe dyspnea and markedly decreased exercise tolerance.
c. Diagnosis
   i. Chest X-ray
      1. Precapillary reveals right ventricular enlargement and prominent pulmonary arteries.
      2. Passive reveals prominent upper lobe pulmonary veins, increased density in the central lung fields, and Kerley B lines.
      3. Reactive reveals right ventricular enlargement and very prominent central pulmonary arteries.
   ii. EKG
      1. Precapillary demonstrates right ventricular hypertrophy or right-axis deviation.
      2. Reactive demonstrates right ventricular hypertrophy.
   iii. Right heart catheterization or pulmonary angiography is needed to confirm diagnosis.
      1. See Table 2-11 for angiography results in pulmonary hypertension.
d. Treatment
   i. Treat underlying cause.
   ii. Acute pulmonary hypertension can be treated with prostaglandin (epoprostenol), nitrous oxide, or adenosine.
   iii. Calcium channel blockers can be helpful in a select group of patients.
   iv. Anticoagulation should be considered in all patients.
   v. Reactive pulmonary hypertension is reversible with correction of underlying cause.
   vi. Final treatment options include heart and heart-lung transplantation.

NOTES

III. Cor pulmonale
  a. General
    i. Enlargement or dysfunction of the right ventricle due to pulmonary hypertension.
    ii. Most common cause is COPD.
      1. Other causes include:
        (a) Cystic fibrosis
        (b) Diseases of pulmonary vasculature
        (c) Primary pulmonary hypertension
        (d) Acute massive PE
        (e) Connective tissue disease
        (f) Morbid obesity
        (g) Malignant disease
        (h) Sleep apnea syndromes
  b. Clinical manifestations
    i. Patients present with symptoms of the underlying cause that leads to the right ventricular hypertrophy and failure.
      1. Typically present with easy fatigability, increased dyspnea, increased sputum production, and peripheral edema.
    ii. Physical examination reveals a dyspneic patient with central cyanosis, distended neck veins, parasternal lift, systolic murmur along left sternal border that changes with inspiration, and peripheral edema.
  c. Diagnosis
    i. Arterial blood gases reveal hypoxia and hypercapnia.
    ii. EKG demonstrates right ventricular hypertrophy and prominent P waves in leads II, III, and aVF.
      1. Indicates right atrial enlargement
    iii. Chest X-ray reveals enlarged central pulmonary vessels and decrease in peripheral vessels.
      1. Described as pruning on chest X-ray.
    iv. Echocardiography, magnetic resonance imaging, or cardiac catheterization may be used to evaluate size and function of the right ventricle.
  d. Treatment
    i. Treatment must focus on the underlying cause.
      1. In patients with COPD, this will include bronchodilators, beta-agonists, and antibiotics.
    ii. Oxygen may be needed but used with caution because many patients with cor pulmonale are CO_2 retainers.
    iii. Vasodilators, such as hydralazine or calcium channel blockers, can be used to decrease pulmonary vascular resistance and increase right ventricular stroke volume.
    iv. Diuretics may be needed for peripheral edema.

RESTRICTIVE PULMONARY DISEASE

I. Idiopathic pulmonary fibrosis
  a. General
    i. A fibrosing interstitial pneumonia.
      1. Course is progressive with increasing fibrosis.
    ii. Presents typically between ages 50 and 70 years.

Table 2-11 • Angiography Results in Pulmonary Hypertension				
	Normal	**Precapillary**	**Passive**	**Reactive**
Pulmonary artery pressure	15 mm Hg	Increased	Increased	Increased
Left atrial pressure	5 mm Hg	Normal	Increased	Increased
Pulmonary artery/left atrial pressure gradient		>12 mm Hg	<12 mm Hg	>12 mm Hg

NOTES

1. Very uncommon to present before age 40 years.
iii. Cigarette smoking is a strong link to disease.
iv. Etiology is unknown.
v. Includes the following disorders.
1. Acute interstitial pneumonia (AIP)
2. Usual interstitial pneumonia (UIP)
3. Nonspecific interstitial pneumonia (NSIP)
4. Bronchiolitis obliterans with organizing pneumonia (BOOP)
5. See Table 2-12 for comparison of various idiopathic interstitial pneumonias.
b. Clinical manifestations
i. Initial symptoms include exertional dyspnea (major symptom) and nonproductive cough.
ii. Physical examination reveals tachypnea, clubbing, and fine bibasilar inspiratory crackles (Velcro rales).
c. Diagnosis
i. Chest X-ray reveals bilateral reticular opacities in the periphery and lower lobes.
ii. Pulmonary function test reveals a restrictive pattern.
iii. Lung biopsy is the gold standard for diagnosis.
d. Treatment
i. There is no proven treatment.
1. Mean survival after diagnosis is 3 years.
ii. Anti-inflammatory medications, mainly corticosteroids, are the mainstay of therapy.
1. Corticosteroids are used to suppress the chronic alveolitis.
2. Therapy must be attempted for 3 months before effectiveness can be assessed.
3. Corticosteroids can be combined with azathioprine or cyclophosphamide to improve response.

Table 2-12 • Comparison of Types of Idiopathic Interstitial Pneumonias

Feature	AIP	UIP	NSIP	BOOP
Onset/age	Acute/50s	Insidous/60s	Subacute/50s	Acute or subacute/50s
Cigarette smoking	Unknown	Two thirds	Not known	One half
Mean survival	1–2 mo	5–6 yr	18 mo	
Steroid response	Poor	Poor	Good	Excellent
Complete recovery possible	Yes	No	Yes	Yes

AIP, acute interstitial pneumonia; BOOP, bronchiolitis obliterans with organizing pneumonia; NSIP, nonspecific interstitial pneumonia; UIP, usual interstitial pneumonia.

Table 2-13 • Side Effects of Medications Used in Idiopathic Pulmonary Fibrosis

Corticosteroids	Cyclophosphamide	Azathioprine
Water retention	Leukopenia	Leukopenia
Hyperglycemia	Thrombocytopenia	Anemia
Depression	Hemorrhagic cystitis	Thrombocytopenia
Osteoporosis	Nausea and vomiting	Nausea and vomiting
Peptic ulcer disease		

NOTES

(a) See Table 2-13 for common side effects of medications used in treatment of idiopathic pulmonary fibrosis.

   iii. Single lung transplantation should be considered in young patients.

II. Pneumoconiosis

  a. General

    i. Chronic lung disease caused by inhalation of dust particles through work exposure.

    ii. Smoking has an added detrimental effect.

    iii. Common disorders and features are described in Table 2-14.

  b. Clinical manifestations

    i. Obtaining occupational history is vital.

    ii. Most patients are asymptomatic.

    iii. As disease progresses, patients develop a mild productive cough and exertional dyspnea that may worsen to dyspnea at rest.

    iv. Physical examination is unremarkable early; patients later develop decreased breath sounds, rhonchi, wheezing, clubbing, cyanosis, and edema.

  c. Diagnosis

    i. Chest X-ray reveals small, round, parenchymal opacities.

      1. Later, these lesions become larger.

    ii. Pulmonary function tests reveal a mixed pattern depending on etiology.

  d. Treatment

    i. Further exposure to material should be avoided and smoking cessation is critical.

    ii. Supportive therapy is the center of therapy; other options include inhaled beta-agonists and oxygen.

Table 2-14 • Comparison of Pneumoconioses

Feature	Asbestosis	Coal Workers Lung	Silicosis	Berylliosis
Material	Asbestos	Coal dust	Silica	Beryllium
Occupations	Asbestos millers Brake lining workers Insulators Construction workers	Coal miners	Foundry workers Glass makers Pottery workers Sandblasters	Aerospace Electronics Foundries Nuclear reactors Nuclear weapons Telecommunications
Chest X-ray	Pleural plaques	Small nodules in lower lung fields	Hilar node calcification (eggshell pattern)	Diffuse interstitial infiltrates and hilar adenopathy
Pulmonary function test pattern	Restrictive	Obstructive	Restrictive	Vary
Complications	Mesotheliomas	Caplan's syndrome	Lung cancer Increased risk for tuberculosis	
Treatment	Supportive care plus steroids	Supportive care plus steroids	Supportive care plus steroids	Supportive care plus steroids, lifelong therapy needed

NOTES

III. Sarcoidosis
  a. General
    i. Multisystem disorder characterized by alveolitis followed by epithelioid granulomas.
      1. Associated with inclusion bodies such as Schaumann's bodies and asteroid bodies.
    ii. Etiology is unknown.
    iii. Disease is more common in young people (<40 years old), blacks, and females.
  b. Clinical manifestations
    i. Symptoms include fatigue, weakness, weight loss, fever, and sweats.
    ii. Most common organ system involved is the lungs.
      1. Present with cough, wheezing, and dyspnea.
    iii. Other systems involved include skin, gastrointestinal, cardiac, ocular, and nervous system.
  c. Diagnosis
    i. Chest X-rays are grouped by stages.
      1. Stage 0: Normal
      2. Stage 1: Bilateral hilar adenopathy
      3. Stage 2: Bilateral hilar adenopathy with diffuse parenchymal infiltrates
      4. Stage 3: Diffuse parenchymal infiltrates without bilateral hilar adenopathy
    ii. Angiotensin-converting enzyme levels are elevated.
    iii. Gallium scanning is positive.
    iv. Diagnosis based on history, chest X-ray findings, and biopsy results.
  d. Treatment
    i. Staging predicts percentage of patients with resolution of disease.
      1. Higher stage means lower percentage of resolution.
    ii. Disease course is unpredictable.
    iii. Anti-inflammatory medications, including glucocorticoids, methotrexate, and cyclophosphamide.

OTHER PULMONARY DISEASE

I. Acute respiratory distress syndrome
  a. General
    i. Form of noncardiac pulmonary edema as a result of acute damage to the alveoli.

> ## QUESTION
>
> Which of the following lab tests is elevated in pulmonary embolism?
>
>   A. Platelets
>   B. Prothrombin time
>   C. Bleeding time
>   D. D-Dimer

    ii. Definition involves three criteria.
      1. Ratio of PaO_2 to $FiO_2 \leq 200$.
      2. Detection of bilateral pulmonary infiltrates on chest X-ray.
      3. Pulmonary wedge pressure ≤ 18 mm Hg or no clinical sign of elevated left atrial pressure.
    iii. Etiologies
      1. Sepsis
      2. Aspiration
      3. Trauma
      4. Multiple transfusions
      5. Drugs
      6. Pneumonia
      7. Burns
      8. Pancreatitis
  b. Clinical manifestations
    i. Signs and symptoms include dyspnea, chest discomfort, and cough.
    ii. Physical exam reveals tachypnea, tachycardia, elevated blood pressure, and crepitations in both lungs.
  c. Diagnosis
    i. Arterial blood gases reveal hypoxia and a respiratory alkalosis.
    ii. Bronchoalveolar lavage shows an increased number of neutrophils and possibly eosinophils.
    iii. Chest X-ray may be normal initially, followed later by bilateral interstitial infiltrates within 24 hours.
      1. White-out of lung fields can be seen in severe cases.
    iv. Presence of pulmonary edema, high cardiac output, and a low pulmonary artery wedge pressure are characteristic.

NOTES

ANSWER D EXPLANATION: *The D-dimer is elevated, and is an excellent test in ruling out pulmonary embolism in low risk patients.*

correct ☐   incorrect ☐

    d. Treatment
      i. Ventilatory support, mechanical ventilation, is typically necessary.
      ii. Treat underlying cause.
      iii. Fluid management is critical.
      iv. Corticosteroids may be helpful in patients with increased eosinophils on bronchoalveolar lavage.
      v. Patients must be treated with some form of deep venous thrombosis and stress ulcer prophylaxis.
      vi. Overall mortality rate is 40% to 60%.

II. Hyaline membrane disease
  a. General
    i. Most common cause of respiratory failure in the first few days of life.
      1. A self-limiting disease.
    ii. Results from collapse of the alveoli and terminal bronchioles due to lack of adequate lung surfactant and immature state of alveolarization of the lung acini.
    iii. Can result in chronic lung disease that may persist for weeks to months.
    iv. Predisposing factors:
      1. Premature birth
      2. Diabetic mother
      3. Positive family history
  b. Clinical manifestations
    i. Present with signs of increased inspiratory effort (accessory muscle use and chest wall retractions) and hypoxemia.
    ii. On physical examination, note tachypnea, grunting respirations, and diminished, harsh, tubular lung sounds
  c. Diagnosis
    i. Arterial blood gases reveal a metabolic and respiratory acidosis.
    ii. Chest X-ray reveals a diffuse reticulogranular pattern of uniform distribution.
      1. Air bronchograms are noted.
    iii. Lecithin-to-sphingomyelin ratio is used to predict risk for disease.
  d. Treatment
    i. Corticosteroids are used to prevent disease in high-risk patients.
    ii. Adequate resuscitation and respiratory support should begin immediately with assisted ventilation or continuous positive end-expiratory pressure.
    iii. Restrict fluids to avoid pulmonary edema.
    iv. Surfactant replacement can be considered as prophylactic therapy or rescue therapy.
      1. Can be used in combination with corticosteroids.
    v. Eighty to 90% of patients survive, most with normal lungs, by 1 month of age.

III. Foreign body aspiration
  a. General
    i. Most cases of foreign body aspiration in children involve preschoolers.
    ii. Most common location of impaction is right main bronchus.
    iii. About one half of cases are due to nuts or peanuts.
      1. Hotdog aspiration is the single most common cause of death.
    iv. Aspiration due to two factors:
      1. Children more likely to place things in their mouth.
      2. Lack of molar teeth development, making it impossible for small children to finely chew foods.
  b. Clinical manifestations
    i. Most common symptom is cough.
    ii. Acute aspiration presents with sudden onset of choking and coughing followed by wheezing, dyspnea, and stridor.
    iii. Symptoms vary depending on location the aspirated material lodges.
      1. See Table 2-15 for common signs and symptoms.
  c. Diagnosis
    i. Sometimes delayed up to 1 month after aspiration.
    ii. Diagnosis suggested based on history.
    iii. Chest X-ray may reveal obstructive asymmetric hyperinflation.

NOTES

Table 2-15 • Most Common Signs and Symptoms of Foreign Body Obstruction

Bronchial	Laryngotracheal
Cough	Dyspnea
Decreased air entry	Cough
Wheezing	Stridor
Dyspnea	Cyanosis

d. Treatment
  i. Varies with age of patient.
    1. Patients younger than 1 year of age are placed face down, and forceful back blows are given.
    2. Patients older than 1 year of age are treated with the Heimlich maneuver.
    3. Blind finger-sweeps are to be avoided because the material could be pushed further back.
  ii. Endoscopy should be performed if material is beyond the oropharynx.

Question 1

Which of the following is a common sign or symptom of croup?

    A. Cervical adenopathy
    B. Pleuritic chest pain
    C. Barking cough
    D. Fever

Question 2

Which of the following pulmonary function test result is typically noted in restrictive lung disease?

    A. Decreased FEV1
    B. Increased VC
    C. Increased RV
    D. Decreased TLC

Question 3

A 60-year-old with a 60-pack year smoking history presents with hemoptysis, chest pain, dyspnea, and weight loss. Laboratory tests reveal a hypo-natremia. Which of the following is the most likely diagnosis?

    A. Tuberculosis
    B. Small cell lung cancer
    C. Sarcoidosis
    D. Non-Hodgkin's lymphoma

Question 4

A 25-year-old male presents with sudden onset of shortness of breath and chest pain. Physical examination reveals absent breath sounds on the entire right side. Which of the following the treatment of choice?

    A. Heparin
    B. Chest tube
    C. Prostaglandin
    D. Incentive spirometry

NOTES

Question 5

Which of the following medications is most beneficial in the treatment of emphysema?

- A. Theophylline
- B. Albuterol
- C. Atrovent
- D. Prednisone

Answer 1

ANSWER **C** EXPLANATION: *Croup most commonly presents with signs of upper respiratory tract infection followed by stridor and a barking cough. Fever is typically absent*

Topic: Croup

correct ☐   incorrect ☐

Question 6

High-risk groups, such as the elderly, patients with COPD, and children age 6-24 months, should routinely receive which of the following vaccines?

- A. Tuberculosis
- B. Tetanus
- C. Pertussis
- D. Influenzae

Answer 2

ANSWER **D** EXPLANATION: *Restrictive lung diseases typically present with decreased vital capacity, residual volume, and total lung capacity. FEV and FEV1 may be normal.*

Topic: Restrictive lung diseases

correct ☐   incorrect ☐

Question 7

Which of the following is a common cause of pneumonia in patients with a recent history of influenzae?

- A. Staphylococcus aureus
- B. Pneumocystis carinii
- C. Klebsiella pneumoniae
- D. Mycobacterium tuberculosis

Answer 3

ANSWER **B** EXPLANATION: *Lung cancer typically develops in patients with a long smoking history and presents with cough, dyspnea, weight loss, chest pain, and change in voice. Hyponatremia is common in small cell lung cancer secondary to inappropriate secretion of antidiuretic hormone.*

Topic: Bronchogenic carcinoma

correct ☐   incorrect ☐

NOTES

Answer 4

ANSWER **B** EXPLANATION: *Pneumothorax typically develops in thin males and presents with decreased or absent breath sounds and sudden onset of dyspnea and pleuritic chest pain. Diagnosis is confirmed by chest x-ray and treated with chest tube placement to re-expand involved lung.*

Topic: Pneumothorax

correct ☐   incorrect ☐

Answer 5

ANSWER **C** EXPLANATION: *First line medical therapy for emphysema consists of the use of anti-cholinergic agents, such as Atrovent. Smoking cessation is the most important intervention and oxygen has shown to improve survival and quality of life.*

Topic: Emphysema

correct ☐   incorrect ☐

Answer 6

ANSWER **D** EXPLANATION: *Influenzae vaccine should be given to high-risk groups. These groups include the elderly, nursing home residents, patients with a history of chronic diseases such as COPD or cardiac disease, pregnancy, children age 6–24 months, and persons in contact with high risk patients.*

Topic: Influenzae

correct ☐   incorrect ☐

Answer 7

ANSWER **A** EXPLANATION: *Staphylococcus aureus, Streptococcus pneumoniae, and Haemophilus influenzae are common causes of pneumonia in patients with a recent history of influenzae.*

Topic: Pneumonia

correct ☐   incorrect ☐

NOTES

Gastroenterology System

EXAM BLUEPRINT TOPICS

Esophagus
Esophagitis
Motor disorders
Mallory-Weiss tear
Neoplasms
Strictures
Varices
Stomach
Gastroesophageal reflux disease
Gastritis
Neoplasms
Peptic ulcer disease
Pyloric stenosis
Gallbladder
Acute/chronic cholecystitis
Cholelithiasis
Liver
Acute hepatitis
Chronic hepatitis
Neoplasms
Cirrhosis
Pancreas
Acute pancreatitis
Chronic pancreatitis
Neoplasms
Small Intestine/Colon
Appendicitis
Constipation
Diverticular disease
Duodenal atresia
Inflammatory bowel disease
Intussusception
Irritable bowel syndrome
Ischemic bowel disease
Malabsorption
Neoplasms
Obstruction

Toxic megacolon
Rectum
Anal fissure
Anorectal abscess/fistula
Fecal impaction
Hemorrhoids
Neoplasms
Pilonidal disease
Polyps
Hernia
Hiatal
Incisional (ventral)
Inguinal
Umbilical
Infectious Diarrhea
Acute infectious diarrhea
Traveler's diarrhea
Nosocomial diarrhea
Nutritional Deficiencies

- Niacin
- Thiamine
- Vitamin A
- Riboflavin
- Vitamin C
- Vitamin D
- Vitamin K

Metabolic Disorders
Phenylketonuria

ESOPHAGUS

I. Esophagitis
  a. Infectious
    i. General

NOTES

1. Occurs principally in immunocompromised patients.
2. Most common agents include:
3. *Candida albicans*
4. Herpes simplex
5. Cytomegalovirus

  ii. Clinical manifestations
1. Odynophagia may be severe.
2. Dysphagia, weight loss, and upper gastrointestinal (GI) bleeding are common.
3. Esophageal candidiasis is associated with oral candidiasis.
4. Herpes esophagitis is associated with oral herpetic lesions.

  iii. Diagnosis
1. Barium swallow
2. "Shaggy" mucosa suggests *Candida*.
3. Many, small, volcanic-shaped ulcers suggest herpes.
4. Large, deep linear ulcers suggest cytomegalovirus.
5. Endoscopy
6. A biopsy is required to make the definitive diagnosis.
7. *Candida* reveals many, small, white-yellow plaques on the mucosa.
8. Herpes reveals many vesicles that ulcerate to form small, shallow, volcanic-shaped ulcers.
9. Cytomegalovirus reveals large, deep, often linear ulcers.

  iv. Treatment
1. *Candida* esophagitis
2. Oral nystatin or clotrimazole in non-AIDS patients.
3. Oral or intravenous (IV) fluconazole in AIDS patients.
4. Herpes esophagitis
5. Oral or IV acyclovir
6. Valacyclovir or famciclovir is also possible, or IV foscarnet for resistant disease.
7. Cytomegalovirus esophagitis
8. First choice is IV ganciclovir or IV foscarnet for resistant disease.

  b. Pill-induced
    i. General
1. Common in elderly patients or any patient not taking medications correctly.
2. Common drugs include:
3. Doxycycline/tetracycline
4. Potassium chloride
5. Vitamin C
6. Nonsteroidal anti-inflammatory agents
7. Quinidine
8. Alendronate
9. Iron

  ii. Clinical manifestations
1. Characterized by odynophagia accompanied by dysphagia

  iii. Treatment
1. Stop the offending agent and treat with sucralfate suspension.

  c. Radiation
    i. General
1. Occurs from radiation to the chest at levels exceeding 3000 cGy.

  ii. Clinical manifestations
1. Can develop severe esophagitis and ulcerations.
2. Concomitant chemotherapy with cytotoxic agents can potentiate the injury.
3. Present with substernal chest pain, odynophagia, and dysphagia.

  iii. Treatment
1. Nutritional supplement
2. Delay radiation if possible
3. Sucralfate suspension

II. Motor disorders
  a. General
    i. May present with chest pain, dysphagia, or both.
    ii. Dysphagia is with solids and liquids.
    iii. Types of dysphagia
1. Oropharyngeal
2. Due to neuromuscular disorders of the oropharynx or skeletal muscle of the esophagus.
3. Difficulty in bolus transfer to esophagus, nasal regurgitation, or coughing with swallowing.
4. Includes stroke, Parkinson's disease, amyotrophic lateral sclerosis, multiple sclerosis, and myasthenia gravis.
5. Procedure of choice for diagnosis is the modified barium swallow with videofluoroscopy.

NOTES

6. Esophageal
7. Due to disease of the smooth muscle of the esophagus.
8. Do not have difficulty with transfer of bolus, regurgitation, or coughing.
9. Includes stricture, cancer, and Schatzki's ring.
10. Dysphagia with only solids.
11. Also achalasia, diffuse esophageal spasm, and scleroderma.
12. Dysphagia with solids and liquids.
13. Procedure of choice for diagnosis is manometry to evaluate peristaltic and sphincter function.
    b. Achalasia
        i. General
            1. Most common esophageal motor disorder.
            2. Etiology is unknown.
            3. Degeneration of nerves in Auerbach's plexus, vagus nerve, and swallowing center.
            4. Leads to increase in lower esophageal sphincter (LES) pressure, incomplete relaxation of the LES with swallowing, and aperistalsis in the esophagus.
        ii. Clinical manifestations
            1. Dysphagia of liquids and solids is the primary problem.
            2. Regurgitation is common.
        iii. Diagnosis
            1. Barium swallow shows a dilated esophagus, air-fluid level, delayed esophageal emptying, and a smooth tapered "birds-beak" deformity at the LES.
            2. Confirm by esophageal manometry.
        iv. Treatment
            1. A muscle relaxant, such as nifedipine, before meals.
            2. Endoscopic injection of botulinum toxin or pneumatic dilation.
    c. Diffuse esophageal spasm
        i. General
            1. Uncommon disorder.
            2. Signs and symptoms are intermittent.
            3. Associated with degeneration of Auerbach's plexus.

QUESTION

A patient presents with severe odynophagia. On examination, white plaques are noted on the oral mucosa. Which of the following is the most likely diagnosis?

A. Herpes esophagitis
B. Candida esophagitis
C. Diffuse esophageal spasm
D. Achalasia

        ii. Clinical manifestations
            1. Presents with chest pain, dysphagia, or both.
        iii. Diagnosis
            1. Barium swallow shows prominent, spontaneous, nonpropulsive, tertiary contractions.
            2. Gives a "corkscrew" esophagus appearance on barium swallow.
        iv. Treatment
            1. Supportive and empirical
            2. Smooth muscle relaxants—nifedipine, isosorbide
            3. Antidepressants—amitriptyline, imipramine
            4. Relaxation exercises, biofeedback, or counseling
III. Mallory-Weiss tear
    a. General
        i. One of the top causes of upper GI bleeding.
        ii. Occur in the distal esophagus at the gastroesophageal (GE) junction.
        iii. Typically occurs after a bout of vomiting or retching.
        iv. Bleeding occurs when tear involves the underlying venous or arterial plexus.
        v. Increase risk in patients with portal hypertension.
    b. Clinical manifestations
        i. Typically middle-aged males who present with hematemesis.
            1. Frequently follows episode of vomiting after drinking alcohol.
    c. Diagnosis
        i. Endoscopy is the procedure of choice.

NOTES

1. Appears as an elongated or elliptical ulcer at the GE junction.
  d. Treatment
    i. Most tears stop bleeding spontaneously.
    ii. Injection and thermal coagulation may be needed.
      1. Avoid thermal coagulation in patients with portal hypertension or esophageal varices.
    iii. Complications include rebleeding.

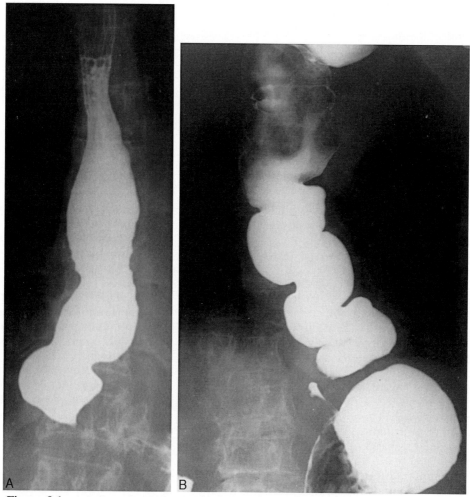

A   B

Figure 3-1 Achalasia. Note the birds beak deformity. (From Feldman M. Sleisenger and Fordtran's Gastrointestinal and Liver Disease, 7th ed. Philadelphia: WB Saunders, 2002: 578, Fig. 32.9.)

NOTES

IV. Neoplasms
   a. General
      i. Predominately affects patients between 60 and 70 years of age.
      ii. Males more common than females.
      iii. Two types of cancer
         1. Adenocarcinoma: typically involves the distal esophagus.
         2. Squamous cell: typically involves the middle or distal esophagus.
         3. See Table 3-1 for esophageal cancer risk factors.
   b. Clinical manifestations
      i. Most common presenting symptom is progressive dysphagia.
         1. First solids, then liquids
      ii. Also present with odynophagia, chest pain, weight loss, and anorexia.
   c. Diagnosis
      i. Initial workup includes barium esophagram, which shows narrowing of the lumen at the tumor site and dilation proximal to the tumor.
      ii. Confirm diagnosis with upper endoscopy with biopsy.
   d. Treatment
      i. Squamous cell treated with chemoradiation and surgery.
      ii. Adenocarcinoma is treated with surgery or chemotherapy because it is not sensitive to radiation.
      iii. Overall 5-year survival rate is 10% to 30%.

Table 3-1 • Esophageal Cancer Risk Factors	
Adenocarcinoma	**Squamous Cell Carcinoma**
Barrett's esophagus and gastroesophageal reflux disease	Smoking
Smoking	Alcohol consumption
Alcohol consumption	History of radiation therapy
History of colon cancer	Achalasia
Obesity	

QUESTION

Which of the following leads to Barrett's esophagus?
   A. Pyloric stenosis
   B. Mallory-Weiss tear
   C. Esophageal stricture
   D. Gastroesophageal reflux disease

V. Strictures
   a. General
      i. Includes esophageal webs and rings, and diverticula.
         1. Webs and rings are thin diaphragm-like structures that interrupt the esophageal lumen.
   b. Disorders
      i. Cervical esophageal webs
         1. More commonly found in females and often associated with iron deficiency anemia (Plummer-Vinson syndrome).
         2. Major complaint is intermittent solid food dysphagia.
         3. Signs of iron deficiency may also be present.
         4. Cine-esophagography is the study of choice for diagnosis.
         5. Web is often ruptured during endoscopic exam; therefore, procedure may be curative.
      ii. Lower esophageal ring (Schatzki's ring)
         1. Common cause of intermittent solid food dysphagia.
         2. Tends to occur when patients are eating quickly.
         3. Barium esophagram is the diagnostic tool.
         4. Treatment includes dilation of the ring.
      iii. Zenker's diverticulum
         1. Outpouching of the esophagus between the inferior pharyngeal constrictor and cricopharyngeal muscles.
         2. Pathogenesis is unknown.
         3. Many are asymptomatic but may present with dysphagia and regurgitation.
         4. Spontaneous regurgitation of food ingested several hours previously is characteristic of a large Zenker's diverticulum.

NOTES

ANSWER **D** EXPLANATION: *Chronic gastroesophageal reflux disease can lead to Barrett's esophagus, which can lead to esophageal cancer.*

correct ☐   incorrect ☐

  5. Barium esophagram is used to make the diagnosis.
  6. Treatment consists of surgery.
VI. Varices
  a. General
    i. Venous collaterals that develop as a result of portal hypertension.
      1. Causes include prehepatic thrombosis, hepatic disease, postsinusoidal disease, alcoholic liver disease, and viral hepatitis.
    ii. Typically have massive upper GI bleeding and history of chronic liver disease and cirrhosis.
  b. Clinical manifestations
    i. Symptoms include hematemesis, melena, hematochezia, and dizziness.
    ii. Manifestations of cirrhosis and portal hypertension may be noted.
    iii. Elevation in liver enzymes and bilirubin with low albumin and cholesterol, and elevated prothrombin time (PT) are noted.
  c. Diagnosis
    i. Endoscopy is the test of choice for diagnosis.
  d. Treatment
    i. Medical therapy
      1. IV vasopressin
      2. IV nitroglycerin
      3. IV octreotide
      4. Balloon tamponade
    ii. Endoscopic therapy
      1. Endoscopic hemostasis is the treatment of choice. Includes:
      2. Endoscopic injection sclerotherapy
      3. Variceal band ligation
    iii. Complications
      1. Bleeding stops spontaneously in more than 50% of patients.
      2. Increased mortality in patients with continued bleeding.
      3. Uncontrolled bleeding can lead to hemorrhage and death.

STOMACH

I. Gastroesophageal reflux disease
  a. General
    i. A process that refers to the effortless movement of gastric contents from the stomach to the esophagus.
    ii. Affects men more than women and is more common in whites than blacks.
    iii. Develops when acid content of the stomach refluxes into the esophagus and remains long enough to overcome the resistance of the esophageal epithelium.
      1. Due to increased frequency of transient LES relaxations.
  b. Clinical manifestations
    i. Recurrent heartburn is the hallmark symptom.
    ii. Alarm symptoms include dysphagia, GI bleeding, or weight loss.
      1. If present consider stricture or adenocarcinoma.
    iii. Extraesophageal symptoms
      1. Include pharyngitis, earache, gingivitis, laryngitis, chronic cough, asthma, and aspiration pneumonia.
  c. Diagnosis
    i. History of recurrent heartburn and a positive response to acid-suppression drugs.
    ii. Specific testing is reserved for patients with alarm symptoms.
      1. Upper GI series
        (a) Detects grossly abnormal reflux
      2. Esophageal pH monitoring
        (a) The gold standard for identifying reflux.
      3. Bernstein's test
        (a) Establishes gastroesophageal reflux disease (GERD) as a cause of symptoms.
  d. Treatment
    i. Consists of lifestyle modifications and drug therapy
    ii. See Table 3-2 for lifestyle modifications.
    iii. See Table 3-3 for drug therapy.
II. Gastritis
  a. General
    i. Inflammation of the gastric mucosa.
    ii. Etiologies

NOTES

Table 3-2 • Lifestyle Modifications with Gastroesophageal Reflux Disease

Elevate head of bed 6 inches
Stop smoking
Stop alcohol consumption
Decrease dietary fat
Decrease meal size
Avoid bedtime snacks
Avoid chocolate, peppermint, coffee, tea, colas, and citrus fruit juices

QUESTION

A 75-year-old male presents with progressive dysphagia to solid foods and weight loss. He denies heartburn or chest pain. Which of the following is the most likely diagnosis?

    A. Achalasia
    B. Scleroderma
    C. Esophageal spasm
    D. Esophageal cancer

       1. *Helicobacter pylori*
       2. Autoimmune
          (a) Pernicious anemia is a late complication of autoimmune gastritis.
       3. Environmental
       4. Chemical—bile, nonsteroidal anti-inflammatory drugs (NSAIDs)
   b. Clinical manifestations
      i. Epigastric pain
      ii. Nausea and vomiting
   c. Diagnosis
      i. *H. pylori*
         1. Detect by serology testing, urea-breath test, or stool antigen testing.

      ii. Endoscopy
         1. Note erosions and petechial hemorrhages.
   d. Treatment
      i. *H. pylori*: antibiotics and proton pump inhibitor.
      ii. Discontinue drugs (NSAIDs).
      iii. Medical therapy with proton pump inhibitor or H_2 antagonists.
III. Neoplasms
   a. General
      i. Predominantly malignant with a majority of them being adenocarcinoma.
      ii. Occurs typically in the 50- to 70-year-old age group, is rare before age 30 years.
      iii. Etiologic factors include:
         1. Environmental
            (a) *H. pylori*

Table 3-3 • Drug Therapy in GERD

Drug Therapy	Mechanism	Example
Antacids	Buffer HCl and increase lower esophageal sphincter pressure	Mylanta
Barriers	Viscous mechanical barrier and buffer HCl	Aluminum hydroxide
H_2 receptor antagonists	Decrease HCl secretion	Cimetidine, famotidine
Prokinetics	Increase lower esophageal sphincter pressure and increase gastric emptying	Bethanechol Metoclopramide
Proton pump inhibitors	Decrease HCl secretion and gastric volume	Omeprazole Lansoprazole, rabeprazole

NOTES

ANSWER D EXPLANATION: *Esophageal cancer is typically noted in the elderly and presents with progressive dysphagia, first solids then liquids, and weight loss.*

correct ☐   incorrect ☐

      (b) Dietary: excess salt, nitrates/nitrites, and deficiency in fresh fruit and vegetables.
    2. Genetic
      (a) Blood group A
    3. Predisposing conditions
      (a) Chronic gastritis
      (b) Pernicious anemia
      (c) Large gastric adenomatous polyps
      (d) Chronic peptic ulcer
  b. Clinical manifestations
    i. Early in disease patient is asymptomatic.
    ii. Later symptoms include bloating, dysphagia, epigastric pain, or early satiety.
      1. Food or antacids do not relieve the epigastric pain.
    iii. Physical examination may be unremarkable.
      1. Later in the disease, patients become cachectic, and an epigastric mass may be noted.
      2. Patient may show signs of metastatic disease.
        (a) Hepatomegaly and jaundice due to liver metastases.
        (b) Lymph node involvement in the left supraclavicular region (Virchow's node) or periumbilical nodes (Saint Mary Joseph's node).
  c. Diagnosis
    i. Upper endoscopy with biopsy.
  d. Treatment
    i. Five-year survival rate is less than 20%.
    ii. Surgical resection provides the highest chance for cure.
    iii. Somewhat responsive to chemotherapy.
    iv. Radiation therapy is ineffective alone, but combined with chemotherapy has shown to improve survival.

IV. Peptic ulcer disease
  a. General
    i. Most common causes are *H. pylori* and NSAIDs.
    ii. Unusual cause is a gastrinoma (Zollinger-Ellison syndrome).
      1. Tumor that secretes excess amounts of gastrin and gastric acid hypersecretion.
      2. Diarrhea is common.
      3. Tumors located in the pancreas and duodenum.
      4. Laboratory studies reveal markedly elevated serum gastrin levels.
      5. Treatment is with proton pump inhibitors and surgery.
  b. Clinical manifestations
    i. Burning, epigastric pain worse on empty stomach or at night.
    ii. May also present with GI bleeding.
    iii. On examination, may note epigastric tenderness with deep palpation.
    iv. Symptoms vary with source, gastric versus duodenal.
      1. See Table 3-4 for comparison of gastric and duodenal ulcers.
  c. Diagnosis
    i. Upper GI endoscopy
      1. Important to biopsy gastric ulcers due to risk for cancer.
      2. Duodenal ulcers are almost never malignant, so biopsy is not needed.
    ii. Barium contrast studies
    iii. Gastrin levels are indicated in intractable ulcer disease or possible Zollinger-Ellison syndrome.
    iv. Tests for *H. pylori*
      1. Rapid urease test: requires endoscopy
      2. Histology: requires endoscopy
      3. Culture: requires endoscopy
      4. Urea breath test: useful for diagnosis and follow-up
      5. Stool antigen test: useful for diagnosis and follow-up
      6. Serologic testing: unsuitable for follow-up
  d. Treatment
    i. Antisecretory drugs
      1. H_2 receptor antagonists
      2. Proton pump inhibitors

NOTES

Table 3-4 • Symptoms in Gastric and Duodenal Ulcers		
Symptom	**Gastric Ulcer**	**Duodenal Ulcer**
Epigastric pain	↑↑↑	↑↑↑
Nocturnal pain	↑	↑↑↑
Pain relief with food	↑	↑↑
Episodic pain	↑	↑↑
Bloating/belching	↑↑	↑↑
Anorexia/weight loss	↑↑	↑
Nausea/vomiting	↑↑↑	↑↑

Table 3-5 • Treatment of *Helicobacter pylori* Infection

Triple therapy
　A proton-pump inhibitor BID, *plus*
　Amoxicillin, 1 g BID, *plus*
　Metronidazole, 500 mg BID, or clarithromycin, 500 mg BID

Three- and four-times-daily triple therapies
　Bismuth subsalicylate 2 tablets QID, *plus*
　Tetracycline, 500 mg QID, *plus*
　Metronidazole, 250 mg TID

Quadruple therapies
　Proton pump inhibitor BID, *plus*
　Bismuth subsalicylate, 2 tablets QID, *plus*
　Tetracycline, 500 mg QID, *plus*
　Metronidazole, 250 mg TID

　　　3. Synthetic prostaglandin
　ii. Antimicrobial therapy
　　　1. Treatment requires multiple drug therapy
　　　2. See Table 3-5 for treatment options.
　iii. Stop NSAIDs if possible
　iv. Surgery
　　　1. Usually seen in cases of intractable or persistent disease.
　　　2. Procedures include:
　　　　(a) Truncal vagotomy and pyloroplasty
　　　　(b) Highly selective vagotomy without pyloroplasty
　v. Complications
　　　1. Hemorrhage
　　　　(a) Peptic ulcer disease is the most common cause of upper gastrointestinal bleeding.
　　　2. Perforation
　　　　(a) Typically present with abrupt onset of severe abdominal pain followed by signs of peritoneal inflammation.
　　　3. Obstruction
V. Pyloric stenosis
　a. General
　　i. Hypertrophy of pyloric circular muscle.
　　ii. Most common etiology is idiopathic.
　　iii. There is male predominance (4:1) and a positive family history in 10% to 15%.

　b. Clinical manifestations
　　i. Onset at about 3 weeks of age, but may be as late as 5 months.
　　ii. Projectile nonbilious vomiting.
　　　1. Vomitus may be blood-tinged.
　　iii. A palpable olive-shaped mass noted in the mid epigastrium.
　c. Diagnosis
　　i. Ultrasound reveals elongated pyloric channel and thickened pyloric wall.
　　ii. Radiographic contrast studies
　　　1. String sign—from elongated pyloric channel
　　　2. Shoulder sign—bulge of pyloric muscle into the antrum
　　iii. Laboratory tests may reveal a hypochloremic alkalosis with hypokalemia.
　d. Treatment
　　i. Surgery, pyloromyotomy, is curative.

GALLBLADDER

I. Acute cholecystitis
　a. General
　　i. Due to sustained obstruction of the cystic duct.
　b. Clinical manifestations

NOTES

    i. Pain is severe, located in the right upper quadrant and will last longer than 6 hours.
    ii. On exam, there is right upper quadrant tenderness with positive Murphy's sign.
    iii. Fever may be present.
    iv. Laboratory tests reveal a leukocytosis and mild elevation in liver function tests.
  c. Diagnosis
    i. Ultrasonography
      1. Detect stones, gallbladder wall thickening, or pericholecystic fluid.
        (a) Pericholecystic fluid is highly specific for acute cholecystitis and not chronic disease.
      2. Hepatobiliary scintigraphy
        (a) Uses a radioactive isotope to detect obstruction of cystic duct.
        (b) Failure of the isotope to appear in the gallbladder in 4 hours is highly specific for acute cholecystitis.
  d. Treatment
    i. Laparoscopic cholecystectomy
    ii. Open cholecystectomy
    iii. Broad-spectrum antibiotics
II. Cholelithiasis
  a. General
    i. Two types of stones
      1. Cholesterol
      2. Pigmented
    ii. Risk factors
      1. Increasing age
      2. Female
      3. Pregnancy
      4. Estrogens
      5. Obesity
      6. Native Americans
      7. Cirrhosis
      8. Hemolytic anemia
  b. Clinical manifestations
    i. Most are asymptomatic.
    ii. In symptomatic patients, the clinical features can vary.
      1. Episodic pain
        (a) Due to intermittent obstruction of the cystic duct.
        (b) Pain is in the upper right quadrant with radiation to right side of back or right shoulder.
          (i) Pain can be nocturnal.

        (c) Pain is described as wavelike, cramping pain that develops between 15 minutes and 2 hours after eating a fatty meal.
        (d) Pain may last up to 4 hours with concomitant nausea and vomiting.
        (e) Physical exam is normal between episodes, and during episode, right upper quadrant tenderness is noted.
      2. Complications
        (a) Acute cholecystitis
        (b) Common bile duct stones
        (c) Pancreatitis
        (d) Cholangitis
  c. Diagnosis
    i. Ultrasonography
      1. Has more than 95% sensitivity in detecting gallstones.
    ii. Oral cholecystography
      1. Useful is providing information on gallbladder function.
    iii. Computed tomography (CT)/magnetic resonance imaging (MRI)
    iv. Endoscopic retrograde cholangiopancreatography (ERCP)
    v. Hepatobiliary scintigraphy
      1. Not useful in detecting stones but useful in patients with acute cholecystitis.
  d. Treatment
    i. If asymptomatic and patient healthy the gallstones should be left alone.
    ii. Surgical therapy
      1. Laparoscopic cholecystectomy
      2. Open cholecystectomy
    iii. Nonsurgical therapy
      1. Ursodeoxycholic acid
        (a) Stones greater than 1.5 cm or pigmented stones are not responsive to treatment via this method.
      2. Extracorporeal shock wave lithotripsy

LIVER

I. Acute hepatitis
  a. General
    i. Caused by five different viruses.
    ii. Routes of spread include fecal–oral, parenteral, and sexual.

NOTES

iii. See Table 3-6 for summary of viral hepatitis.
b. Clinical manifestations
  i. Incubation period: virus can be detected, but laboratory tests are normal. Asymptomatic.
  ii. Preicteric phase: symptoms include malaise, nausea, decreased appetite, and vague abdominal pain.
    1. Viral specific antibodies start to appear.
    2. Serum transaminases start to elevate.
  iii. Icteric phase: symptoms worsen, and jaundice appears.
    1. Serum transaminases reach their peak.
      (a) Ten times the upper limit of normal.
    2. Urine darkens in color, and stool becomes lighter in color.
c. Diagnosis
  i. Serology results vary with each virus.
  ii. See Table 3-7 for summary of serology testing in acute hepatitis.
d. Treatment
  i. Symptomatic treatment, with avoidance of alcohol and sexual contact.
  ii. Virus specific:
    1. Hepatitis A
      (a) Hepatitis A virus (HAV) vaccine
      (b) Postexposure prophylaxis with immune globulin for household and intimate contacts.

Table 3-6 • Comparison of Causes of Acute Viral Hepatitis

Hepatitis Virus	Genome	Spread	Incubation Period	Fatality Rate	Chronic Rate	Antibody
A	RNA	Fecal–oral	25 days	1%	None	Anti-HAV
B	DNA	Parenteral Sexual	75 days	1%	5%	Anti-HBs Anti-HBc Anti-HBe
C	RNA	Parenteral	50 days	<0.1%	80%	Anti-HCV
D	RNA	Parenteral Sexual	30–150 days	2%–10%	5%	Anti-HDV
E	RNA	Fecal–oral	35 days	1%	None	Anti-HEV

Table 3-7 • Serology Testing for Acute Hepatitis

Diagnosis	Screening Assays	Duration	Antibodies	Note
Hepatitis A	Anti-HAV immunoglobulin M	4 wk to 10 mo	Anti-HAV	HAV in stool before onset of symptoms
Hepatitis B	HBsAg Anti-HBc immunoglobulin M	5–25 wk 6–52 wk	HBeAg Anti-HBe	
Hepatitis C	Anti-HCV	Onset 8 wk		
Hepatitis D	HBsAg		Anti-HDV	Seen only in presence of hepatitis B
Hepatitis E	History		Anti-HEV	

NOTES

(c) HAV vaccine and immune globulin can be used concurrently.
2. Hepatitis B
  (a) Hepatitis B virus (HBV) vaccine
    (i) Recommended at birth.
  (b) Postexposure prophylaxis with hepatitis B immune globulin (HBIG).
    (i) Recommended for newborns and patients with parenteral exposure.
3. Hepatitis C
  (a) Pegylated interferon-alpha and ribavirin beneficial in chronic hepatitis C
4. Hepatitis D
  (a) No specific treatment, but hepatitis B vaccine can prevent infection with hepatitis D.
5. Hepatitis E
  (a) No specific treatment.
II. Chronic hepatitis
  a. General
    i. All have chronic inflammatory injury of the liver that can lead to cirrhosis and end-stage liver disease.
    ii. There are multiple causes.
      1. Chronic hepatitis B, D, and C
      2. Autoimmune hepatitis
      3. Drug-induced chronic hepatitis
      4. Wilson's disease
  b. Clinical manifestations
    i. Clinical symptoms are typically nonspecific, intermittent, and mild.
    ii. The most common symptom is fatigue.
    iii. On physical examination, the most common finding is liver tenderness.
  c. Diagnosis
    i. Laboratory results reveal elevated serum transaminases and little or no elevation in alkaline phosphatase.
      1. Serum transaminases are elevated 1 to 5 times normal.
    ii. See Table 3-8 for diagnostic testing for chronic hepatitis.
    iii. Diagnosis is based on histologic appearance of the liver.
  d. Treatment
    i. Varies with specific cause.
      1. Chronic hepatitis B

Table 3-8 • Diagnostic Tests for Chronic Hepatitis

Diagnosis	Screening Test
Chronic hepatitis B	HBsAg
Chronic hepatitis C	Anti-HCV
Chronic hepatitis D	Anti-HDV
Autoimmune hepatitis	ANA
Drug-induced disease	History
Wilson's disease	Ceruloplasmin

      (a) Pegylated interferon-alpha
      (b) Oral nucleoside analogs such as lamivudine and adefovir dipivoxil.
      (c) Avoid all immunosuppressive drugs.
    2. Chronic hepatitis D
      (a) Therapy is difficult, but prolonged treatment with interferon-alpha results in some improvement.
    3. Chronic hepatitis C
      (a) Interferon-alpha and ribavirin.
    4. Autoimmune
      (a) Will have a rapid clinical response to corticosteroids.
        (i) Prednisone or azathioprine can be used.
    5. Drug induced
      (a) Discontinue the involved drug.
    6. Wilson's disease
      (a) Copper chelation improves survival but does not reverse cirrhosis.
III. Neoplasms
  a. General
    i. Metastatic tumors are the most common malignant tumor of the liver.
      1. Most frequent primary tumors to spread to the liver include: gastrointestinal (colon, stomach, and pancreas), lung, and breast.
      2. Prognosis is poor, with mean survival only 6 months.

NOTES

ii. Most common primary malignancy of the liver is hepatocellular carcinoma.
  1. A complication of chronic liver disease and cirrhosis.
    (a) Causes include hepatitis C infection, alcohol usage, and hemochromatosis.
b. Clinical manifestations
  i. Present with abdominal pain, palpable abdominal mass, and constitutional symptoms.
  ii. Can also have signs of obstructive jaundice.
  iii. Primary hepatocellular carcinoma can metastasize to the lymph nodes and lung.
c. Diagnosis
  i. Alpha-fetoprotein is elevated in hepatocellular carcinoma.
  ii. CT scan will reveal the lesions of both primary and metastatic liver carcinoma.
  iii. Diagnosis is confirmed by biopsy.
d. Treatment
  i. Prevention is most important.
  ii. For primary disease, resection or transplantation may be indicated.
    1. Systemic chemotherapy and radiation therapy are of limited value.
IV. Cirrhosis
a. General
  i. Liver cirrhosis represents the end stage of chronic liver disease.
    1. Due to chronic wound healing in the liver after chronic damage.
  ii. See Table 3-9 for causes of cirrhosis.
b. Clinical manifestations
  i. Symptoms include weakness, fatigue, weight loss, anorexia, and abdominal pain.
  ii. Physical examination reveals jaundice, edema, and dermatologic changes.
    1. Dermatologic changes include spider angiomas, telangiectasias, palmar erythema, purpura, and signs of feminization.
  iii. Laboratory results vary depending on cause.
    1. Screening tests include: liver function tests, iron studies, renal function, ceruloplasmin, complete blood count (CBC), viral hepatitis serology markers, antinuclear antibodies, alpha-fetoprotein, and ammonia level.

QUESTION

Which sign is indicative of acute cholecystitis?

A. Cullen's
B. Chadwick's
C. Hegar's
D. Murphy's

---

  2. See Table 3-10 for utilization of liver function tests.
c. Diagnosis
  i. Abdominal ultrasound to evaluate liver size, shape, and composition.
  ii. CT scan with liver biopsy.
d. Treatment
  i. Treat underlying cause and prevent and treat complications.
    1. Abstain from alcohol.

Table 3-9 • Causes of Cirrhosis
Alcohol abuse

Viral hepatitis
  Hepatitis B
  Hepatitis D
  Hepatitis C

Metabolic disorders
  Hemochromatosis
  Wilson's disease
  Alpha-1-antitrypsin deficiency
  Cystic fibrosis

Autoimmune hepatitis

Biliary disorders
  Sclerosing cholangitis
  Primary biliary cirrhosis

Drugs and toxins
  Carbon tetrachloride
  Dimethylnitrosamine
  Methotrexate
  Amiodarone

NOTES

ANSWER **D** EXPLANATION: *Murphy's sign, increase pain in right upper quadrant with inspiration, is typical of acute cholecystitis.*

correct ☐   incorrect ☐

2. Autoimmune hepatitis: treat with immunosuppressive therapy (corticosteroids and azathioprine).
3. Hemochromatosis: frequent phlebotomies.
4. Wilson's disease: a chelating agent (penicillamine).
5. Primary biliary cirrhosis: a bile acid, ursodeoxycholic acid.

ii. Liver transplantation is the treatment of choice for end-stage liver disease.
iii. Complications include the following:
1. Jaundice: due to failure to metabolize bilirubin.
2. Variceal bleeding: due to portal hypertension.
3. Ascites: due to portal hypertension and hypoproteinemia.
4. Spontaneous bacterial peritonitis

5. Encephalopathy
6. Hypersplenism: leads to mainly thrombocytopenia, but also anemia and neutropenia.

PANCREAS

I. Acute pancreatitis
  a. General
    i. Inflammatory disease of the pancreas.
    ii. Etiology
      1. Alcohol
      2. Gallstones
      3. Pancreatic obstruction
      4. Drugs/toxins
        (a) Major drugs involve the immunosuppressants (azathioprine), ddI, furosemide, angiotensin-converting enzyme inhibitors, and estrogens.
      5. Metabolic: hypertriglyceridemia
    iii. Due to activation of digestive enzymes and autodigestion.
  b. Clinical manifestations
    i. Typically present with abdominal pain, nausea, and vomiting.
    ii. Pain is constant, located in the epigastric region with radiation to the mid back.

Table 3-10 • Liver Function Tests

Name	Normal Range	Utilization
Aspartate aminotransferase (AST)	0–40 IU/L	Hepatocellular damage
Alanine aminotransferase (ALT)	0–40 IU/L	Hepatocellular damage
Alkaline phosphatase	25–100 IU/L	Cholestatic hepatobiliary disease
γ-Glutamyl transferase	5–30 U/L	Cholestatic hepatobiliary disease
Total bilirubin	0.5–1.2 mg/dL	Metabolite clearance
Ammonia	10–65 µmol/L	Metabolite clearance
Prothrombin time	18–22 sec	Hepatic synthesis function
Albumin	3.5–4.5 g/dL	Hepatic synthesis function
Alpha-fetoprotein	<20 ng/dL	Tumor marker for hepatocellular carcinoma

NOTES

    iii. Abdominal examination results vary from minimal tenderness to marked generalized rebound tenderness with guarding.

    iv. Bowel sounds may be diminished.

    v. In severe necrotizing pancreatitis, may note large ecchymoses on the flanks (Grey Turner's sign) or periumbilical (Cullen's sign).

  c. Diagnosis

    i. Laboratory results

QUESTION

Which of the following hepatitis viruses never causes chronic hepatitis?

    A. Hepatitis A

    B. Hepatitis B

    C. Hepatitis C

    D. Drug-induced hepatitis

Table 3-11 • Metabolic Diseases of the Liver

Disease	Inheritance	Clinical	Laboratory	Treatment
Alpha-1-antitrypsin	Recessive	Chronic obstructive pulmonary disease Cirrhosis	$\downarrow$ Alpha-1-antitrypsin level Phenotyping	Transplantation
Wilson's disease	Autosomal recessive	Kayser-Fleischer rings Cirrhosis	$\uparrow$ Copper level $\downarrow$ Ceruloplasmin	Copper chelation with penicillamine
Hemochromatosis	Autosomal recessive	Abdominal pain Hepatomegaly Cirrhosis	$\uparrow$ Ferritin $\uparrow$ Hepatic iron index	Phlebotomy Iron chelation with deferoxamine

Table 3-12 • Disorders of Bilirubin Metabolism

Feature	Crigler-Najjar Syndrome Type I	Crigler-Najjar Syndrome Type II	Gilbert's Syndrome	Dubin-Johnson Syndrome	Rotor's Syndrome
Incidence	Very rare	Uncommon	Up to 12% of population	Uncommon	Rare
Total bilirubin (mg/dL)	15–45	5–25	≤4	2–5	3–7
Liver function tests	Normal	Normal	Normal	Normal	Normal
Pharmacologic response	No response to phenobarbital	Phenobarbital reduces bilirubin by ≤ 75%	Phenobarbital reduces bilirubin to normal	Increased bilirubin with estrogens	
Clinical features	Kernicterus in infancy	Kernicterus with fasting	None	Occasional hepatosplenomegaly	None
Inheritance	Recessive	Recessive	Recessive	Recessive	Recessive
Treatment	Phototherapy	Phenobarbital	None	Avoid estrogens	None

NOTES

ANSWER **A** EXPLANATION: *Hepatitis A and E do not cause chronic hepatitis.*

correct ☐   incorrect ☐

1. Elevated serum amylase and lipase
   (a) Elevated serum amylase noted the first 2 to 12 hours with a decrease in levels over 3 to 5 days.
   (b) Elevated serum lipase noted first 12 hours with decreasing levels over 7 to 10 days.
   (c) Amylase and lipase are also elevated in intestinal injury/obstruction, biliary stone, and renal failure.
2. Other laboratory test findings
   (a) Leukocytosis
   (b) Mild hyperglycemia
   (c) Hypocalcemia
   (d) Elevated serum bilirubin, alkaline phosphatase, and transaminases.
ii. Ultrasound/CT scan
   1. Ultrasound may note presence of gallstones and pancreatic edema.
   2. CT scan is used to evaluate the extent and local complications.
iii. ERCP
   1. Not useful in diagnosing acute pancreatitis but is useful for the diagnosis and treatment of persistent bile duct stones.
   2. ERCP may also increase the risk for developing pancreatitis.

d. Treatment
   i. Must establish severity of pancreatitis to predict course and risk for complications.
   ii. Ranson's criteria are commonly used.
      1. Fewer than two criteria have a 1% mortality rate.
      2. Presence of three of more of the criteria predicts a complicated clinical course.
      3. See Table 3-13 for summary of Ranson's criteria.
   iii. Treatment
      1. Main goal is supportive care.
         (a) Maintain fluid balance
         (b) No oral fluids or food until abdominal pain resolved.
         (c) Pain control
      2. If gallstones present cholecystectomy is indicated.
      3. Abstain from alcohol.
   iv. Complications
      1. Local
         (a) Pancreatic necrosis
            (i) Noted in patients who worsen after initial improvement.
            (ii) Will develop signs of sepsis: fever, marked leukocytosis, and positive blood cultures.
            (iii) Treatment includes CT guided aspiration of fluid and antibiotics.
               (1) Antibiotics include imipenem, fluoroquinolones, and metronidazole.

Table 3-13 • Ranson's Criteria	
On Admission	**48 hours after Admission**
Age > 55 yr	Hematocrit decrease by > 10%
White blood cell count > 16,000/μL	Blood urea nitrogen increase by > 5 mg/dL
Aspartate aminotransferase > 250 U/L	Calcium < 8 mg/dL
Lactate dehydrogenase > 350 U/L	Arterial PO_2 < 60 mm Hg
Glucose > 200 mg/dL	Base deficit > 4 mEq/L Fluid sequestration > 6 L

NOTES

(b) Pseudocysts
 (i) Noted in patients who show evidence of persistent pancreatitis.
 (ii) Diagnosis made with ultrasound or CT scan.
 (iii) Small cysts will resolve without treatment, larger cysts require surgical drainage.

2. Systemic
 (a) Renal failure
  (i) As a result of hypovolemia and decreased renal perfusion.
 (b) Respiratory failure
  (i) May develop acute respiratory distress syndrome.

II. Chronic pancreatitis
 a. General
  i. Permanent and progressive damage to the pancreas.
   1. Intermittent attacks of acute pancreatitis.
  ii. Major cause is alcohol consumption.
 b. Clinical manifestations
  i. Abdominal pain is the major symptom.
   1. Pain may improve as severity of pancreatitis worsens.
  ii. Other symptoms include weight loss, diarrhea and steatorrhea (secondary to malabsorption), and diabetes mellitus.
 c. Diagnosis
  i. Suggested by history and confirmed by measurement of pancreatic function.
   1. Assessment of pancreatic exocrine function
    (a) 72-hour fecal fat
    (b) Secretin or cholecystokinin stimulation tests
   2. Assessment of pancreatic structure
    (a) Plain abdominal X-ray to evaluate for calcification of the pancreas.
    (b) See Figure 3-2 for X-ray in chronic pancreatitis.
    (c) Ultrasound
    (d) ERCP is the most sensitive and specific test for the diagnosis of chronic pancreatitis.
 d. Treatment
  i. Avoidance of alcohol.
  ii. Pain control
   1. Opiates may be needed for pain control.
  iii. Management of pancreatic insufficiency

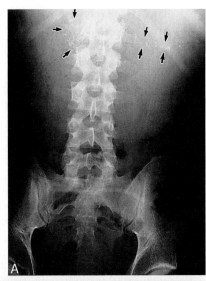

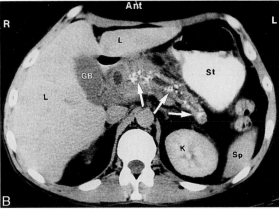

Figure 3-2 A (Abdominal X-ray in a patient with chronic pancreatitis. Note the calcifications. B) Abdominal CT scan of patient with chronic pancreatitis. Note calcifications in the pancrea. (From Mettler FA. Essentials of Radiology, 2nd ed. Philadelphia: Elsevier Saunders, 2005:171, Fig. 6-13.)

   1. Pancreatic enzyme replacement used to control steatorrhea.
   2. Reduction in dietary fat should also be done.
III. Neoplasms
 a. General
  i. Most common is ductal adenocarcinoma.
   1. Most common location is head of the pancreas.
  ii. Fourth most common cause of cancer death.
  iii. Five-year survival rate is less than 5%.

NOTES

iv. Risk factors include smoking, obesity, chronic pancreatitis, high intake of animal fat, and prolonged exposure to petroleum products.
b. Clinical manifestations
  i. Early symptoms include nonspecific abdominal discomfort, nausea, vomiting, anorexia, and malaise.
  ii. Most common presenting symptoms are epigastric pain, obstructive jaundice, and weight loss.
    1. Typically found late in disease and associated with advanced disease.
  iii. On physical exam, a palpably distended, nontender gallbladder may be noted (Courvoisier's sign).
c. Diagnosis
  i. CT scan of the abdomen is the test of choice for evaluation of possible pancreatic cancer.

ii. Tumor marker CA-19-9 is elevated in pancreatic cancer.
d. Treatment
  i. Surgical resection is the treatment of choice if no metastatic disease is present.
  ii. After resection chemotherapy is indicated (5-fluorouracil).
  iii. If not resectable, biliary and gastric bypass may benefit patients.

SMALL INTESTINE/COLON

I. Appendicitis
  a. General
    i. Acute inflammation of the appendix, typically due to obstruction by a fecalith.
    ii. Most common in ages 10 to 30 years.

Table 3-14 • Abdominal Causes of Acute Abdomen Pain

Disease	Location	Mode of Onset	Referred Pain	Nausea/Vomiting	Fever	Evaluation
Appendicitis	RLQ	Gradual		Yes	Yes	CT scan Ultrasound
Diverticulitis	LLQ	Gradual		No	Yes	CT scan
Ectopic pregnancy	RLQ LLQ	Sudden		No	No	Beta-HCG Ultrasound
Endometriosis	RLQ LLQ	Intermittent		No	No	
Gallbladder	RUQ	Gradual	Right shoulder/ scapula	Yes	No	Ultrasound
Biliary tract		Intermittent				Liver function tests
Gastritis	LUQ	Gradual		No	No	Clinical endoscopy
Hepatic abscess	RUQ	Gradual	Right shoulder	No	Yes	Ultrasound CT scan
Hepatitis	RUQ	Gradual		No	No	Serology

NOTES

b. Clinical manifestations
    i. First present with abdominal pain, colicky in nature, in the periumbilical or epigastric area.
    ii. Pain then becomes constant, more severe, and localizes to the right lower quadrant.
    iii. Anorexia and nausea are frequent. Vomiting may be present.
        1. Fever occurs late in the presentation or after perforation.
    iv. On physical examination, tenderness is noted at McBurney's point, and rebound tenderness is present.
        1. Rovsing's, psoas, and obturator signs are positive.

QUESTION

A 45-year-old female with a history of alcoholism presents with nausea, vomiting, and epigastric pain. She states the pain radiates to her back. Lab results reveal a markedly elevated lipase and mild elevation in AST and ALT. The remaining labs are normal. Which of the following is the most likely diagnosis?

    A. Cholecystitis
    B. Diverticulitis
    C. Pancreatitis
    D. Peptic ulcer disease

Table 3-14 • Abdominal Causes of Acute Abdomen Pain—cont'd

Disease	Location	Mode of Onset	Referred Pain	Nausea/ Vomiting	Fever	Evaluation
Intestinal obstruction	Diffuse RLQ	Sudden—high intestine Gradual—low intestine		Yes	No	Abdominal X-ray CT scan
Mesenteric thrombus	Diffuse	Sudden		Yes	No	CT scan
Pancreatitis	Epigastric RUQ	Gradual	Back–midline	No	Yes	Amylase Lipase Ultrasound CT scan
Peptic ulcer disease	RUQ	Intermittent, Gradual		No	No	Endoscopy
Peritonitis	Diffuse	Sudden		Yes	Yes	Clinical
Renal stone	RLQ LLQ	Sudden	Groin Genitalia	Yes	No	Abdominal X-ray CT scan
Salpingitis (pelvic inflammatory disease)	RLQ LLQ	Intermittent	Gradual	No	Yes	Ultrasound
Splenic rupture	LUQ	Sudden	Left shoulder/ scapula	No	No	CT scan

CT, computed tomography; beta-HCG, beta-human chorionic gonadotropin; LLQ, left lower quadrant; LUQ, left upper quadrant; RLQ, right lower quadrant; RUQ, right upper quadrant.

NOTES

ANSWER C EXPLANATION: *Pancreatitis, most commonly due to alcohol or gallstones, presents with epigastric pain with radiation through to the back, nausea, vomiting, and elevated lipase and amylase.*

correct ❑   incorrect ❑

c. Diagnosis
   i. Laboratory tests reveal a leukocytosis with a left shift.
   ii. Urinalysis is typically normal; a few white and red blood cells may be noted.
   iii. Ultrasound or CT scan of the appendix will reveal a dilated appendix and thickened wall.
d. Treatment
   i. Surgical removal of the appendix.
   ii. Broad-spectrum antibiotics needed with perforation.
II. Constipation
   a. General
      i. Perception of abnormal bowel movements.
         1. Two or fewer bowel movements per week are considered abnormal.
      ii. Is more common in women and with advancing age.
      iii. See Table 3-16 for causes of constipation.
   b. Clinical manifestations
      i. Include bloating, abdominal pain or discomfort, stools difficult to pass, anal pain, and nausea.
   c. Diagnosis
      i. Screening for systemic disease with CBC, chemistry profile, and thyroid function.
      ii. Further testing should be reserved for severe disease and patients who have failed conservative treatment.
         1. Colonic transit study
         2. Pelvic floor function
   d. Treatment
      i. Limit use of medications that cause constipation.
      ii. Regular exercise and adequate hydration are also beneficial.
      iii. Dietary modifications by increasing fiber intake.

Table 3-15 • Nonabdominal Causes of Acute Abdomen Pain
Myocardial infarction
Pneumonia
Herpes zoster virus

Metabolic
  Diabetic ketoacidosis
  Uremia
  Addisonian crisis

Sickle cell crisis
Leukemia
Aortic aneurysm

Toxins
  Drugs
  Venoms
  Lead poisoning

   iv. Drug therapy
      1. Osmotic laxatives: used to soften the stool.
         (a) Work within 3 hours of administration.
         (b) Nonabsorbable sugars: lactulose or sorbitol.
            (i) May lead to cramping and bloating.
         (c) Saline laxatives: magnesium hydroxide
            (i) Watch use in patients with renal failure due to risk of hypermagnesemia.
      2. Emollient laxatives: docusate sodium or mineral oil.
         (a) Work to promote stool softening.
         (b) Risk for aspiration pneumonitis with mineral oil.
      3. Stimulant laxatives: senna or bisacodyl.
         (a) Useful in acute constipation.
         (b) Work within 12 hours with oral administration and 60 minutes with rectal administration.

NOTES

III. Diverticular disease
  a. Diverticulosis
    i. General
      1. Occur when the vasa recta penetrate the circular muscle layers between the taenia coli.
    ii. Clinical manifestations
      1. Typically asymptomatic or may present with intermittent cramping abdominal pain in the left lower quadrant.
      2. Physical examination may reveal mild left lower quadrant tenderness.
      3. Laboratory studies are normal, and fecal occult blood is negative.

QUESTION

An 18-year-old presents with 24-hour history of peri-umbilical pain. In the last 12 hours, the pain has moved to the right lower quadrant and they have developed nausea and started vomiting. On examination, there is tenderness at McBurney's point. What is the most likely diagnosis?

  A. Cholecystitis
  B. Diverticulitis
  C. Pancreatitis
  D. Appendicitis

Table 3-16 • Causes of Constipation

Lifestyle	Medications	Structural	Systemic Disease
Low fiber	*Anticholinergics* Antidepressants Antihistamines Antiparkinson drugs	Perianal disease	Metabolic/endocrinologic Hypothyroidism Hypercalcemia Renal failure (chronic) Diabetes
Decreased fluid intake	*Antihypertensives* Calcium channel blockers Clonidine	Obstruction lesions	Neurologic Spinal cord lesions Multiple sclerosis Parkinson's disease Hirschsprung's disease Autonomic neuropathy
Poor toilet habits	*Cation-containing agents* Iron Calcium Antacids	Colon strictures	Other Amyloidosis Depression Dementia Dermatomyositis
Inability to toilet	*Opiates* Morphine Codeine		
Decreased exercise			

NOTES

ANSWER **D** EXPLANATION: *Appendicitis starts with periumbilical pain that migrates to the right lower quadrant. Nausea, vomiting, and anorexia are also noted. Tenderness is noted at McBurney's point. Rovsing's, psoas, and obturator signs are also positive.*

correct ☐   incorrect ☐

   iii. Diagnosis
      1. Barium enema demonstrates multiple diverticula, typically involving the descending and sigmoid colon.
      2. Avoid endoscopic examination if diverticulitis is suspected.
   iv. Treatment
      1. Pain control and promoting regular bowel activity.
         (a) Increase in dietary fiber and decrease in dietary fat are recommended.
         (b) Avoidance of nuts and seeds is not indicated.
      2. Surgery is not indicated in uncomplicated diverticulosis.
   b. Acute diverticulitis
      i. General
         1. Perforation of a diverticulum causing acute infection.
         2. Occurs in about 20% of patients with diverticulosis.
      ii. Clinical manifestations
         1. Present with gradual onset of left lower quadrant pain.
            (a) Pain persists and is accompanied by colonic spasms and loose bowel movements.
         2. Anorexia, nausea, and vomiting may occur.
         3. On physical examination, fever is noted with left lower quadrant tenderness.
      iii. Diagnosis
         1. Laboratory results reveal a leukocytosis, and urinalysis may show red and white blood cells.
         2. Barium enema
            (a) Note spasm and a sawtooth pattern of the involved segment.
            (b) Barium enema is a relative contra-indication in acute diverticulitis.

      3. CT scan
         (a) Note inflammation of surrounding tissues, thickening of the bowel wall, abscess formation, and diverticula.
      4. Endoscopic evaluation is contraindicated in acute diverticulitis.
   iv. Treatment
      1. Medical therapy
         (a) Pain control
         (b) Rehydration
         (c) Broad-spectrum IV antibiotics
      2. Surgical therapy
         (a) Colectomy indicated in recurrent disease.
      3. Complication
         (a) Fistula formation
         (b) Colonic obstruction
         (c) Abscess formation
         (d) Peritonitis
         (e) Hemorrhage
   c. Diverticular hemorrhage
      i. General
         1. About 10% of patients with diverticulosis will develop an acute hemorrhage.
         2. Diverticular hemorrhage accounts for 50% of the causes of lower GI bleeding.
      ii. Clinical manifestations
         1. Present with dark to bright red blood per rectum in moderate to large amounts.
         2. Typically, bleeding is painless.
         3. Hemoglobin and hematocrit may be normal at start.
      iii. Diagnosis
         1. Red blood cell scans
         2. Endoscopic evaluation
      iv. Treatment
         1. Most diverticular hemorrhages will stop spontaneously.
         2. Medical therapy
            (a) Supportive with IV fluid administration.
            (b) Blood transfusions are typically needed.
         3. Surgical therapy
            (a) Colectomy indicated after failed medical therapy

NOTES

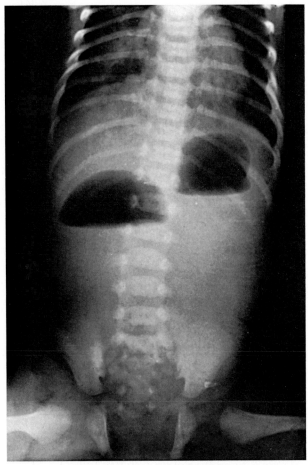

Figure 3-3 Duodenal atresia. Note the double bubble sign. (From Behrman RE. Nelson Textbook of Pediatrics, 17th ed. Philadelphia: WB Saunders, 2004:1233, Fig. 311-1.)

IV. Duodenal atresia
  a. General
    i. Due to failure to recanalize lumen after solid phase of intestinal development.
    ii. A history of polyhydramnios is common.
    iii. Down's syndrome seen in about one fourth of the cases.
    iv. Associated with other anomalies such as malrotation, esophageal atresia, and congenital heart disease.
  b. Clinical manifestations
    i. On first day of life, patient presents with bilious vomiting without abdominal distention.

    c. Diagnosis
      i. X-ray of abdomen reveals a double-bubble sign.
    d. Treatment
      i. Decompression of GI tract and IV fluids.
      ii. Surgery, duodenoduodenostomy, is indicated.
V. Inflammatory bowel disease
  a. Ulcerative colitis
    i. General
      1. Inflammation confined to the mucosa and submucosa.
      2. Confined to the colon.
      3. Equal distribution between males and females.
      4. Peak age of onset between 15 and 25 years and 55 and 65 years.
    ii. Clinical manifestations
      1. Major symptom is bloody diarrhea.
      2. May have rectal or lower quadrant abdominal pain with fever.
      3. Urgency and fecal incontinence are also noted.
      4. Laboratory studies reveal leukocytosis, anemia, and an elevated erythrocyte sedimentation rate.
      5. May have extraintestinal manifestations
        (a) Arthritis
        (b) Ankylosing spondylitis
        (c) Hepatitis/cirrhosis
        (d) Sclerosing cholangitis
        (e) Pyoderma gangrenosum
        (f) Erythema nodosum
        (g) Uveitis

NOTES

ANSWER D EXPLANATION: *Diverticulitis presents with gradual onset of left lower quadrant pain, fever, anorexia, nausea, and vomiting. A leukocytosis and hematuria are also present. CT scan of the abdomen shows bowel wall thickening,*

correct ☐   incorrect ☐

iii. Diagnosis
  1. Pathology
     (a) Inflammation begins in the rectum and extends proximally a certain distance and then stops.
     (b) A clear separation between inflamed and noninflamed tissue is noted.
  2. Radiographic
     (a) Barium enema reveals loss of haustra markings, narrowing of the lumen, and straightening of the colon.
  3. Endoscopy
     (a) Note diffuse erythema with edema and loss of vascular pattern in the rectum.
     (b) Inflammation begins in the rectum and extends proximally.
iv. Treatment
  1. General supportive care
     (a) Antidiarrheal agents and nutritional support play a small role in ulcerative colitis.
  2. Aminosalicylates
     (a) Not systemically absorbed but work in the lumen.
     (b) Can be given orally or topically in the rectum.
  3. Corticosteroids
  4. Immunomodulator
     (a) Work by blocking lymphocyte proliferation and activation.
  5. Surgery
     (a) Colectomy may be curative.
  6. Complications
     (a) Toxic megacolon
     (b) Increased risk for colon cancer.
b. Crohn's disease
  i. General

  1. Inflammation extends through the intestinal wall from mucosa to serosa.
  2. Can appear in any part of the GI tract, but distal small bowel and colon are commonly affected.
  3. Equal distribution between males and females.
  4. Peak age of onset between 15 and 25 years and 55 and 65 years.
ii. Clinical manifestations
  1. The major presenting symptoms are abdominal pain, diarrhea, and weight loss.
  2. On physical examination, aphthous ulcer may be noted on the oral mucosa.
  3. Abdomen may be tender and perianal disease is common.
  4. Laboratory studies reveal leukocytosis, anemia, and an elevated erythrocyte sedimentation rate.
  5. May have extraintestinal manifestations
     (a) Arthritis
     (b) Ankylosing spondylitis
     (c) Hepatitis/cirrhosis
     (d) Sclerosing cholangitis
     (e) Pyoderma gangrenosum
     (f) Erythema nodosum
     (g) Uveitis
iii. Diagnosis
  1. Pathology
     (a) Inflammation leads to thickening of the bowel wall and cobblestone appearance on the mucosa.
     (b) Typically have rectal sparing from inflammation.
     (c) Typically areas of inflammation are separated by normal tissue (skip lesions).
  2. Radiographic
     (a) Barium enema shows aphthous ulcers. When they deepen and enlarge, they give a cobblestone appearance.
     (b) Fistulas and strictures are common.
  3. Endoscopy
     (a) Aphthous ulcers are noted giving the mucosa a cobblestone appearance.
     (b) Areas of normal mucosa are noted between areas of inflammation.

NOTES

iv. Treatment
1. General supportive care
(a) Antidiarrheal agents and nutritional support play a small role in ulcerative colitis.
2. Aminosalicylates
(a) Are not systemically absorbed but work in the lumen.
(b) Can be given orally or topically in the rectum.
3. Corticosteroids
4. Immunomodulator
(a) Work by blocking lymphocyte proliferation and activation.
(b) Azathioprine and 6-mercaptoprine are effective in treating Crohn's disease.
(c) Drugs may cause leukopenia and increase risk for lymphoma.
5. Antibiotics
(a) Used in the management of complications, such as abscess and perianal disease.
6. Infliximab
(a) Antibody directed against tumor necrosis factor.
(b) Reserved for patients who have failed with the immunomodulator.
7. Surgery
(a) Used more conservatively because it is not curative; recurrence is common.
(b) Segmental resection is most commonly done.
8. Complications
(a) Abscesses and fistulas
(b) Intestinal obstruction
(c) Perianal disease
(d) Colon cancer
(i) Risk is less than that of ulcerative colitis, but greater than that of the general population.

VI. Intussusception
a. General
i. Defined as invagination of one part of the bowel into itself.
ii. The most frequent cause of intestinal obstruction during the first 2 years of life.
iii. More common in males (3:1) than females.

iv. Most common cause is idiopathic.
v. Most common location is ileocolic.
b. Clinical manifestations
i. Develop paroxysmal colicky abdominal pain followed by vomiting and diarrhea.
ii. Diarrhea becomes bloody with mucus (currant jelly stool).
iii. On exam, abdomen is distended and tender.
iv. On palpation, a sausage-shaped mass is noted in the upper mid-abdomen.
v. Some patients may show signs of altered consciousness, lethargy, and seizures.
c. Diagnosis
i. Abdominal film shows a paucity of bowel gas.
ii. Ultrasound reveals a single or hypoechoic ring with hyperechoic center (target or donut sign).
iii. Barium enema is diagnostic and therapeutic.
d. Treatment
i. Decompression of the intestine.
ii. Correct dehydration if present.

Table 3-17 • Comparison of Ulcerative Colitis and Crohn's Disease

Feature	Ulcerative Colitis	Crohn's Disease
Pathologic		
Rectal involvement	Always	Common
Fissures and fistulas	Never	Common
Skip lesions	Never	Always
Perianal disease	Never	Common
Granulomas	Occasional	Common
Clinical		
Rectal bleeding	Always	Occasional
Malaise, fever	Occasional	Common
Abdominal pain	Occasional	Common
Abdominal mass	Never	Common
Fistulas	Never	Common
Endoscopic		
Aphthous ulcers	Never	Common
Friable mucosa	Common	Occasional
Rectal involvement	Always	Common
Cobblestoning	Rare	Common

NOTES

iii. Surgery may be indicated if reduction is not possible or not successful.

VII. Irritable bowel disease
   a. General
      i. Greater incidence in females than males.
      ii. Typically present for care between ages 30 and 50 years.
      iii. Due to abnormality in motor function (smooth muscle) and disturbed sensation (visceral hypersensitivity).
   b. Clinical manifestations
      i. Chronic or recurrent abdominal pain is the major symptom.
         1. Described as postprandial cramps or discomfort.
         2. Pain is relieved by defecation.
      ii. Irregular defecation (diarrhea, constipation, or alternating between the two) is common.
      iii. Bloating, heartburn, and nausea without vomiting are also noted.
      iv. Physical examination may reveal abdominal tenderness.
   c. Diagnosis
      i. Based on history and after ruling out other causes of the symptoms. Criteria include 3 months of the following:
         1. Abdominal pain relieved by defecation or associated with a change in frequency and/or consistency of stool.
         2. And/or disturbed defecation
            (a) Two or more of the following
               (i) Altered stool frequency
               (ii) Altered stool form
               (iii) Altered stool passage
               (iv) Passage of mucus
         3. Bloating or abdominal distention.
   d. Treatment
      i. Counseling and discussion of the disease with the patient are vital.
      ii. Avoid unnecessary medications that can cause constipation or diarrhea.
      iii. Dietary changes include increasing fiber and decreasing fat intake.
      iv. Antispasmodics may be helpful.
      v. Antidepressants are helpful in resistant cases.

VIII. Ischemic bowel disease
   a. General
      i. Symptoms vary with location of the ischemia.
      ii. Blood flow to the GI tract.
         1. Celiac trunk supplies the liver, biliary tract, spleen, stomach, duodenum, and pancreas.
         2. Superior mesenteric artery supplies the duodenum, pancreas, small intestine, ascending colon, and part of the transverse colon.
         3. Inferior mesenteric artery supplies the part of the transverse colon, descending colon, and rectum.
   b. Acute arterial mesenteric ischemia
      i. General
         1. Patient typically has a history of heart disease and arrhythmias, congestive heart failure, recent myocardial infarction, or hypotension.
      ii. Clinical manifestations
         1. Sudden abdominal pain with abdominal tenderness on exam.
      iii. Diagnosis
         1. Laboratory results reveal a leukocytosis, metabolic acidosis, and elevated amylase.
         2. Abdominal X-rays show formless loops of small intestine, ileus, or "thumbprinting" of the small bowel or right colon secondary to submucosal bleeding.
         3. CT scan, ultrasound, or angiogram may be helpful.
      iv. Treatment
         1. Treat underlying cause.
         2. Laparotomy is required to restore blood flow to organ.
         3. Survival rate is low unless diagnosed early.
   c. Ischemic colitis
      i. General
         1. The most common ischemic injury to the GI tract.
         2. Most patients are older than 60 years.
         3. Cause or trigger of most episodes is unknown.

NOTES

ii. Clinical manifestations
  1. Present with sudden, mild, crampy, left lower abdominal pain, urge to defecate, and passage of bright red blood mixed with stool.
  2. Physical examination typically reveals only mild abdominal tenderness over the involved area of bowel.
iii. Diagnosis
  1. If no signs of peritonitis, a colonoscopy should be performed.
  2. Barium studies reveal "thumbprinting."
iv. Treatment
  1. Most symptoms resolve in 24 to 48 hours.
  2. If no signs of peritonitis, then bowel rest, antibiotics, and supportive care.
  3. Resection of the colon is indicated if signs of peritonitis or gangrene are present.

IX. Malabsorption
  a. General
    i. Refers to impaired transport across the mucosa.
    ii. Pathophysiologically due to:
      1. Impaired luminal hydrolysis
      2. Impaired mucosal function
      3. Impaired removal of nutrients from the mucosa
  b. Clinical manifestations
    i. Typically present with steatorrhea.
      1. Stools are pale in color, bulky, greasy.
      2. Diarrhea is watery and stools tend to float.
    ii. Abdominal distention and increased flatus.
    iii. Weight loss is common in severe malabsorption.
    iv. Other symptoms related to vitamin and mineral deficiency.
  c. Diagnosis
    i. Tests for fat absorption
      1. Qualitative or quantitative fecal fat.
        (a) Elevated in fat malabsorption disorders.
    ii. Tests for carbohydrate absorption
      1. D-Xylose test.
        (a) Low levels suggest mucosal dysfunction.
    iii. Tests for small bowel bacterial overgrowth
      1. Glucose breath hydrogen test
      2. Quantitative culture of jejunum aspirate

iv. Routine blood test
  1. Includes CBC, chemistry profile, PT, vitamin B_{12}, folate, iron, and carotene.
v. Radiology
  1. Small bowel follow-through and CT scan are helpful in the evaluation, and results vary depending on the etiology.
vi. Pathology
  1. Biopsy of the small intestine is important in the evaluation process.
d. Specific disorders
  i. Celiac sprue
    1. Due to abnormal immune response to gluten.
      (a) Gluten found in wheat, barley, rye, and oats.
    2. Biopsy shows atrophy of the villi in the small intestine.
    3. Laboratory tests reveal presence of antigliadin and antiendomysial antibodies.
    4. Evaluation includes exclusion of gluten from the diet and then rechallenge the patient with gluten.
    5. Treatment consists of a gluten-free diet.
  ii. Small bowel bacterial overgrowth
    1. Bacteria have effect on fat absorption by interfering with bile acids, and protein and carbohydrate absorption are affected secondary to mucosal damage.
    2. Diagnosis made by showing evidence of malabsorption and bacterial overgrowth.
    3. Treatment consists of antibiotics.
  iii. Disaccharidase deficiency
    1. Classic disease is lactase deficiency.
    2. As patient ages, there is loss of lactase activity.

QUESTION

Which of the following best describes the pathogenesis of irritable bowel syndrome?

A. Chronic infection of the bowel
B. Chronic anxiety disorder
C. Bowel motility disorder
D. Food intolerance

NOTES

ANSWER C EXPLANATION: *Irritable bowel syndrome is due to abnormality in motor or motility function (smooth muscle) and disturbed sensation (visceral hypersensitivity.)*

correct ☐   incorrect ☐

3. Diarrhea is profuse, and an osmotic gap may exist.
4. Treatment is avoidance of the offending agent.

X. Neoplasms
  a. General
    i. Adenocarcinoma makes up 98% of malignancies of the large intestine.
    ii. Peak incidence is between ages 60 and 80 years.
    iii. Risk factors include first-degree relative with colon cancer, inflammatory bowel disease, and diets high in fat and low in fiber.
    iv. See Table 3-18 for inherited colorectal cancer syndromes.
    v. Screening
      1. Fecal occult blood testing, flexible sigmoidoscopy, and colonoscopy are major approaches to cancer screening.
        (a) Starting at age 50 years, the average-risk patient should have occult blood testing done yearly, flexible sigmoidoscopy every 5 years, and colonoscopy every 10 years.
        (b) High-risk patients should have a colonoscopy done every 5 years.
  b. Clinical manifestations
    i. May remain clinically silent for years.
    ii. Major symptoms suggestive of colon cancer are rectal bleeding, pain, and change in bowel habits.
    iii. Laboratory tests reveal occult blood positive stools and anemia.
    iv. Symptoms related to metastatic disease may also be present (hepatomegaly, bowel obstruction, and pulmonary complaints).
  c. Diagnosis
    i. Colonoscopy with biopsy
  d. Treatment
    i. Surgical resection of tumor is the treatment of choice.
    ii. Radiation therapy and chemotherapy (5-fluorouracil) are also helpful in reducing local recurrence and distant metastasis.
    iii. Monitor response to treatment with carcinoembryonic antigen levels.

XI. Obstruction
  a. Small intestine
    i. General
      1. Mechanical obstruction implies a physical barrier to the movement of intestinal contents.
        (a) Paralytic ileus (adynamic ileus) refers to a disorder that has neurogenic

Table 3-18 • Inherited Colorectal Cancer Syndromes					
Syndrome	Histology	Distribution	Age Onset	Risk for Colon Cancer	Other
Familial polyposis	Adenoma	Large intestine	8–30 years	100%	Have 100s to 1000s of polyps in the large intestine
Gardner's syndrome	Adenoma	Large and small intestine	8–30 years	100%	Have extraintestinal manifestations
Peutz-Jeghers syndrome	Hamartoma	Large and small intestine	First decade	Slightly above average	Mucocutaneous pigmentation

NOTES

disruption of peristalsis as the cause
of failure to move intestinal contents
forward. There is not mechanical
obstruction.
  2. Most common cause is adhesions,
followed by neoplasms, hernias,
intussusception, and volvulus.
    (a) Volvulus is due to rotation of bowel
loops around a fixed point.
      (i) Typically due to congenital
abnormalities or adhesions.
      (ii) Onset of obstruction is abrupt,
and strangulation occurs
rapidly.
  ii. Clinical manifestations
    1. Signs and symptoms vary with location of
the obstruction.
      (a) High: frequent vomiting, intermittent
pain, and no distention.
      (b) Middle: moderate vomiting,
moderate distention, and
intermittent crescendo, colicky
abdominal pain.
      (c) Low: feculent vomiting late in the
course, marked distention, and
variable pain.
    2. If patient has signs of shock consider
strangulation obstruction.
  iii. Diagnosis
    1. Abdominal X-rays show a stepwise
pattern of dilated small intestine with
air-fluid levels.
      (a) The colon typically shows lack of
intestine gas.
      (b) See Figure 3-4 for abdominal X-ray
findings in bowel obstruction.
  iv. Treatment
    1. Partial obstruction can be treated with
decompression via a nasogastric tube.
    2. Surgery should be considered
with complete or strangulation
obstructions.
  b. Large intestine
  i. General
    1. Most common location is the sigmoid
colon.
    2. Etiologies include carcinoma,
diverticulitis, fecal impaction, and
inflammatory disorders.

QUESTION

Which of the following is a risk factor for the development of colon cancer?

  A. Daily aspirin use
  B. High fiber diet
  C. History of GERD
  D. Inflammatory bowel disease

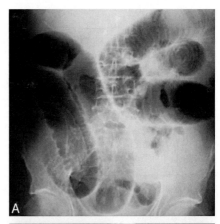
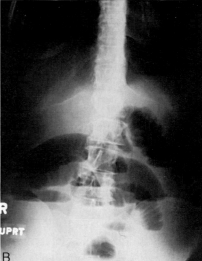

Figure 3-4 Bowel obstruction. Note air-fluid levels in bowel.
(From Feldman M. Sleisenger and Fordtran's Gastrointestinal
and Liver Disease, 7th ed. Philadelphia: WB Saunders,
2002:2116, Fig. 109-2.)

NOTES

ANSWER D EXPLANATION: *Risk factors for colon cancer include a first-degree relative with colon cancer, familial polyposis, colon polyps, smoking, history of inflammatory bowel disease, and diets high in fat and low in fiber. Aspirin may lower risk of colon cancer.*

correct ☐   incorrect ☐

    ii. Clinical manifestations
       1. Deep, visceral, cramping pain is noted that is referred to the hypogastrium.
       2. Constipation is common in complete obstruction.
       3. Vomiting may occur late in the course.
       4. Physical examination reveals abdominal distention and tympany.
          (a) High-pitched tinkles with gurgles are noted on auscultation.
   iii. Diagnosis
       1. Abdominal X-ray shows dilated large intestine.
       2. Barium enema will confirm diagnosis and identify the location.
   iv. Treatment
       1. First goal is decompression.
       2. Surgery to remove the obstruction is also important.

XII. Toxic megacolon
  a. General
    i. A rare life-threatening form of ulcerative colitis.
  b. Clinical manifestations
    i. Signs of toxic colitis, including fever, tachycardia, abdominal distention, and signs of peritonitis.
  c. Diagnosis
    i. Laboratory results reveal a leukocytosis.
    ii. Abdominal X-ray shows a dilated colon, greater than 6 cm.
  d. Treatment
    i. Aggressive fluid management.
    ii. IV steroids and broad-spectrum antibiotics.
    iii. If fail to improve in 24 to 48 hours or signs of perforation, then surgery is indicated.

RECTUM

I. Anal fissure
  a. General
    i. Due to a split in the anoderm.
      1. An ulcer is a chronic fissure.
      2. A skin tag (sentinel pile) is associated with a mature ulcer.
    ii. Fissures are most commonly caused during defecation of a large firm stool.
  b. Clinical manifestations
    i. Present with severe anal pain and bleeding with defecation.
    ii. Blood is noted on the stool or toilet paper.
    iii. On physical examination, a linear tear with a white ulcerated base.
  c. Diagnosis
    i. Diagnosis based on physical exam
  d. Treatment
    i. Stool softeners, bulking agents, and sitz baths are successful in healing fissures.
    ii. Internal anal sphincterotomy is required when conservative measures are not successful.

II. Anorectal abscess/fistula
  a. General
    i. Arise from infected anal glands.
  b. Clinical manifestations
    i. Causes severe continuous throbbing anal pain that is worse with ambulation and straining.
    ii. On rectal examination, the patient has a very tender mass palpable externally in the perianal area.
  c. Diagnosis
    i. Diagnosis is made on physical examination.
  d. Treatment
    i. Requires surgical drainage.
    ii. Complications
      1. Infection may spread resulting in tissue loss.
      2. May develop fistula-in-ano.

III. Fecal impaction
  a. General
    i. May lead to large bowel obstruction.
    ii. Predisposing conditions include severe psychiatric disease, prolonged bed rest,

NOTES

neurogenic disease of the colon, spinal cord disease, and constipating medications.
  b. Clinical manifestations
    i. May present with pelvic pain, diarrhea, nausea, vomiting, and abdominal distention.
    ii. On rectal exam, hard, dry stool is noted.
  c. Treatment
    i. Enemas or digital disimpaction.
    ii. Long-term care includes maintaining soft stools.
IV. Hemorrhoids
  a. General
    i. Internal hemorrhoids arise above the dentate line.
    ii. External hemorrhoids arise below the dentate line.
    iii. Major risk factor is prolonged straining with defecation.
    iv. Internal hemorrhoids are classified based on the following:
      1. First degree: bleeding only
      2. Second degree: bleeding and prolapse that reduces spontaneously.
      3. Third degree: bleeding and prolapse that requires manual reduction.
      4. Fourth degree: bleeding with incarceration that cannot be reduced.
  b. Clinical manifestations
    i. Internal hemorrhoids do not cause pain, but cause bright red blood per rectum, mucous discharge, and rectal fullness.
    ii. External hemorrhoids cause sudden severe perianal pain and a perianal mass.
  c. Diagnosis
    i. Diagnosed with anoscopy.
    ii. Rarely cause anemia, if anemia present must rule out malignancy.
  d. Treatment
    i. Medical management consists of dietary changes, stool softeners, bulking agents, and increased fluids.
    ii. Excisional hemorrhoidectomy may be needed for large hemorrhoids.
V. Neoplasms
  a. General
    i. Neoplasms of the anus are rare.
    ii. Located in anal canal or anal margin.
    iii. Risk factors include anogenital warts, history of pelvic cancer, and smoking.
    iv. Histologic types vary with location

QUESTION

A 45-year-old male presents with abdominal pain, nausea, and vomiting. Examination of the patient reveals high-pitched bowel sounds. X-ray of the abdomen reveals air-fluid levels. What is the most likely diagnosis?

  A. Paralytic ileus
  B. Small bowel obstruction
  C. Crohn's disease
  D. Ulcerative colitis

      1. Anal margin: squamous cell, basal cell, Bowen's disease, and Paget's disease.
      2. Anal canal: epidermoid carcinoma
  b. Clinical manifestations
    i. May note rectal mass, bleeding, pain, discharge, itching, and tenesmus.
  c. Diagnosis
    i. Diagnosis is made by biopsy.
  d. Treatment
    i. Wide local excision of the mass.
    ii. Radiation and chemotherapy may be needed for large tumors or metastatic disease.
VI. Pilonidal disease
  a. General
    i. Increase disease in white males ages 15 to 40 years.
    ii. May be congenital or acquired.
      1. Increased risk in hirsute obese individuals.
  b. Clinical manifestations
    i. Present with small midline pits or abscesses near the midline of the coccyx or sacrum.
    ii. On exam, a suppurative or draining abscess is noted with hair protruding from the openings.
  c. Diagnosis
    i. Based on physical examination.
  d. Treatment
    i. Drainage and deroofing of the abscess.
    ii. Maintaining hygiene is important until the abscess heals.
VII. Polyps
  a. General
    i. Adenomatous polyps are common in the distal colon and rectum.
    ii. Neoplastic with malignant potential.

NOTES

ANSWER **B** EXPLANATION: *Small bowel obstruction presents with diffuse abdominal pain, nausea, and vomiting. Abdominal x-rays reveal a stepwise pattern of dilated small intestine with the presence of air-fluid levels.*

correct ☐   incorrect ☐

1. Malignancy potential related to polyp size and level of dysplasia.
   iii. Common in elderly people.
   b. Clinical manifestations
      i. Patients are typically asymptomatic.
      ii. May have positive stool for occult blood or hematochezia.
   c. Diagnosis
      i. Diagnosis made on endoscopic examination or barium studies.
      ii. Colonoscopy with biopsy is the gold standard.
   d. Treatment
      i. Goal is removal or destruction of the polyp.
      ii. Follow-up colonoscopy is recommended in 3 years, or earlier if multiple or large polyps have been noted.

HERNIA

I. Hiatal
   a. General
      i. Two types: paraesophageal and sliding.
      ii. In paraesophageal hernias, all or part of the stomach herniates into the thorax.
         1. This occurs to the left of the nondisplaced gastroesophageal junction.
      iii. Sliding hiatal hernias are due to decreased resting pressure in LES.
   b. Clinical manifestations
      i. Paraesophageal hernias are typically asymptomatic.
         1. If symptoms do occur, it is due to obstruction.
      ii. Sliding
         1. Reflux is common and often worse when lying down.
         2. Nausea and vomiting are uncommon in adults but common in children.
         3. Dysphagia may also be noted.
   c. Diagnosis
      i. Diagnosis made on upper GI series.
   d. Treatment
      i. Surgical repair is indicated in paraesophageal hernias.
         1. In sliding hiatal hernias, surgery is indicated in persistent or recurrent symptoms.
            (a) Nissen fundoplication is the most effective surgery.
      ii. Medical treatment is indicated in sliding hiatal hernias.
         1. Prokinetic drugs, H_2 receptor blockers, or proton pump inhibitors are indicated.

II. Incisional (ventral)
   a. General
      i. History of prior abdominal surgery.
      ii. Risk factors include poor surgical technique, wound infection, age, obesity, and placement of drains.
   b. Clinical manifestations
      i. Mass noted at site of prior surgery.
   c. Diagnosis
      i. Diagnosis made on clinical findings
   d. Treatment
      i. Surgical repair to eliminate risk for obstruction.

III. Inguinal
   a. General
      i. Indirect inguinal hernias are congenital hernias and typically present during the first year of life.
         1. May not appear until patient older when the increased intra-abdominal pressure and dilated internal inguinal ring allow abdominal contents to enter the cavity.
      ii. Direct inguinal hernias are acquired as a result of weakness of the transversalis fascia in Hesselbach's triangle.
   b. Clinical manifestations
      i. Most hernias produce no symptoms until a lump is noted in the groin.
      ii. With indirect hernias, some patients may note a dragging sensation or radiation of pain into the scrotum.

NOTES

iii. On physical examination, different results are noted.
    1. Direct
        (a) When standing the hernia appears as a symmetric, circular swelling at the external ring.
        (b) Disappears when the patient is supine.
    2. Indirect
        (a) Descend into the scrotum.
        (b) Present as an elliptical swelling that does not reduce easily.
iv. Tissue must be noted in the inguinal ring with coughing for the diagnosis of a hernia.
c. Diagnosis
  i. Based on clinical findings.
d. Treatment
  i. Indirect hernias are more likely to become incarcerated or strangulate.
  ii. Surgical repair is indicated.

IV. Umbilical
a. General
  i. More common in adult females than males.
  ii. In adults, due to gradual loosening of the tissue around the umbilical ring.
    1. In children, due to the umbilical ring not closing.
  iii. Predisposing factors include multiple pregnancies, ascites, obesity, and large intra-abdominal tumors.
b. Clinical manifestations
  i. Present as increasing mass at the umbilical ring.
c. Diagnosis
  i. Based on clinical findings.
d. Treatment
  i. In children, will obliterate spontaneously by 12 months of age.
  ii. Surgical repair indicated to avoid incarceration and strangulation.

INFECTIOUS DIARRHEA

I. Acute infectious diarrhea
a. General
  i. Acute diarrhea is sudden change in bowel habits, passage of increased number of stools, or decreased form for less than 2 weeks.

ii. See Table 3-19 for comparison of inflammatory and noninflammatory diarrhea.
iii. See Table 3-20 for causes of infectious diarrhea.
b. Clinical manifestations
  i. History very important. Should include:
    1. Travel history
    2. Foods eaten
    3. Recent hospitalizations
    4. Recent antibiotic usage
    5. Exposure to others affected
    6. Sexual history
    7. Shellfish ingestion
    8. Exposure to farm animals
    9. Systemic disease
    10. Immune status
  ii. Physical exam to include vitals with orthostatics, skin turgor, and abdominal and rectal examination.
c. Diagnosis
  i. Evaluation should include fecal white blood cell count, stool culture, stool for ova and parasites, *Clostridium difficile* toxin, and possible endoscopy.
d. Treatment
  i. Oral rehydration with WHO-ORS or similar product.
  ii. Empiric antibiotic therapy
    1. Most cases of infectious diarrhea resolve in 3 days without antibiotics.
    2. Antibiotics may prolong duration of fecal excretion of the pathogen.

NOTES

ANSWER D EXPLANATION: *Perirectal abscesses arise from infected anal glands and present with continuous pain that worsens with straining or defecation. On rectal examination a tender mass is palpable.*

correct ☐   incorrect ☐

iii. Symptomatic therapy
    1. Antimotility agents such as diphenoxylate or loperamide.
    2. Avoid these agents if presence of fever or bloody diarrhea.

Table 3-19 • Inflammatory versus Noninflammatory Diarrhea

	Inflammatory Diarrhea	Noninflammatory Diarrhea
Clinical	Small-volume bloody diarrhea Lower abdominal pain Fecal urgency	Large-volume watery diarrhea Upper abdominal pain Nausea and vomiting
Fecal leukocytes	Present	Absent
Etiologies	*Shigella* species *Campylobacter* species *Salmonella* species *Entamoeba histolytica* *Yersinia* species *Clostridium difficile* Enteroinvasive *Escherichia coli*	*Vibrio* species *Giardia* species Entertoxigenic *Escherichia coli* Rotavirus Norwalk agent *Staphylococcus aureus* *Clostridium perfringens*

Table 3-20 • Causes of Infectious Diarrhea

Organism	Vehicle	Presentation	Treatment
Viral			
Rotavirus	Person to person	Vomiting followed by watery diarrhea Duration, 5–7 days	Volume replacement
Norwalk agent	Person to person	Duration, 1–2 days	Volume replacement
Bacterial			
Staphylococcus aureus	Mayonnaise-containing foods Cream-filled pies	Symptoms occur within 1–6 hours Nausea, vomiting, abdominal pain, and then diarrhea Fever is rare	Supportive No role for antibiotics
Bacillus cereus	Fried rice Poorly refrigerated prepared foods	Symptoms occur in 1–6 hr for emetic form and 8–16 hr for diarrheal form	Supportive

NOTES

Table 3-20 • Causes of Infectious Diarrhea—cont'd

Organism	Vehicle	Presentation	Treatment
Clostridium perfringens	Canned foods	Onset within 24 hrs Present with watery diarrhea and epigastric pain Resolves in 24 hours	Supportive
Vibrio cholerae	Water Seafood	Severe diarrhea and fluid loss Death can occur in 3–4 hours Stools described as rice water	Fluid and electrolyte replacement Antibiotics, including tetracycline or doxycycline, are agents of choice
Vibrio parahaemolyticus Pathogenic *Escherichia coli*	Shellfish Water (foreign travel)	Diarrhea lasting 5 days Watery diarrhea, nausea, and abdominal cramping Diarrhea improves in 24 hours	Supportive Supportive Antibiotics, including trimethoprim-sulfamethoxazole or fluoroquinolones
Shigella species	Poultry Seafood Day care centers	Abdominal pain, fever, and multiple small-volume bloody diarrheas Length of disease, 7 days	Supportive Antibiotics, including trimethoprim-sulfamethoxazole or fluoroquinolones, will shorten duration of disease
Salmonella species	Poultry Eggs Reptiles	Bacteremia common High fever, headache, and abdominal pain	Antibiotics, including third-generation cephalosporins or fluoroquinolones
Campylobacter species	Poultry	Diarrhea and fever are common	Supportive Antibiotics (erythromycin) may be indicated in severe cases
Enterohemorrhagic *E. coli* (O157:H7)	Undercooked beef	Can lead to development of hemolytic-uremic syndrome (HUS) in children. Severe diarrhea, abdominal pain, and nausea and vomiting	Supportive Antibiotics may increase risk for HUS.
Aeromonas species	Water	Watery diarrhea, vomiting, and mild fever	Trimethoprim-sulfamethoxazole is the drug of choice
Protozoal *Entamoeba histolytica*	Water	Tissue invasive and can infect other sites such as liver	Metronidazole

(continued)

NOTES

113

Table 3-20 • Causes of Infectious Diarrhea—cont'd

Organism	Vehicle	Presentation	Treatment
Giardia lamblia	Water with animal vector such as beaver	Diarrhea with mucus but no blood	Metronidazole
Cryptosporidium parvum	Water Day care	Associated with HIV Watery diarrhea, with nausea, abdominal cramps, and low-grade fever	Supportive Paromomycin may be considered

II. Traveler's diarrhea
   a. General
      i. Passage of three loose stools in a 24-hour period, with nausea and vomiting, tenesmus, or passage of blood or mucus in stool.
      ii. Transmitted by fecal–oral route.
      iii. Can occur up to 1 week after returning from travel.
      iv. Most cases are bacterial in etiology.
         1. Includes enterotoxigenic *Escherichia coli* and Shigella, *Campylobacter, Aeromonas, Salmonella,* and *Vibrio* species.
   b. Clinical manifestations
      i. Symptoms vary with etiology.
      ii. May have high fever, bloody stools, nausea and vomiting, and leukocytosis.
   c. Diagnosis
      i. Evaluation should be based on location of travel and possible etiologic agents.
         1. Could include fecal white blood cell count, stool culture, stool for ova and parasites, *C. difficile* toxin, and possible endoscopy.
      ii. Prevention
         1. Instruct patients to refrain from drinking local water or eating fresh fruits and vegetables.
         2. Prophylactic measures include bismuth subsalicylate and the fluoroquinolones.
   d. Treatment
      i. Fluid replacement is vital. Monitor vital signs.
      ii. Antibiotics are used in moderate or severe disease
         1. Antibiotics of choice are the fluoroquinolones.
      iii. Antidiarrheal agents can also be used to control symptoms.
III. Nosocomial diarrhea
   a. General
      i. Most common etiology is *C. difficile.*
         1. A Gram-positive anaerobic organism.
         2. Is a toxin-producing organism.
      ii. Occurs most commonly after antibiotic usage.
         1. Can appear up to 6 weeks after the antibiotic use.
      iii. A severe inflammatory response that can lead to pseudomembrane formation.
   b. Clinical manifestations
      i. Present with watery diarrhea and crampy abdominal pain.
      ii. On physical examination, can note a distended abdomen and diffuse tenderness.
   c. Diagnosis
      i. Positive for fecal leukocyte.
      ii. Positive for *C. difficile* toxin.
      iii. Endoscopic examination reveals colitis to pseudomembranes.
   d. Treatment
      i. Discontinue the offending agent.
      ii. Avoid antimotility agents.
      iii. Antibiotics are typically required.
         1. Vancomycin or metronidazole is the drug of choice.

NOTES

Table 3-21 • Nutritional Deficiencies

Vitamin	Fat Soluble	Function	Deficiency	Toxicity	Source	Note
Niacin (vitamin B$_3$)	No	NAD/NADP	Pellagra coenzyme	Flushing Hyperglycemia Liver damage	Fish, liver, meat, poultry, grains, eggs, milk	Lowers low-density and increases high-density lipoprotein cholesterol
Thiamine (vitamin B$_1$)	No	Neural conduction	Beriberi	Lethargy Ataxia	Pork liver, organ meats, legumes, grains, wheat germ	
Vitamin A	Yes	Visual pigments, cell differentiation, gene regulation	Night blindness	Hepatocellular necrosis Intracranial hypertension	Liver, dairy, yellow and dark green leafy vegetables	Teratogenic early in pregnancy Toxic in large amounts
Riboflavin	No	Coenzyme	Cheilosis Glossitis Angular stomatitis	None	Milk and dairy, organ meats, green leafy vegetables	
Vitamin C	No	Antioxidant	Scurvy	Nausea Diarrhea	Citrus fruits Tomato	Decreased levels impair wound healing
Vitamin D	Yes	Calcium homeostasis, bone metabolism	Rickets Osteomalacia	Renal damage Hypercalcemia	Milk, liver, egg, salmon, tuna	Toxic in large amounts
Vitamin K	Yes	Blood clotting	Hemorrhage	With IV administration, dyspnea and cardiovascular collapse can occur	Liver, oils, green leafy vegetable Synthesize by intestinal tract bacteria	Interferes with warfarin Toxic in large amounts

NUTRITIONAL DEFICIENCIES

See Table 3-21 for summary of nutritional deficiencies.

METABOLIC DISORDERS

I. Phenylketonuria
   a. General
      i. An inborn error of metabolism.

NOTES

ii. An autosomal recessive disorder with decreased activity of phenylalanine hydroxylase.

iii. Incidence of 1 in 10,000 live births.

b. Clinical manifestations

i. Patients untreated develop severe mental retardation, hyperactivity, seizures, light complexion, and eczema.

ii. The urine has a mouselike odor

c. Diagnosis

i. Early diagnosis through early infancy screening.

ii. Screening test must be completed between 24 hours and 3 weeks of age.

d. Treatment

i. Limit dietary intake of phenylalanine to permit normal growth and development.

ii. Dietary changes must be followed throughout life.

Drugs used in Gastroenterology

Drug Name	Mechanism of Action	Therapeutic Use	Side Effects
Cimetidine	H2 receptor antagonist	PUD GERD Zollinger Ellison Syndrome	Headache Dizziness Diarrhea Gynecomastia
Famotidine	H2 receptor antagonist	PUD GERD Zollinger Ellison Syndrome	Headache Dizziness Diarrhea Gynecomastia
Nizatidine	H2 receptor antagonist	PUD GERD Zollinger Ellison Syndrome	Headache Dizziness Diarrhea Gynecomastia
Ranitidine	H2 receptor antagonist	PUD GERD Zollinger Ellison Syndrome	Headache Dizziness Diarrhea Gynecomastia
Misoprostol	Analog of prostaglandin E1	NSAID induced ulcers	Diarrhea Nausea Contraindicated in pregnancy.
Lansoprazole	Binds to H^+/K^+-ATPase (proton pump) and suppresses H^+ secretion.	Esophagitis PUD Zollinger Ellison Syndrome	Gastric carcinoid tumor. No drug interactions.

NOTES

Drugs used in Gastroenterology—cont'd

Drug Name	Mechanism of Action	Therapeutic Use	Side Effects
Omeprazole	Binds to H^+/K^+-ATPase (proton pump) and suppresses H^+ secretion.	Esophagitis PUD (H. pylori) Zollinger Ellison Syndrome	Gastric carcinoid tumor. Multiple drug interactions: warfarin, phenytoin, and diazepam.
Sucralfate	Binds with particles to form a barrier.	Duodenal ulcers	Do not give with a H2 antagonist
Prochlorperazine	Phenothiazine-blocks dopamine receptors.	Antiemetic	Hypotension Restlessness Extrapyramidal symptoms
Domperidone	Butyrophenones-blocks dopamine receptors.	Chemotherapy induced nausea and vomiting.	Tardive dyskinesia Extrapyramidal symptoms Neuroleptic malignant syndrome
Droperidol	Butyrophenones-blocks dopamine receptors.	Chemotherapy induced nausea and vomiting.	Tardive dyskinesia Extrapyramidal symptoms Neuroleptic malignant syndrome
Haloperidol	Butyrophenones-blocks dopamine receptors.	Chemotherapy induced nausea and vomiting.	Tardive dyskinesia Extrapyramidal symptoms Neuroleptic malignant syndrome
Alprazolam	Enhance affinity for GABA receptors.	Anticipatory vomiting	Drowsiness Ataxia Confusion
Lorazepam	Enhance affinity for GABA receptors.	Anticipatory vomiting	Drowsiness Ataxia Confusion
Granisetron	Blocks 5-HT3 receptors in periphery and brain.	Chemotherapy and post-operative nausea and vomiting.	Headache

(continued)

NOTES

Drugs used in Gastroenterology—cont'd

Drug Name	Mechanism of Action	Therapeutic Use	Side Effects
Ondansetron	Blocks 5-HT3 receptors in periphery and brain.	Chemotherapy and post-operative nausea and vomiting.	Headache
Diphenoxylate	Opioid-like action on bowel and decreases peristalsis.	Antidiarrheal	Drowsiness Abdominal cramps Dizziness Toxic megacolon
Loperamide	Opioid-like action on bowel and decreases peristalsis.	Antidiarrheal	Drowsiness Abdominal cramps Dizziness Toxic megacolon
Bismuth Subsalicylate	Decrease fluid secretion in bowel	Antidiarrheal	Salicylate toxicity Black stools
Castor oil	Irritating to gut and promotes increased peristalsis, stimulates colon activity.	Laxative	Atonic colon
Senna	Irritating to gut and promotes increased peristalsis, stimulates colon activity.	Laxative	Atonic colon
Magnesium sulfate	Saline cathartic	Laxative	
Polyethylene glycol	Osmotic laxative	Colonic lavage	Nausea Vomiting Abdominal cramps
Lactulose	Osmotic laxative	Laxative	
Docusate sodium	Stool softener, surface active agent	Laxative	
Mineral oil	Stool softener, surface active agent	Laxative	Lipid pneumonitis Decreased absorption of fat-soluble vitamins.

NOTES

Drugs used in Gastroenterology—cont'd			
Drug Name	**Mechanism of Action**	**Therapeutic Use**	**Side Effects**
Bethanechol	Cholinergic agonist, increased tone and motility of the bowel.	Post-operative ileus	Cramping Diarrhea Salivation Sweating Urinary incontinence
Metoclopramide	Enhances motility and tone by stimulating acetylcholine release. Antiemetic by blocking dopamine receptors.	Antiemetic Gastroparesis Parkinsonism	GI cramping Diarrhea

Question 1

Which of the following is the most common presenting symptom of esophageal cancer?

A. Dysphagia
B. Regurgitation
C. Hoarseness
D. Lymphadenopathy

Question 2

A positive fecal leukocyte suggests which of the following disorders?

A. Salmonella infection
B. Giardia infection
C. Viral infection
D. Vibrio infection

Question 3

A 4-week-old infant presents with projectile vomiting and failure to gain weight. The mother states that the infant does not appear ill and feeds again immediately after vomiting. On physical examination a palpable mass is noted in mid-epigastric region. Which of the following the most likely diagnosis?

A. Pyloric stenosis
B. Lactose intolerance
C. Intussusception
D. Meckel's diverticulum

Question 4

An 80-year-old patient presents with a 1-year history of constipation. Workup has been negative. What management option should be recommended to this patient?

A. Regular enemas and low protein diet
B. Daily laxative and high fat diet
C. Increased physical activity and daily multi-vitamin
D. Increased fluid intake and high fiber diet

NOTES

Question 5

What is the mechanism of action of omeprazole (Prilosec)?

A. Blocks H_2 histamine receptors
B. Block cholinergic receptors
C. Stimulates prostaglandin receptors
D. Inhibits H^+/K^+-ATPase proton pump

Question 6

Barrett's esophagus is a common sequela of which of the following?

A. Pyloric stenosis
B. Mallory-Weiss tear
C. Esophageal stricture
D. Gastroesophageal reflux disease

Question 7

A 10-year-old develops fever, headache, and abdominal pain after playing with a pet snake. Later develops a bloody diarrhea. Which of the following is the most likely agent causing these symptoms?

A. Campylobacter sp.
B. Shigella sp.
C. Salmonella sp.
D. Vibrio sp.

Answer 1

ANSWER **A** EXPLANATION: *The most common presenting symptom for esophageal cancer is dysphagia, first to solids and then liquids. Patients may also present with odynophagia, chest pain, weight loss, and anorexia.*

Topic: esophageal neoplasm

correct ☐   incorrect ☐

Answer 2

ANSWER **A** EXPLANATION: *Presence of fecal leukocytes indicates the presence of inflammation in the colon. Causes of inflammatory diarrhea include Shigella, Salmonella, Campylobacter, E. histolytica, Yersinia, C. difficile, and enteroinvasive E. coli.*

Topic: Infectious diarrhea

correct ☐   incorrect ☐

Answer 3

ANSWER **A** EXPLANATION: *Pyloric stenosis typically develops around the age of 3-5 weeks and presents with projectile, non-bilious vomitus and on physical examination a palpable olive-shaped mass is noted in the mid-epigastrium region.*

Topic: Pyloric stenosis

correct ☐   incorrect ☐

NOTES

Answer 4

ANSWER **D** EXPLANATION: *Constipation, with no underlying cause, should be treated with conservative measures. These measures include regular exercise, adequate fluid intake, and increasing dietary fiber.*

Topic: Constipation

correct ☐   **incorrect** ☐

Answer 6

ANSWER **D** EXPLANATION: *Prolonged exposure of the esophagus to gastric acid as in gastric esophageal reflux disease can lead to epithelial damage and Barrett's esophagus.*

Topic: Gastric esophageal reflux disease

correct ☐   **incorrect** ☐

Answer 5

ANSWER **D** EXPLANATION: *Omeprazole is a proton-pump inhibitor and works by binding to H^+/K^+-ATPase and suppresses H^+ secretion.*

Topic: Peptic ulcer disease

correct ☐   **incorrect** ☐

Answer 7

ANSWER **C** EXPLANATION: *Salmonella infection presents with bloody diarrhea, high fever, headache, and abdominal pain. The vehicle of infection is poultry, eggs, and reptiles.*

Topic: Infectious diarrhea

correct ☐   **incorrect** ☐

NOTES

Musculoskeletal System

4

EXAM BLUEPRINT TOPICS

Disorders of the Shoulder
Dislocations
Rotator cuff disorders
Separations
Disorders of the Forearm/Wrist/Hand
Dislocations
Gamekeeper's thumb
Nursemaid's elbow
Sprains
Tenosynovitis

- Carpal tunnel syndrome
- De Quervain's tenosynovitis
- Epicondylitis

Disorders of the Back/Spine
Ankylosing spondylitis
Back strain/sprain
Cauda equina syndrome
Herniated disk pulposus
Kyphosis/Scoliosis
Low back pain
Spinal stenosis
Disorders of the Hip
Aseptic necrosis
Dislocations
Slipped capital femoral epiphysis
Disorders of the Knee
Bursitis
Dislocations
Meniscal injuries
Osgood-Schlatter disease
Sprains/Strains
Disorders of the Ankle/Foot
Dislocations
Sprains/Strains
Fractures
Ankle/Foot

Forearm/Wrist/Hand

- Boxer's
- Colles'
- Humeral
- Radial
- Scaphoid

Hip
Knee
Shoulder
Infectious Diseases
Osteomyelitis
Septic arthritis
Neoplastic Disease
Bone cysts
Bone tumors
Ganglion cysts
Osteosarcoma
Osteoarthritis
Osteoporosis
Rheumatologic Conditions
Fibromyalgia
Gout/Pseudogout
Juvenile rheumatoid arthritis
Polyarteritis nodosa
Polymyositis
Polymyalgia rheumatica
Reiter syndrome
Rheumatoid arthritis
Systemic lupus erythematosus
Scleroderma
Sjögren syndrome

DISORDERS OF THE SHOULDER

I. Dislocations
  a. General
    i. Dislocation can be anterior or posterior.

NOTES

ii. Mechanism of action.
   1. Anterior: due to trauma from a fall or forceful throwing motion.
   2. Posterior: posteriorly directed force when the arm is in adduction and internal rotation.
b. Clinical manifestations
   i. Note sensation of shoulder slipping out of joint when arm is abducted and externally rotated.
      1. Note severe pain with any movement of the shoulder.
   ii. With anterior dislocation patient supports the arm in a neutral position.
      1. Apprehension test positive in anterior dislocation.
   iii. With posterior dislocation patient holds the arm in adduction and internal rotation.
      1. Jerk test positive in posterior dislocation.
   iv. Evaluate for possible axillary nerve injury.
c. Diagnosis
   i. Anteroposterior (AP) and axillary shoulder X-rays should be obtained.
      1. Compression fracture of the posterior humeral head is evidence of an anterior dislocation.
      2. Axillary view needed to diagnose posterior dislocation.
   ii. Magnetic resonance imaging (MRI) or arthrogram may be needed for diagnosis.
d. Treatment
   i. Dislocation should be reduced and physical therapy begun to strengthen the rotator cuff muscles.
   ii. Surgery may be needed to correct recurrent dislocations.

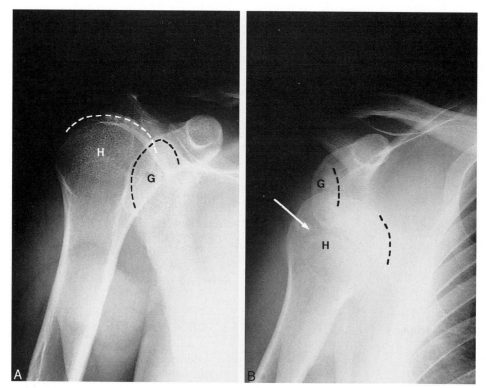

Figure 4-1 Shoulder dislocation. (From Mettler FA: Essentials of Radiology, 2nd ed. Philadelphia, Elsevier Saunders, 2005, p. 287, Fig. 8-49.)

NOTES

II. Rotator cuff disorders
  a. General
    i. Rotator cuff is composed of four muscles.
      1. Supraspinatus
      2. Infraspinatus
      3. Subscapularis
      4. Teres minor
    ii. Disorders include rotator cuff tendinitis or tear.
    iii. Tendinitis is a common cause of shoulder pain in middle-aged patients.
      1. Etiology is loss of microvascular blood supply and repeated mechanical insult to the tendon.
    iv. Tear is more common in patients over age 40.
      1. Etiology is acute injury, age-related degeneration, or altered blood supply to the tendon.
      2. Tears in young patients are secondary to physical activity or repeated trauma.
  b. Clinical manifestations
    i. Tendinitis
      1. Gradual onset of pain exacerbated by overhead activity.
      2. Night pain is common.
      3. Palpation over the greater tuberosity and subacromial bursa elicits tenderness and crepitus with shoulder motion.
    ii. Tear
      1. Atrophy of muscles at the top and back of the shoulder may be noted.
      2. Recurrent shoulder pain with history of a specific injury triggering pain.
      3. Weakness, catching, and grating are noted when lifting arm overhead.
      4. Passive range of motion is normal, but active range of motion is limited.
      5. Difficulty holding arm elevated when lifted parallel to the floor.
        (a) A positive drop arm test is noted in severe tears.
  c. Diagnosis
    i. Tendinitis
      1. X-ray of the shoulder is normal.
    ii. Tear
      1. X-ray may reveal a high riding humerus.
      2. MRI is the test of choice to evaluate tear.

  d. Treatment
    i. Tendinitis
      1. Rest from offending activity and nonsteroidal anti-inflammatory drugs (NSAIDs).
      2. Steroid injection can be considered if above is not successful.
    ii. Tear
      1. First treatment option is NSAIDs, sling, physical therapy, and strengthening exercises.
      2. Steroid injection can provide short-term relief from pain and inflammation.
      3. Surgery is only indicated with significant symptoms and failed rehabilitation.

III. Separations
  a. General
    i. Result from a fall onto the tip of the shoulder.
    ii. Three types.
      1. Type 1
        (a) Acromioclavicular (AC) joint ligaments are partially or completely disrupted, but the joint capsule is intact.
      2. Type 2
        (a) AC ligaments are torn and the joint capsule is damaged.
      3. Type 3
        (a) Coracoclavicular ligaments are completely disrupted and clavicle is completely separated from the acromion.
        (b) Bruising is often present.
  b. Clinical manifestations
    i. Pain is noted over AC joint and pain is noted on lifting the arm.
    ii. Patient supports arm in an adducted position and any motion causes pain.
  c. Diagnosis
    i. AP X-ray will confirm type 2 or 3 separations.
      1. Weighted X-rays, with a 10-pound weight, may increase separation on the X-ray.
  d. Treatment
    i. Type 1 and 2 are treated with a sling for a few days.
      1. Ice is helpful the first 48 hours along with pain medications.
    ii. Type 3 may require surgery.

NOTES

DISORDERS OF THE FOREARM/WRIST/HAND

I. Dislocations
  a. Elbow
    i. General
      1. Elbow dislocation results from a fall on an outstretched hand with the elbow extended.
      2. Most are posterior and can be complete or perched.
      3. Concomitant fractures, of the radial head in adults or medial epicondyle in children, are common.
    ii. Clinical manifestations
      1. Present with severe pain, swelling, and inability to bend elbow.
      2. Must evaluate brachial artery, median nerve, and ulnar nerve for injury.
    iii. Diagnosis
      1. AP and lateral X-ray assist in the diagnosis.
    iv. Treatment
      1. Reduction of the elbow should be performed as soon as possible.
        (a) Hold elbow flexed at 45 degrees and apply slow, steady, downward traction on the forearm.
      2. After reduction the arm should be splinted.
  b. Hand
    i. General
      1. Common injury due to hyperextension injury.
        (a) Involves complete tear of the volar capsule.
        (b) PIP joint is most commonly affected.
    ii. Clinical manifestations
      1. Note joint deformity immediately after the injury.
      2. Joint instability is also noted.
    iii. Diagnosis
      1. X-rays are needed to rule out fracture.
    iv. Treatment
      1. Closed reduction is required for PIP and distal interphalangeal (DIP) joint dislocations.
      2. Buddy taping to adjacent finger will stabilize joint.

II. Gamekeeper's thumb
  a. General
    i. Injury to ulnar collateral ligament of the thumb.
    ii. Due to a fall on thumb that forcibly deviates it radially.
      1. Frequently due to forced abduction of thumb against a ski pole (skier's thumb).
  b. Clinical manifestations
    i. Pain and swelling occurs shortly after the injury.
    ii. Swelling is noted on the inside of the thumb metacarpophalangeal (MCP) joint.
    iii. Note weakness with pinching the thumb and index finger.
  c. Diagnosis
    i. Based on physical exam findings.
  d. Treatment
    i. Surgical treatment is required for complete tears.
    ii. Partial tears can be treated with thumb spica splint or cast.

III. Nursemaid's elbow (Subluxation of the radial head)
  a. General
    i. Common elbow injury in children under age 5.
    ii. Due to increased ligament laxity.
    iii. Mechanism of injury is a pull on the forearm when the elbow is extended and forearm pronated.
    iv. Annular ligament slips proximally and becomes trapped between the radius and ulna.
  b. Clinical manifestations
    i. Pain noted immediately after injury.
    ii. Child then reluctant to use arm and extremity is held by the side with elbow slightly flexed and forearm pronated.
    iii. Tenderness noted over radial head.
  c. Diagnosis
    i. X-ray is normal.
    ii. Based on clinical findings.
  d. Treatment
    i. Reduction is done by placing thumb over the radial head and supinating the forearm.
    ii. If successful child will begin using arm immediately.

NOTES

IV. Sprains (Fingers)
  a. General
    i. Typically a result of either radial or ulnar collateral ligament injury to the PIP or DIP joints.
    ii. Etiologies include sports, falls, work-related trauma, or direct blows.
    iii. Grades
      1. Grade 1
        (a) Damage to the ligament but no joint instability.
      2. Grade 2
        (a) Stretching and partial tearing of the ligament.
      3. Grade 3
        (a) Complete disruption of the ligament.
  b. Clinical manifestations
    i. Grade 1
      1. Swelling and tenderness to palpation, but no functional abnormality.
    ii. Grade 2
      1. Swelling with bruising is noted with some joint laxity.
    iii. Grade 3
      1. Joint is painful and feels unstable.
  c. Diagnosis
    i. Based on clinical findings.
  d. Treatment
    i. Grades 1 and 2 are treated by buddy taping injured finger to adjacent finger.
    ii. Grade 3 is buddy taped and referred for surgery.
V. Tenosynovitis
  a. Carpal tunnel syndrome
    i. General
      1. Entrapment of the median nerve at the wrist.
      2. Common neuropathy of the upper extremity.
        (a) More common in middle-aged or pregnant women.
      3. Common precipitating causes include repetitive use trauma, tumors, pregnancy, thyroid disease, or diabetes.
    ii. Clinical manifestations
      1. Present with a vague ache that radiates into the thenar area.
      2. Paresthesias and numbness are noted on the thumb and index, long, and radial half of the ring fingers.

      3. May note frequently dropping items or cannot twist lids.
      4. Often awakened at night with pain or numbness.
      5. Thenar atrophy may occur.
      6. Phalen test and Tinel sign are positive.
        (a) Phalen test is performed by placing wrists in flexion and noting aching or numbness in the median nerve distribution in 60 seconds.
        (b) Tinel sign is positive if tingling is noted in median nerve distribution with tapping over the median nerve.
    iii. Diagnosis
      1. Electromyograph and median nerve conduction velocity studies are abnormal.
    iv. Treatment
      1. Splinting and NSAIDs are used in the treatment of mild cases.
        (a) Injection of steroids can be used if above fails.
      2. Surgery is needed for those patients with muscle atrophy, weak thenar muscles, or decreased sensation.
  b. De Quervain's tenosynovitis
    i. General
      1. Inflammation of the sheath around the abductor pollicis longus and extensor pollicis brevis tendons on the thumb side of the wrist.
    ii. Clinical manifestations
      1. Note pain, swelling, and a locking of the tendon with movement of the thumb.
      2. Patients note pain and swelling over the radial styloid, made worse with movement of the thumb.

NOTES

ANSWER D EXPLANATION: *Shoulder separation result from a fall on the tip of the shoulder. Present with pain at the AC joint and with any movement. Treatment involves placement of injured shoulder in a sling.*

correct ☐   incorrect ☐

3. Finkelstein test is positive.
   (a) Pain with full flexion of the thumb into the palm followed by ulnar deviation of the wrist.
iii. Diagnosis
   1. Based on clinical findings.
iv. Treatment
   1. Thumb spica splint to immobilize thumb and wrist, and use of NSAIDs are initial treatment.
   2. Steroid injection can be used if above treatment fails.
   3. If no improvement surgery may be needed.
c. Epicondylitis
   i. General
      1. Lateral (Tennis elbow)
         (a) Pain and tenderness at the site of origin of the extensor carpi radialis brevis muscle, lateral epicondyle of the humerus.
         (b) Typical patient is between ages 35–50.
      2. Medial (Golfer's elbow)
         (a) Pain and tenderness at the site of origin of the flexor and pronator muscles, just distal to the medial epicondyle.
   ii. Clinical manifestations
      1. Lateral
         (a) Note gradual onset of pain in lateral elbow and forearm during activities involving wrist extension (turning a screwdriver or backhand in tennis).
         (b) On exam tenderness is noted 1 cm distal to the lateral epicondyle.
         (c) Pain produced with resisted extension of the wrist with the elbow in extension.

   (d) No numbness or tingling is noted.
   (e) Patients note pain with lifting with the palm down.
      2. Medial
         (a) Pain noted with active wrist flexion and forearm pronation (taking a golf swing, baseball pitching, or swimming).
         (b) Area of tenderness is distal to the medial epicondyle.
         (c) Pain produced by pronating forearm and flexing the wrist against resistance.
         (d) Patients note pain when lifting with the palm up.
   iii. Diagnosis
      1. Based on clinical findings.
   iv. Treatment
      1. Modification or elimination of the activity causing symptoms.
      2. NSAIDs and physical therapy may be helpful.
      3. Tennis elbow wrap worn two finger widths below the lateral epicondyle may be helpful.

DISORDERS OF BACK/SPINE

I. Ankylosing spondylitis (Fig. 4-2)
   a. General
      i. A systemic, seronegative spondyloarthropathy.
      ii. Affects the sacroiliac (SI) joint, spine, and hips.
         1. SI joint involvement is necessary to make diagnosis.
      iii. More common in males and there is a direct relationship with presence of HLA-B27.
   b. Clinical manifestations
      i. Early symptoms include morning stiffness and general back pain.
         1. Pain is improved with bending forward.
      ii. As disease progresses spinal range of motion (ROM) is lost.
      iii. Spinal fragility increases and minor trauma may lead to significant neurologic deficit.

NOTES

iv. Physical examination will reveal a decreased chest expansion.

c. Diagnosis
  i. Spine X-ray reveals a bamboo spine.
  ii. Laboratory tests reveal anemia, elevated erythrocyte sedimentation rate (ESR), and elevated creatine phosphokinase (CPK).

d. Treatment
  i. Anti-inflammatory medications for pain relief and physical therapy to maintain mobility of the spine.

II. Back strain/sprain
  a. General
    i. Due to injury to the paravertebral spinal muscles, ligamentous injuries of the facet joints, or anulus fibrosis.
      1. Sprain refers to damage to a ligament.
      2. Strain refers to damage to a muscle.
    ii. Precipitated by repeated lifting and twisting.
    iii. Risk factors include poor fitness, smoking, and hypochondriasis.
  b. Clinical manifestations
    i. Symptoms are typically of limited duration.

QUESTION

A 43-year-old female who works as a tailor presents with a 3-month history of pain, weakness, and numbness of the right hand. Exam reveals hypoesthesia and atrophy of the thenar eminence. Which of the following nerves is most likely compression?

  A. Axillary
  B. Median
  C. Radial
  D. Ulnar

    ii. Pain radiates into the buttocks and posterior thigh.
    iii. Patient may have trouble standing erect.
    iv. Physical examination reveals diffuse tenderness in the lower back or SI region.
    v. ROM is decreased, especially flexion.
    vi. Sensory exam and deep tendon reflexes are normal.

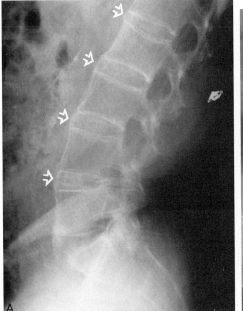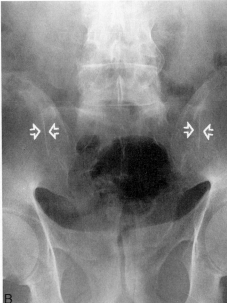

Figure 4-2 Ankylosing spondylitis. (From Mettler FA: Essentials of Radiology, 2nd ed. Philadelphia, Elsevier Saunders, 2005, p. 282, Fig. 8-39A.)

NOTES

ANSWER **B** EXPLANATION: *Carpal tunnel is due to entrapment of the median nerve. Symptoms include pain and numbness in the distribution of the median nerve. Phalen test and Tinel sign are positive.*

correct ☐   incorrect ☐

c. Diagnosis
   i. X-rays only needed if atypical symptoms present.
      1. Includes pain at rest, pain at night, or significant trauma.
d. Treatment
   i. Short period of bed rest (1–2 days).
   ii. Cold therapy is started first followed by heat therapy after 48–72 hours.
   iii. Pain medications with NSAIDs or other non-narcotics.
   iv. Muscle relaxants may be helpful first 3–5 days.
   v. After pain has resolved, strengthening and conditioning should be started.

III. Cauda equina syndrome
   a. General
      i. Distal end of the spinal cord, conus medullaris, ends at the L1-L2 level.
         1. L2-L5 area is filled with nerve roots, the cauda equina.
      ii. Cauda equina syndrome is due to reduction in volume of lumbar spinal canal, causing compression and paralysis.
      iii. Etiologies include central disk herniation, epidural abscess, hematoma, or fracture.
   b. Clinical manifestations
      i. Radicular pain and numbness involving both legs.
      ii. Leg weakness is present.
      iii. Difficulty with urinary and anal sphincter control.
      iv. Physical examination may reveal difficulty walking, inability to walk on toes or heels, and loss of sensory function (perianal numbness).
   c. Diagnosis
      i. Myelogram or MRI is diagnostic.

d. Treatment
   i. Requires emergency surgery for nerve decompression.

IV. Herniated disk pulposus
   a. General
      i. Due to herniation of the nucleus pulposus into the lumbar spinal canal.
      ii. Most commonly occurs at L4-L5 or L5-S1 levels with irritation of the L5 or S1 nerve root.
   b. Clinical manifestations
      i. Abrupt onset of symptoms.
         1. Pain is severe and exaggerated by sitting, walking, standing, or coughing.
         2. Pain radiates from the buttock down the posterior or posterolateral leg to the ankle or foot.
      ii. Low back pain is accompanied by unilateral radicular leg pain.
      iii. Physical examination reveals a positive straight leg raise, tenderness in the sciatic notch, and limited ROM.
      iv. Neurologic symptoms vary with location of nerve impingement.
         1. See Table 4-1 for summary of neurologic findings.
   c. Diagnosis
      i. MRI is very useful in diagnosing herniation.
   d. Treatment
      i. NSAIDs are used in the acute phase with 1–3 days of bed rest.
         1. Muscle relaxants and/or narcotics may be helpful.
      ii. Oral steroids or epidural injection may reduce pain.
      iii. Muscle strengthening exercises are begun after acute attack is over.
      iv. Surgery may be needed if no improvement.
         1. Consider laminectomy, microscopic disk excision, or percutaneous disk excision.

V. Kyphosis/Scoliosis
   a. Kyphosis
      i. General
         1. Also called "round back."
         2. Two major types of kyphosis.
            (a) Congenital

NOTES

(i) Due to failure of formation or a failure of segmentation of the spine.
(ii) Can lead to paralysis.
(b) Scheuermann's
(i) Idiopathic nonflexible kyphosis.
(ii) Have end-plate abnormalities and wedging of three or more vertebral bodies noted on lateral spine X-ray.
ii. Clinical manifestations
1. Kyphosis greater than 40 degrees is abnormal.
iii. Diagnosis
1. Based on physical exam and X-ray findings.
iv. Treatment
1. Bracing is indicated if kyphosis measures more than 45 degrees.
b. Scoliosis
i. General
1. Lateral curvature of the spine.
2. May be structural or functional in nature.
(a) Structural
(i) Have vertebral body rotation.
(ii) Caused by congenital malformation, degenerative or metabolic conditions, or idiopathic.
(b) Functional

(i) Lateral curvature with no structural change or vertebral rotation.
(ii) Secondary to inequality in leg length, local inflammation, or nerve root irritation.
ii. Clinical manifestations
1. Typically diagnosed during adolescence.
2. Shoulder, pelvis, and waist asymmetry are noted on exam.
3. Scapular prominence may also be noted.
iii. Diagnosis
1. Confirmed by standing AP spinal X-ray.
2. Degree of curvature measured by the Cobb method.
iv. Treatment
1. Treatment varies with degree of curvature.
(a) Observation for curvature less than 20 degrees.
(b) Surgical intervention for curvature greater than 40 degrees.
(c) Bracing is used for curvatures between 20 and 40 degrees.
VI. Low back pain
a. Etiologies
i. Originating from the spine
1. Mechanical
(a) Make up over 95% of cases.
(b) Causes include:
(i) Lumbar spondylosis

Table 4-1 • Examination Findings of Cervical and Lumbar Radiculopathies			
Nerve Root	**Motor Weakness**	**Decreased Reflex**	**Decreased Sensation**
C5	Deltoid, biceps	Biceps	Deltoid region
C6	Biceps, wrist extensors	Biceps, brachioradialis	Dorsolateral aspect thumb and index finger
C7	Triceps, finger extensors	Triceps	Index, long fingers, dorsum of hand
L4	Anterior tibialis	Patellar tendon	Shin
L5	Extensor hallucis longus	None	Top of foot, first web space
S1	Gastrocsoleus	Achilles tendon	Lateral foot

NOTES

                    (ii) Disk herniation
                    (iii) Spondylolisthesis
                    (iv) Spinal stenosis
                    (v)   Fractures
                    (vi) Idiopathic
        2. Neoplastic
            (a) Unusual cause of low back pain.
            (b) Metastatic cancer from prostate, lung,
                breast, and thyroid are common.
        3. Infectious
            (a) Includes vertebral osteomyelitis,
                epidural abscess, and septic diskitis.
        4. Inflammatory
            (a) Include the spondyloarthropathies.
        5. Metabolic
            (a) Includes compression fracture from
                osteoporosis.
    ii. Originating from viscera
        1. Includes abdominal aortic aneurysm,
           pyelonephritis, kidney stones, chronic
           prostatitis, endometriosis, ovarian cysts,
           and inflammatory bowel disease.
VII. Spinal stenosis
    a. General
        i. Narrowing of the lumbar spinal canal with
           compression of the nerve roots.
        ii. Etiologies

        1. Congenital
        2. Acquired
            (a) Due to degenerative changes and
                more common in patients over age 60.
            (b) Obesity may be a predisposing factor.
        3. Iatrogenic
        4. Other
            (a) Paget's disease
                (i)   Disorder of bone metabolism.
                (ii) More common in people over
                      age 55.
                (iii) Most frequently involves the
                      pelvis, lumbar spine, and
                      femur.
                (iv) Present with bone pain,
                      fractures, deafness, and
                      enlargement of bone.
                (v)   Laboratory testing reveals an
                      elevated alkaline phosphatase.
                (vi) Treatment consists of calcitonins
                      and bisphosphonates.
            (b) Acromegaly
    b. Clinical manifestations
        i. Symptoms may develop following minor
           trauma or be indolent.
        ii. Present with low back pain and stiffness.

Table 4-2 • Comparison of Neurogenic and Vascular Claudication

Feature	Neurogenic	Vascular
Claudication distance	Varies	Fixed
Relief of pain	Sitting	Standing
Walking up hill	No discomfort	Discomfort
Type of pain	Numbness, ache	Tightness
Pulses	Present	Absent
Skin	Normal	Loss of hair
Weakness	Occasional	Rare
Back pain	Common	Uncommon

NOTES

iii. Neurogenic claudication causing radicular complaints in one or both lower extremities.
    1. Symptoms progress from proximal to distal direction.
iv. Note fatigue or weakness of the legs with walking or prolonged standing.
v. May note short-term relief of discomfort with leaning forward.
vi. See Table 4-2 for comparison of neurologic and vascular claudication.
vii. Physical examination reveals muscle weakness in the legs, impaired proprioception, decreased reflexes, and possible decrease in urinary and anal sphincter tone.

c. Diagnosis
    i. Computed tomography (CT) scan, MRI, or myelogram is used to evaluate for stenosis.
d. Treatment
    i. NSAIDs, physical therapy, and activity modification are initial treatment.
    ii. Surgery may be required.

DISORDERS OF THE HIP

I. Aseptic necrosis (Osteonecrosis)
a. General
    i. Result of bone tissue death in the femoral head.
    ii. Etiologies include trauma to vascular supply or decrease in circulation.
        1. Risk factors include hip trauma, steroid use, alcoholism, sickle cell disease, rheumatoid arthritis (RA), and systemic lupus erythematosus (SLE).
    iii. Increased incidence in patients age 30–50.
b. Clinical manifestations
    i. Present with acute onset of dull or throbbing pain in groin, buttock, or lateral hip and a limp.
    ii. On physical examination pain with internal or external rotation of the hip and decreased range of motion.
c. Diagnosis
    i. X-ray (AP and frog leg views) of the hip reveals a flattened femoral head with joint space narrowing.

QUESTION

A patient with low back pain presents with weakness of the foot dorsiflexors and great toe extensors. No change in knee or ankle jerk is noted. At what level is the possible nerve root compression?

   A. L3-L4
   B. L4-L5
   C. L5-S1
   D. S1-S2

ii. MRI and bone scan may reveal early changes.
d. Treatment
    i. Protective weight bearing should be started until definitive treatment is established.
    ii. Referral for surgery is indicated in most cases.
        1. If collapse has occurred then hip arthroplasty is indicated.

II. Dislocations
a. General
    i. Occur when femoral head is displaced from the acetabulum.
    ii. Typically occur due to high-energy trauma, such as a motor vehicle accident.
    iii. Two types.
        1. Posterior
        2. Anterior
b. Clinical manifestations
    i. Posterior
        1. Hip is short and fixed in flexion, adduction, and internal rotation position.
        2. Sciatic nerve injuries are common.
    ii. Anterior
        1. Hip is in mild flexion, abduction, and external rotation position.
        2. Femoral artery and obturator nerve injury may be present.
c. Diagnosis
    i. X-ray of a posterior dislocation reveals the affected femoral head appearing smaller than the opposite side.
    ii. X-ray of an anterior dislocation reveals the affected femoral head appearing larger than the opposite side.

d. Treatment
  i. Avascular necrosis can occur due to vascular compromise.
    1. More common in posterior dislocations.
  ii. Reduction should occur as soon as possible, after a fracture has been ruled out.
  iii. After reduction, crutch-assisted ambulation with limited weight bearing until pain-free.

III. Slipped capital femoral epiphysis
  a. General
    i. Separation of the proximal femoral epiphysis through the growth plate.
    ii. Femoral head is typically displaced medially and posteriorly relative to the femoral neck.
    iii. More common in blacks than whites.
  b. Clinical manifestations
    i. Noted most commonly in obese adolescent males.
    ii. Cause is unknown.
      1. Trauma is not a cause.
    iii. Patients note pain referred to the thigh and medial side of the knee, and a limp.
      1. Any child with knee pain should have hip pathology ruled out.
    iv. On physical examination internal rotation of the hip is limited, hip flexion contracture, and local tenderness around the hip.
  c. Diagnosis
    i. Based on clinical findings and X-ray.
      1. X-ray views include AP and Lauenstein (frog) lateral views that show epiphyseal displacement.
  d. Treatment
    i. Surgical repair with pinning.
    ii. Long-term complications include avascular necrosis.

DISORDERS OF THE KNEE

I. Bursitis
  a. General
    i. Bursae lie between the skin and bony prominences or between tendons, ligaments, and bone.
    ii. Chronic pressure of friction leads to thickening of the lining, excess fluid formation, swelling, and pain.
    iii. Prepatellar bursitis.
      1. Lies between the skin and bony patella.
      2. Most common bursitis of the knee.
      3. Develops secondary to chronic kneeling (Housemaid's knee).
  b. Clinical manifestations
    i. Prepatellar bursitis presents with dome-shaped swelling over the anterior aspect of the knee.
      1. Early in disease course note pain with activity or direct pressure.
      2. Movement of the knee does not increase pain.
  c. Diagnosis
    i. Aspiration of the bursa will assist in separating inflammatory, hemorrhagic, or septic bursitis.
      1. Inflammatory bursitis presents with slightly yellow fluid.
      2. Hemorrhagic bursitis presents with bloody fluid.
      3. Septic bursitis presents with cloudy fluid.
  d. Treatment
    i. Nonoperative treatment includes NSAIDs, ice, and activity modifications.
    ii. Aspiration may be therapeutic.
    iii. Steroid injection may be needed.

II. Dislocations
  a. General
    i. Severe injury resulting from violent trauma.
    ii. Typically have three to four major ligaments injured with dislocation.
      1. Vascular and nerve injuries are common.
    iii. Classification based on direction of dislocation: anterior, posterior, lateral, medial, and rotatory.

NOTES

1. Anterior dislocation is due to hyperextension of the knee.
2. Posterior dislocation is due to a direct blow to the anterior tibia with the knee flexed 90 degrees.
    iv. Patella dislocation is due to a twisting injury on an extended knee.
      1. More common in females.
  b. Clinical manifestations
    i. Obvious deformity may be noted.
      1. Dimple sign on the anteromedial surface is noted in posterolateral dislocation.
    ii. Neurovascular complications are common and status must be evaluated in all patients.
      1. Complications involve popliteal artery and peroneal nerve.
    iii. Patella dislocation presents with the patella displaced laterally over the lateral condyle.
  c. Diagnosis
    i. X-rays are required to determine the direction of the dislocation and presence of any fracture.
  d. Treatment
    i. Reduction should be undertaken immediately.
      1. After reduction the knee should be immobilized.
    ii. If reduction is not possible or vascular injury is present, immediate surgical intervention is required.
    iii. Flexing the hip, hyperextending the knee, and sliding the patella back into place reduce patella dislocation.
      1. Have immediate relief of pain.
III. Meniscal injuries
  a. General
    i. Menisci are fibrocartilage pads that function as shock absorbers between the femur and tibia.
    ii. Mechanism of injury is a significant twisting knee injury.
  b. Clinical manifestations
    i. After acute injury patient can typically ambulate and knee swelling and stiffness develop over the next 2–3 days.
    ii. Patients note pain on the medial or lateral side of the knee.

QUESTION

Which of the following is the most common complication of a displaced femoral neck fracture?

  A. Osteomyelitis
  B. Avascular necrosis
  C. Pulmonary emboli
  D. Nonunion

---

      1. Locking or catching of the knee joint may occur.
      2. Climbing stairs brings about more pain than descending stairs.
    iii. On physical examination note tenderness over the medial or lateral joint line.
      1. Large effusion or hemarthrosis may be present.
      2. Range of motion is limited due to presence of effusion.
    iv. McMurray test and Apley's compression tests are positive.
  c. Diagnosis
    i. MRI is very sensitive for evaluation of meniscal injury.
  d. Treatment
    i. Initial treatment is rest, ice, compression, and elevation (RICE).
    ii. Surgical débridement or repair is indicated.
IV. Osgood-Schlatter disease
  a. General
    i. Microfracture at location of patellar tendon insertion into the tibia tubercle.
    ii. More common in boys age 12–15 and girls 11–13 years of age.
  b. Clinical manifestations
    i. Pain may curtail normal activities.
    ii. Physical examination reveals swelling, tenderness, and increased prominence of the tibia tubercle.
  c. Diagnosis
    i. Based on history and physical examination.
    ii. X-rays are often needed to rule out other possible disorders.

NOTES

ANSWER B EXPLANATION: *Avascular necrosis is most commonly cause by trauma, including hip fracture. Other etiologies include chronic steroid use, alcohol, and hemoglobinopathies, such as sickle cell.*

correct ☐   incorrect ☐

      1. May note irregularities of the tubercle contour.
  d. Treatment
    i. Rest, restriction of activities, and at times immobilization are needed.
      1. Complete healing occurs in 12–24 months.
    ii. Casting may be required in severe cases.
    iii. Anti-inflammatory medications are typically not helpful.
V. Sprains/Strains
  a. Medial collateral ligament injury
    i. General
      1. Mechanism of injury is direct blow to the lateral portion of the knee.
    ii. Clinical manifestations
      1. Patients typically report hearing or feeling a pop over the medial knee.
      2. Medial knee pain and swelling is noted.
      3. On physical examination the ligament is tender to palpation.
      4. Degree of injury is evaluated by applying valgus stress to the knee when fully extended and in 20–30 degrees of flexion.
    iii. Diagnosis
      1. Based on history and physical examination.
    iv. Treatment
      1. Conservative therapy with RICE.
      2. Bracing may be helpful.
  b. Lateral collateral ligament injury
    i. General
      1. Mechanism of injury is a direct blow to the medial knee or anteromedial tibia with the knee flexed and foot planted.
    ii. Clinical manifestations
      1. Pain, stiffness, and localized swelling are noted.

      2. Varus stressing of the knee reveals increased laxity.
      3. If peroneal nerve damage is present weakness of foot dorsiflexion and eversion is noted.
    iii. Diagnosis
      1. Based on history and physical exam.
    iv. Treatment
      1. Surgical repair is indicated.
  c. Anterior cruciate ligament injury
    i. General
      1. Mechanism of injury is direct blow or indirect stress.
        a. Requires a sudden change in direction of the weight-bearing knee.
    ii. Clinical manifestations
      1. Note immediate swelling and pain after injury.
      2. Knee is very unstable and weight bearing is difficult.
      3. On physical examination pain and tenderness is noted in the posterolateral area of the knee or near the tibial plateau.
      4. A positive anterior drawer or Lachman test is noted.
    iii. Diagnosis
      1. Based on history and physical exam.
    iv. Treatment
      1. Referral is needed for possible surgery.
  d. Posterior cruciate ligament injury
    i. General
      1. Mechanism of injury is hyperextending the knee or a direct blow to the anterior proximal tibia with the knee flexed and foot planted.
    ii. Clinical manifestations
      1. Patient may note a dull aching pain and stiffness.
        (a) Swelling is not typical.
      2. Physical exam may reveal only a mild effusion and posterior drawer test is positive.
    iii. Diagnosis
      1. Based on history and physical exam findings.

NOTES

2. MRI may be used to evaluate for possible ligament damage.
  iv. Treatment
    1. Conservative treatment and physical therapy (PT) may be successful.
    2. Surgical intervention is the treatment of choice.

DISORDERS OF THE ANKLE/FOOT

I. Dislocations
  a. General
    i. Can occur in one of four planes and are commonly associated with a fracture.
    ii. Posterior dislocation occurs when a backward force is applied when the foot is plantar flexed.
    iii. Anterior dislocation occurs when force applied to anterior aspect of the tibia with the foot dorsiflexed.
  b. Clinical manifestations
    i. Pain, swelling, and deformity are noted at site of injury.
    ii. Patient is unable to bear weight and range of motion is decreased.
    iii. Neurovascular compromise can occur.
      1. Peroneal nerve is at risk.
  c. Diagnosis
    i. X-ray reveals widening of joint spaces.
  d. Treatment
    i. All dislocations of the ankle should be referred.
    ii. Closed reduction should be performed immediately to limit risk of ischemia.
      1. Open reduction and external fixation (ORIF) and posterior splint are typically required.
II. Sprains/Strains
  a. General
    i. Injury to the lateral ligaments is most common.
      1. Injury to the syndesmosis (anterior tibiofibular ligament) is less common and called a high ankle sprain.
    ii. Mechanism of injury is increased rotational stress.

QUESTION

A 10-year-old obese male presents with right knee and anteromedial thigh pain. The patient states the pain improves with rest. On examination, the physician assistant notes a slight limp. X-rays of both knees are normal. What is the most likely diagnosis?

  A. Osteomyelitis
  B. Osgood-Schlatter disease
  C. Slipped capital femoral epiphysis
  D. Acute suppurative arthritis

---

    1. Inversion injury is most common for lateral ankle sprain.
    2. Eversion injury leads to medial ankle sprain.
    3. Forceful external rotations lead to syndesmosis injury.
   iii. Grading of injury
    1. Grade I
      (a) Ligaments stretched, but no tear.
      (b) Ankle painful, but stable and has normal function.
    2. Grade II
      (a) Some ligament tearing with moderate swelling and pain.
      (b) Some function limitations.
    3. Grade III
      (a) Complete tear of the ligament with marked swelling, bruising, and joint instability.
  b. Clinical manifestations.
    i. Pain, swelling, and loss of function are common.
    ii. On physical examination note ecchymosis and swelling around the entire ankle.
    iii. Injury to the syndesmosis is noted by a positive squeeze test and external rotation test.
    iv. Lateral ankle sprain will have a positive anterior drawer test and talar tilt test.
      1. Anterior drawer evaluates the anterior talofibular ligament.
      2. Talar tile test evaluates the calcaneofibular ligament.

NOTES

ANSWER C EXPLANATION: *Slipped capital femoral epiphysis is most commonly noted in obese adolescent males who present with a limp and hip pain that is referred to the thigh and medial side of the knee. X-ray of the hip reveals epiphyseal displacement and normal knee x-ray.*

correct ☐   incorrect ☐

c. Diagnosis
   i. AP, lateral, and mortise views required to rule out fracture.
d. Treatment
   i. Initial treatment is NSAIDs and RICE.
   ii. Brace and air brace provide support and promote soft-tissue healing.

FRACTURES

I. General
   a. Definition
      i. Fracture is a break in the continuity of bone or cartilage.
      ii. Pathologic fractures occur through abnormal bone.
      iii. Greenstick fractures are incomplete angulated fractures of long bones in children.
   b. Descriptors
      i. Closed fracture: skin and soft tissue overlying the fracture are intact.
      ii. Open fracture: fracture exposed to the outside environment.
      iii. Types of fractures
         1. Transverse
            (a) Fracture occurs at a right angle to the long axis of the bone.
         2. Oblique
            (a) Fracture runs oblique to the long axis of the bone.
         3. Spiral
            (a) Fracture encircles the shaft of the bone in a spiral fashion.
         4. Comminuted
            (a) Fracture where there are more than two fragments present.

c. Epiphyseal fractures
   i. Salter-Harris classification
      1. Type I
         (a) Fracture extends through the epiphyseal plate, resulting in displacement.
      2. Type II
         (a) As above, plus a triangular segment of metaphysis is fractured.
      3. Type III
         (a) Fracture runs from the joint surface through epiphyseal plate and epiphysis.
      4. Type IV
         (a) Fracture as in type III but also through the adjacent metaphysis.
      5. Type V
         (a) Crush injury of the epiphysis.
      6. See Figure 4-3 for Salter-Harris classification.
d. Accompanying nerve injuries
   i. Certain nerve injuries may accompany certain fractures.
   ii. See Table 4-3 for summary of nerve injuries.
II. Types
   a. Ankle/Foot
      i. Ankle fractures involve the lateral, medial, or posterior malleolus.
         1. Mechanism of injury is result of eversion or lateral rotation on the talus.
      ii. Foot fractures involve the talus, calcaneus, metatarsal, and phalanges.
         1. Talus fracture due to a twisting injury, fall, or high-energy impact.
         2. Calcaneus fracture due to high-energy direct axial compression.
         3. Metatarsal fracture due to direct trauma or twisting force applied to a fixed forefoot.
         4. Phalangeal fracture due to direct trauma, such as dropping a heavy object or stubbing toes.
      iii. Deformity depends on extent of bone displacement.
      iv. Diagnosis made by X-ray.
         1. Standard AP and lateral views plus AP view 15 degrees internally rotated needed to diagnosis ankle fracture.
         2. Foot fractures diagnosed by standard foot and ankle X-rays.

NOTES

3. Ottawa Ankle Rules are used to determine if X-ray needed for ankle or foot injuries.
    (a) See Table 4-4 for summary of Ottawa Ankle Rules.
  v. Treatment
    1. Elevation and ice to control swelling.
    2. Casting with short leg cast.
    3. Referral is indicated with severe displacement.
b. Forearm/Wrist/Hand
  i. Boxer's
    1. Mechanism of injury is direct blow of a closed fist against another object.

QUESTION

A football player is tackled and hyperextends his right knee. He states he heard a pop when he was hit. On examination, the knee is swollen and a positive Drawer test is noted. Which of the following is the most likely site of injury?

A. Medial collateral ligament
B. Posterior cruciate ligament
C. Patellar dislocation
D. Medial meniscus

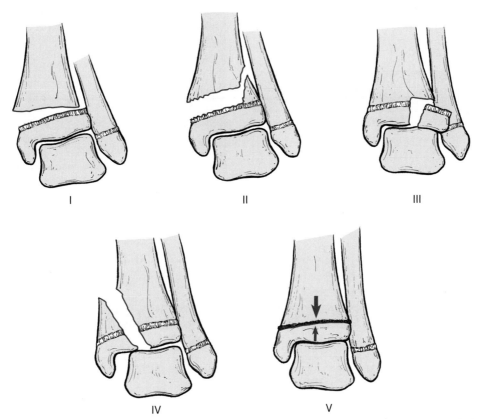

Figure 4-3 Salter-Harris classification of physeal injury. (From Green NE: Skeletal Trauma in Children, 3rd ed. Philadelphia, Elsevier Saunders 2003, p. 21, Fig. 2-3.)

ANSWER **B** EXPLANATION: *The mechanism of injury and positive drawer test indicate an injury to the posterior cruciate ligament.*

correct ☐   incorrect ☐

2. Fracture occurs at the distal end of the fifth metacarpal.
   (a) See Figure 4-4 for Boxer's fracture X-ray.
3. Angulation of fracture greater than 30 degrees should be treated to limit deformity.
4. Treatment is splinting the joint in flexion or percutaneous pinning.

ii. Colles'
1. Mechanism of injury is due to fall on an outstretched hand.

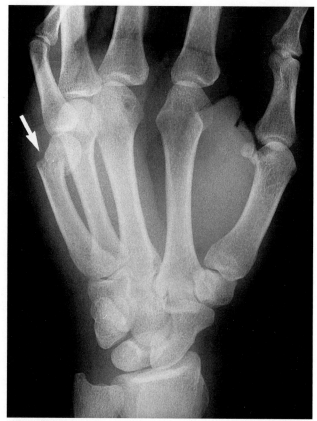

Figure 4-4   Boxer's fracture. (From Mettler FA: Essentials of Radiology, 2nd ed. Philadelphia, Elsevier Saunders, 2005, p. 307, Fig. 8-78.)

Table 4-3 • Nerve Injuries Associated with Fractures

Fracture	Nerve Injury
Humeral shaft	Radial
Sacral	Cauda equina
Acetabulum	Sciatic
Femoral shaft	Peroneal
Lateral tibial plateau	Peroneal

Table 4-4 • Ottawa Ankle Rules

Ankle X-ray	Foot X-ray
Required if pain in malleolar zone and:	Required if pain in midfoot zone and:
1. Bone tenderness at posterior edge or tip of lateral malleolus **or**	1. Bone tenderness base of fifth metatarsal **or**
2. Bone tenderness at posterior edge or tip of medial malleolus **or**	2. Bone tenderness at navicular **or**
3. Inability to bear weight at time of injury and in ER	3. Inability to bear weight at time of injury and in ER

NOTES

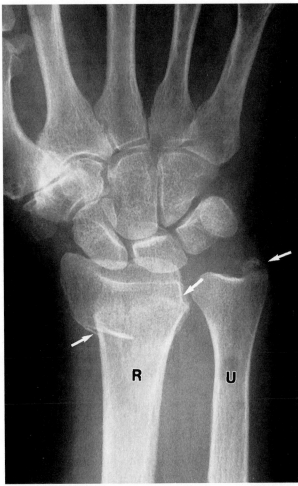

Figure 4-5 Colles' fracture. (From Mettler FA: Essentials of Radiology, 2nd ed. Philadelphia, Elsevier Saunders, 2005, p. 300, Fig. 8-68A.)

QUESTION

A 35-year-old presents to the ER after severe eversion of the right ankle. Pain is noted in the malleolar region and the patient is not able to bear weight. Which of the following is the next best step in the care of this patient?

    A. Elevate and apply heat to the ankle
    B. NDAIDS and start weight bearing
    C. MRI of the ankle
    D. X-ray the ankle

2. Transverse fracture of the distal radial metaphysis with dorsal displacement of the distal fragment.
    (a) Fracture is located within 2 cm of the articular surface.
    (b) See Figure 4-5 for Colles' fracture X-ray.
3. Physical examination reveals a "dinner fork" deformity of the wrist.
    (a) Due to dorsal displacement and angulation of the fracture.

4. Posterior-anterior (PA) and lateral X-ray of the wrist reveals a fracture through the radial metaphysis.
5. Treatment is fracture reduction and sugar tong splinting with the wrist in flexion.
iii. Humeral
    1. Humeral shaft fractures
      (a) Mechanism of injury is due to direct trauma or severe twisting of the arm.
      (b) On physical exam localized pain is noted with swelling.
        (i) The arm may be shortened or rotated.
      (c) Complications include radial nerve injury.
    2. Supracondylar fractures
      (a) Fracture of the distal humerus proximal to the epicondyles.
      (b) Typically an injury of the immature skeleton and due to a fall on the outstretched arm when the elbow is fully extended or hyperextended.
      (c) Present holding the upper extremity in extension to the side with swelling in the area of the elbow.
    3. Epicondyle fracture
      (a) Typically involves the medial epicondyle.
      (b) Mechanism of injury is due to repetitive valgus stress.
    4. Treatment consists of simple immobilization with a splint, cast, sugar tong, or sling and swathe.

NOTES

ANSWER D EXPLANATION: *Ankle injuries with bone tenderness at the posterior edge or tip of the medial or lateral malleolus or the inability to bear weight on the ankle are indications for routine bone x-rays to rule out fracture.*

correct ☐   incorrect ☐

    (a) If significant displacement is noted, a hanging cast may be required.
  iv. Radial
    1. Due to a fall on an outstretched hand.
    2. On physical examination note localized tenderness over the radial head or pain with passive rotation of the forearm.
    3. X-ray may be difficult to interpret.
      (a) Tenderness and a positive fat pad sign may be the only finding.
      (b) See Figure 4-6 for radial fracture X-ray.
    4. Treatment consists of sling support.
  v. Scaphoid
    1. Most common carpal bone fracture and most typically seen in young adults.
    2. Mechanism of injury is fall on an outstretched hand.

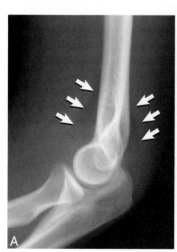 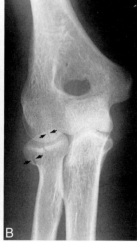

Figure 4-6 Positive fat pad in radial fracture. (From Mettler FA: Essentials of Radiology, 2nd ed. Philadelphia, Elsevier Saunders, 2005, p. 294, Fig. 8-58.)

    3. Patient is tender in the anatomic snuffbox or with resisted supination, and has limited range of motion of the wrist and thumb.
    4. X-ray is often negative.
      (a) May require special scaphoid views or repeat X-ray in 10–14 days after treatment.
    5. Treatment is thumb spica and referral.
      (a) Improper treatment may lead to avascular necrosis.
 c. Hip
  i. General
    1. Incidence of hip fracture doubles each decade of life after age 50.
    2. Women affected more often than men.
    3. Mortality rate is high.
      (a) Deep vein thrombosis (DVT) and pulmonary embolism (PE) are serious complications.
  ii. Clinical manifestations
    1. Pain is the major feature along with inability to bear weight.
    2. On physical exam the affected leg is shortened and externally rotated.
  iii. Diagnosis
    1. X-ray reveals fracture.
  iv. Treatment
    1. Surgical repair, hip arthroplasty, is indicated.
 d. Knee
  i. General
    1. Result of significant trauma.
      (a) Patellar fracture due to direct blow.
      (b) Tibial plateau fracture due to impact, direct axial load, or shearing force.
  ii. Clinical manifestations
    1. Present with knee pain and difficulty walking.
    2. Physical examination reveals swelling and bruising.
    3. Point tenderness over site of injury.
  iii. Diagnosis
    1. Present with large hemarthrosis with fat globules.
    2. X-ray reveals fracture.
  iv. Treatment
    1. Analgesics are required.
    2. The extremity should be immobilized and made nonweight-bearing.

NOTES

e. Shoulder
  i. Clavicle
    1. Very common fracture during childhood.
    2. Mechanism of injury is typically direct force to lateral aspect of shoulder from a fall or sporting injury.
    3. Present with pain over the fracture site and the affected extremity is held close to the body.
    4. Shoulder is typically slumped downward, forward, and inward.
    5. Typically heal without difficulty.
      (a) If displaced may cause pressure on subclavian vessels or brachial plexus.
    6. Treatment is immobilization with a figure eight dressing.
    7. Healing should be adequate in 6 weeks.

QUESTION

In which of the following fractures is a positive fat pad sign noted on x-ray?

  A. Fifth metacarpal
  B. Hamate
  C. Epicondyle
  D. Radial

  ii. Scapula
    1. Uncommon fracture noted primarily in men 30–40 years of age.
    2. Mechanism of injury is typically violent direct trauma.

Table 4-5 • Common Fractures

Fracture	Description	Mechanism
Barton's	intra-articular fracture dislocation of the wrist.	High-velocity impact across radiocarpal joint with wrist in flexion or dorsiflexion.
Bennett's	Oblique fracture through base of first metacarpal.	Produced by direct force.
Boxer's	Fracture neck of fourth and fifth metacarpal.	Produced by striking clenched fist against an object.
Galeazzi's	Fracture of shaft of radius with dislocation of distal radioulnar joint.	Due to fall on outstretched hand with wrist in extension and forearm forcibly pronated.
Hangman's	Fracture and dislocation of atlas and axis.	Due to extreme hyperextension during abrupt deceleration.
March	Stress fracture of the metatarsal.	Due to repetitive trauma.
Monteggia's	Fracture of the junction of the proximal and middle third of the ulna with anterior dislocation of the radial head.	Due to fall on outstretched hand with forced pronation of forearm.
Nightstick	Fracture of ulna, radius, or both.	Due to direct trauma.
Smith's	Extra-articular fracture of distal radius with volar displacement of distal fragment.	Due to fall with force to back of hand.

NOTES

ANSWER D EXPLANATION: *A positive fat pad is noted in fractures of the radius. A fat pad sign may also be noted with fractures of the scaphoid.*

correct ☐   incorrect ☐

3. Typically no displacement.
   (a) May have associated injury to the ribs, chest wall, or shoulder girdle.
4. On examination the shoulder is adducted and the arm held close to the body.
   (a) Increased pain with any movement.
5. Treatment is immobilization with a sling and swathe dressing.
   (a) If significant displacement the patient should be referred.

INFECTIOUS DISEASES

I. Osteomyelitis
   a. General
      i. Infection of the bone that may occur from a variety of methods.
         1. Contiguous spread
         2. Hematogenous spread
      ii. Organisms
         1. *Staphylococcus aureus*
         2. *Escherichia coli*
         3. *Pseudomonas aeruginosa*
         4. *Salmonella*
            (a) Common in children with sickle cell disease.
         5. Anaerobes
      iii. Acute versus chronic
         1. Acute disease evolves over days to weeks.
         2. Chronic disease evolves over weeks to months.
   b. Clinical manifestations
      i. Local pain and tenderness noted at site of infection.
         1. Most commonly affects long bones and vertebral bodies.
      ii. Signs of overlying infection may be present.
      iii. In chronic infection sinus tracts may be present.

iv. Fever may or may not be noted.
   1. Fever and chills more common in acute infection.
c. Diagnosis
   i. White blood cell (WBC) count is normal and may note anemia of chronic disease.
   ii. Diagnosis is made by X-ray.
      1. May be normal early, until substantial bone is lost.
      2. CT scan is more sensitive than plain X-rays.
   iii. Diagnosis and organism are confirmed by blood culture.
   iv. Bone scan can detect and localize early disease.
d. Treatment
   i. Treat with intravenous (IV) antibiotics or antifungals for 4–6 weeks.
      1. After IV treatment, oral antibiotics are used long term to decrease risk of flare up of disease.
      2. See Table 4-6 for summary of treatment options.
   ii. Antibiotics are selected based on organism.
   iii. Monitor response to therapy by following ESR values.

II. Septic arthritis
   a. General
      i. Arises due to hematogenous spread of bacteria to the synovial membrane lining a joint.
         1. Sources of infection include:
            (a) Urinary tract infection (UTI)
            (b) IV drug abuse
            (c) IV catheters
            (d) Soft-tissue infections
      ii. Common organisms include:
         1. *S. aureus*
         2. *Neisseria gonorrhea*
         3. Gram-negative bacilli
         4. Parvovirus B19
         5. Hepatitis B
         6. Mumps
   b. Clinical manifestations
      i. Typical presentation includes swelling and pain in a single joint accompanied by fever.
      ii. Joint is warm to touch and pain is noted with any movement.
      iii. Most commonly affected joints in adults include the knee, hip, shoulder, wrist, ankle, and elbow.

NOTES

1. In children the most commonly affected joint is the hip, followed by the knee.
c. Diagnosis
    i. Analysis of the synovial fluid is critical.
        1. WBC count is greater than 50,000/mm^3 with a predominance of neutrophils.
        2. Gram stain and blood cultures may be positive.
d. Treatment
    i. Joint drainage is very important.
    ii. Systemic antibiotics are required for 3–4 weeks.
        1. Selection is based on most likely organism.

NEOPLASTIC DISEASE

I. Bone cysts
a. General
    i. Common pseudotumor of the bone and most frequent cause of pathologic fractures in children.

ii. Typically age of onset is ages 5–15 years and more common in boys than girls.
iii. Most frequently noted in proximal humerus or upper femur.
b. Clinical manifestations
    i. Patients are typically asymptomatic, unless pathologic fracture present.
c. Diagnosis
    i. X-ray reveals a solitary cyst located in the metaphyseal area with thinning of the adjacent cortical bone.

Table 4-6 • Treatment of Osteomyelitis

Organism	First Choice	Second Choice
Staphylococcus aureus	Penicillin G	Second-generation cephalosporin Clindamycin Vancomycin
S. aureus, penicillin-resistant	Nafcillin	Second-generation cephalosporin Clindamycin Vancomycin
S. aureus, methicillin-resistant	Vancomycin	Teicoplanin
Streptococcus spp.	Penicillin G	Clindamycin Erythromycin Vancomycin
Escherichia coli	Quinolone	Third-generation cephalosporin
Pseudomonas aeruginosa	Piperacillin and gentamicin	Third-generation cephalosporin or quinolone
Anaerobes	Clindamycin	Ampicillin-sulbactam
Mixed	Ampicillin-sulbactam	Imipenem

NOTES

ANSWER C EXPLANATION: *While all the above organisms can be an etiology of osteomyelitis, salmonella is common in patients with sickle cell disease.*

correct ☐   incorrect ☐

d. Treatment
  i. Treatment depends on location of the cysts.
  ii. In weight-bearing bones treatment should be aggressive.
    1. Consists of aspiration and injection of bone marrow.
    2. Curettage and bone grafting may be needed.

II. Bone tumors
  a. General
    i. Benign disease is nonaggressive with very little tendency to metastasize.
    ii. Malignant disease is invasive, destructive, and tends to metastasize.
    iii. Benign tumors include:
      1. Osteoid-forming tumors
        (a) Osteoid osteoma
        (b) Osteoblastoma
      2. Chondroid-forming tumors
        (a) Enchondroma
        (b) Osteochondroma
        (c) Chondroblastoma
    iv. Malignant tumors include:
      1. Osteoid-forming tumors
        (a) Osteosarcoma (see below).
      2. Chondroid-forming sarcomas
        (a) Primary chondrosarcoma
        (b) Secondary chondrosarcoma
      3. Ewing's family of tumors
        (a) Ewing's sarcoma
    i. Found in patients between ages 5–25 years.
    ii. Pelvis is most common location, followed by femur, tibia, and humerus.
    iii. X-ray of the tumor reveals a typical onion-skin appearance.
    iv. Treatment involves radiation therapy.
    v. Metastasis of primary malignancy to bone is common.
      1. Common primary sources include prostate, breast, kidney, thyroid, and lung.
      2. See Table 4-7 for common sites of bone metastasis.

Table 4-7 • Common Sites of Bone Metastasis in Order of Frequency
Spine
Pelvis
Femur
Ribs
Proximal humerus
Skull

  b. Clinical manifestations
    i. Symptoms vary from being asymptomatic to dull, aching pain.
  c. Diagnosis
    i. Initial evaluation of bone tumors is plain X-rays.
  d. Treatment
    i. Varies from use of aspirin and NSAIDs to surgery.

III. Ganglion cysts
  a. General
    i. Encapsulated, mobile mass found near a joint or tendon sheath.
    ii. Risk factors include repetitive movements or arthritic conditions.
  b. Clinical manifestations
    i. Typically cause no clinical problem unless impinging nearby tissue.
    ii. Appear spontaneously and are more common on dorsum or palmar aspect of the wrist.
  c. Diagnosis
    i. Based on history and clinical findings.
  d. Treatment
    i. Cysts can be manually reduced or aspiration can be performed.
    ii. Surgical excision is also an option.
    iii. Ganglion can recur.

IV. Osteosarcoma
  a. Diagnosis
    i. One of the most common primary malignant tumors of bone.

NOTES

ii. Typically noted in ages 10–30 years and more common in males.

iii. Typically found in the metaphyseal areas of long bones.

b. Clinical manifestations

i. Present with pain.

c. Diagnosis

i. X-ray reveals lytic destruction.

d. Treatment

i. Consists of chemotherapy and surgical treatment.

1. Chemotherapeutic agents include methotrexate, doxorubicin, cisplatin, and ifosfamide.

2. Surgical treatment consists of limb-sparing surgery.

OSTEOARTHRITIS

I. General

a. Most common rheumatic disease.

b. Incidence increases with age, obesity, and joint wear and tear.

c. Classified as primary or secondary.

i. Primary

1. No underlying etiologic factor.

ii. Secondary

1. Have presence of underlying etiologic factor.

(a) Previous trauma

(b) Congenital hip dysplasia

(c) Avascular necrosis

(d) Metabolic disorders

II. Clinical manifestations

a. History of deep pain of gradual onset that worsens with activity and is relieved by rest.

b. Morning stiffness lasts less than 30 minutes.

c. On exam note pain with range of motion, tenderness, crepitus, and deformity of the following joints:

i. Hand deformities

1. Heberden's nodes

(a) Enlarged DIP joints

2. Bouchard's nodes

(a) Enlarged PIP joints

ii. Knee

1. Genu valgus or varus

QUESTION

A 24-year-old patient presents with a mass on his right wrist. The mass is about 2 cm in size and is a firm, non-tender, cystic lesion. Which of the following is the most likely diagnosis?

A. Ganglion cyst

B. Baker's cyst

C. Neuroma

D. Bursitis

iii. Hip

1. Loss of internal rotation and extension.

iv. Foot

1. Affects first metatarsophalangeal joint.

v. Spine

1. Commonly affects L3-4 intervertebral disk space.

III. Diagnosis

a. Laboratory results

i. ESR is normal.

ii. Synovial fluid examination reveals mild inflammation, good mucin clot formation, and no crystals.

iii. X-rays reveal joint space narrowing, osteophytes, and subchondral cysts.

IV. Treatment

a. Weight reduction, physical therapy, and support devices are used for joint preservation.

b. NSAIDs are very beneficial for pain and inflammation control.

c. Systemic steroids are typically not indicated.

i. Intra-articular steroid injections are used for acute flare-ups.

d. In severe disease joint replacement may be needed.

OSTEOPOROSIS

I. General

a. Characterized by decreased bone mass with normal bone structure.

b. Disease is predominately noted in white females.

c. Estrogen is protective.

NOTES

ANSWER A EXPLANATION: *Ganglion cysts are encapsulated, mobile cysts located near joints or tendon sheaths. Patients are typically asymptomatic.*

correct ☐   incorrect ☐

Table 4-8 • Bone Density Test Interpretation	
Classification	**Density Results**
Normal	Less than –1 SD below normal
Osteopenia	Greater than –1 SD but less than –2.5 SD below normal
Osteoporosis	Greater than – 2.5 SD below normal
Severe osteoporosis	Greater than – 2.5 SD below normal and presence of a fracture

   d. Etiologies
      i. Primary
         1. Postmenopausal
         2. Senile
         3. Idiopathic
      ii. Secondary
         1. Endocrine
            (a) Diabetes mellitus type I, Addison's disease, thyroid disease
         2. Neoplasia
            (a) Multiple myeloma
         3. Gastrointestinal
            (a) Malabsorption
         4. Rheumatologic
         5. Drugs
            (a) Steroids, anticonvulsants, anticoagulants, lithium
II. Clinical manifestations
   a. Vertebral compression and femur fractures are common.
   b. Low back pain may be only symptom.
III. Diagnosis
   a. X-rays reveal decreased bone density.
   b. X-ray of spine may reveal wedge-shaped deformities with compression fractures.
   c. Bone density testing reveals decreased bone density.
      i. See Table 4-8 for interpretation of bone-density testing.
IV. Treatment
   a. Estrogen replacement therapy can prevent or slow rate of osteoporosis.
      i. Contraindicated in women with high risk of endometrial or breast cancer.
   b. Calcium supplement is important to maintain bone mass and slow or prevent disease.
   c. Bisphosphonates, alendronate, and risedronate increase bone density and prevent bone loss.
   d. Calcitonin inhibits osteoclastic bone resorption.
   e. Weight-bearing and active lifestyle may help prevent osteoporosis.

RHEUMATOLOGIC CONDITIONS

I. Fibromyalgia
   a. General
      i. May coexist with SLE or rheumatoid arthritis.
      ii. Etiology of pain is unknown.
   b. Clinical manifestations
      i. Present with widespread pain for greater than 3 months.
         1. Light touch or breeze may be unpleasant.
      ii. Morning stiffness may be prominent.
      iii. Poor sleep is almost always present.
      iv. Pain is elicited by manual pressure at 11 or more defined tender points.
      v. Laboratory testing typically reveals no abnormal findings.
   c. Diagnosis
      i. Based on clinical history and tender point exam.
   d. Treatment
      i. Nonpharmacologic
         1. Exercise and cognitive-behavioral therapy.
      ii. Pharmacologic
         1. Treatment of chronic pain includes:
            (a) Tricyclic antidepressants
               (i) May be combined with selective serotonin reuptake inhibitors or central-acting muscle relaxant.
            (b) Gabapentin
            (c) Anxiolytics
         2. Above medications can also be used to treat associated depression and improve sleep.

NOTES

II. Gout/Pseudogout
  a. Gout
    i. General
      1. Secondary to purine metabolism disorders.
      2. Most commonly affects middle-aged men.
      3. Etiologies
        (a) Under-excretion of uric acid
          (i) Makes up 90% of cases.
          (ii) Typically a result of:
            (1) Renal disease secondary to volume depletion.
            (2) Drugs, such as aspirin, that decrease uric acid secretion.
        (b) Overproduction of uric acid
          (i) Typically a result of:
            (1) Purine metabolism enzyme deficiency.
            (2) Increased nucleic acid turnover.
    ii. Clinical manifestations
      1. Two clinical stages
        (a) Asymptomatic
          (i) Increased serum uric acid in asymptomatic patient.
        (b) Acute gouty arthritis
          (i) Lower extremity, monoarticular arthritis.
            (1) Typically affects first metatarsophalangeal joint.
          (ii) Joint tender, erythematosus, warm, and swollen.
      2. Acute attacks may be triggered by trauma, alcohol, stress, and acute illness.
    iii. Diagnosis
      1. Laboratory tests reveal a mild leukocytosis and elevated ESR.
      2. Elevated serum uric acid.
      3. Synovial fluid examination reveals monosodium urate crystals.
        (a) Crystals are needle-shaped, negatively birefringent in polarized light.
    iv. Treatment
      1. Acute treatment
        (a) NSAIDs (indomethacin) are useful in relieving pain.

QUESTION

Which of the following diagnostic studies would best predict the risk of vertebral compression fractures in a female patient with a long history of steroid use for asthma?

  A. Bone scan
  B. Bone densitometry
  C. Thoracic lumbar spinal films
  D. Serum calcium and alkaline phosphatase levels

          (i) Aspirin should be avoided due to decreasing uric acid secretion.
        (b) Colchicine is used in acute attacks.
      2. Prophylaxis
        (a) Uricosuric drugs
          (i) Decrease tubular uric acid reabsorption.
          (ii) Examples include probenecid and sulfinpyrazone.
        (b) Allopurinol
          (i) Xanthine oxidase inhibitor lowers serum uric acid levels.
          (ii) Side effects include leukocytosis and decreased renal function.
      3. Complications include acute obstructive uropathy leading to acute renal failure.
  b. Pseudogout
    i. General
      1. Also known as calcium pyrophosphate dihydrate deposition (CPPD) disease.
      2. Etiologies include:
        (a) Hereditary
          (i) Autosomal dominant
        (b) Idiopathic
  c. Associated with other metabolic diseases
    i. Hyperparathyroidism
    ii. Clinical manifestations
      1. Acute attacks present with warmth, erythema, swelling, and tenderness.
        (a) Typically affects the knee and first metatarsophalangeal joint.
      2. Attacks last for days and are typically self-limiting.

NOTES

ANSWER B EXPLANATION: *Risk factors for osteoporosis include chronic steroid use, postmenopausal, endocrine disorders, and neoplasia. While bone x-rays may reveal decreased bone mass, bone densitometry studies are the best predictor for risk of fracture.*

correct ☐   incorrect ☐

iii. Diagnosis
1. CPPD crystals are noted in the synovial fluid.
2. X-rays reveal chondrocalcinosis.
(a) Calcific deposits in the tendons, ligaments, and cartilage.
iv. Treatment
1. NSAIDs and intra-articular steroids are useful in acute attacks.
III. Juvenile rheumatoid arthritis
a. General
i. Characterized by chronic synovitis.
1. Also note villous hypertrophy, hyperplasia of the synovial lining, edema, hyperemia, and increased lymphocytes and plasma cells.
ii. More common in girls with age of onset less than 16 years old.
iii. Risk factors include a positive family history or other rheumatologic disorders.
b. Clinical manifestations
i. May present polyarticular, oligoarthritic, or systemic.
ii. Specific symptoms include morning stiffness, night pain, refusal to bear weight, and joint deformity.
iii. Systemic symptoms include fatigue, anorexia, low-grade fever, rash, and hepatosplenomegaly.
iv. Laboratory results reveal anemia and leukocytosis.
v. Examination of the synovial fluid reveals an elevated WBC count.
c. Diagnosis
i. Based on specific criteria.
1. Age of onset less than 16 years.
(a) Many are affected between the ages of 1–3.

2. Arthritis in one or more joints.
(a) Note swelling or effusion of two or more of the following:
(i) Limitation of range of motion
(ii) Tenderness
(iii) Pain on motion
(iv) Increased heat
3. Duration of disease 6 weeks or longer.
4. Exclusion of other disorders.
d. Treatment
i. Control of inflammation with NSAIDs, immunosuppressive drugs, and steroids.
ii. Physical therapy is vital in maintaining joint function.
IV. Polyarteritis nodosa
a. General
i. Vasculitic disease involving medium-sized arteries.
ii. Primarily affects middle-aged men.
iii. Commonly affects the skin, joints, nerves, and kidneys.
b. Clinical manifestations
i. Systemic symptoms include fever, malaise, and weight loss.
ii. Renal involvement and peripheral neuropathy are common.
iii. Examination of the skin reveals palpable purpura.
iv. Nondeforming arthritis, involving any joint, may be noted.
c. Diagnosis
i. Laboratory tests reveal elevated ESR, leukocytosis, anemia, and thrombocytosis.
ii. Urinalysis is positive for protein and blood if kidneys are involved.
iii. Diagnosed by tissue biopsy.
d. Treatment
i. Consists of steroid and immunosuppressive therapy.
ii. May develop aneurysms and areas of occlusion.
V. Polymyositis
a. General
i. An acquired, systemic connective tissue disease.
ii. Peak prevalence ages 7–15 and 30–50 years.
b. Clinical manifestations
i. Present with symmetric, proximal muscle weakness.

NOTES

1. Patients will have difficulty arising from chairs, reaching overhead, or combing hair.
   ii. A photosensitive rash may also be present.
   iii. Systemic symptoms include fatigue, arthralgias, weight loss, and muscle pain.
c. Diagnosis
   i. Laboratory results reveal elevated creatine phosphokinase (CPK) and lactate dehydrogenase (LDH).
      1. Antinuclear antibody (ANA) is negative.
   ii. Evidence of chronic inflammation noted on muscle biopsy.
   iii. Electromyelogram (EMG) results show the following patterns:
      1. Short duration, low-amplitude
      2. Fibrillation, even at rest
      3. Bizarre, high-frequency discharges
d. Treatment
   i. Center of treatment is the decreasing of inflammation with steroids, methotrexate, or cyclophosphamide.
   ii. Physical therapy is important to maintain range of motion and avoid contractures.

VI. Polymyalgia rheumatica
a. General
   i. Cause of polymyalgia rheumatica (PMR) is unknown.
      1. Inflammation of the synovial lining of the bursa and joints is noted.
   ii. Most commonly affected areas are neck, shoulders, and hips.
   iii. Women are twice as likely as men to have PMR.
   iv. Associated with the same HLA genes as rheumatoid arthritis.
b. Clinical manifestations
   i. Note pain and stiffness in the neck, shoulders, and hip-girdle area that is worse in the morning.
   ii. On physical examination note only decreased active or passive range of motion.
   iii. MRI or ultrasound of the shoulders or hips reveals inflammation of the bursa.
   iv. Laboratory testing reveals an elevated ESR and anemia.
c. Diagnosis
   i. Diagnostic criteria include:
      1. Age greater than 50.

2. Aching and stiffness for greater than 1 month.
3. Affects at least two of three areas: shoulders, neck, or pelvic girdle.
4. Morning stiffness lasting greater than 1 hour.
5. ESR greater than 40 mm/hour.
6. Exclusion of other diseases
7. Rapid response to treatment with steroids.
d. Treatment
   i. NSAIDs and prednisone are cornerstones of therapy.

VII. Reiter syndrome
a. General
   i. Also known as reactive arthritis.
   ii. Occurs secondary to chlamydial urethritis or gastrointestinal (GI) infections caused by *Shigella, Salmonella, Yersinia,* and *Campylobacter.*
   iii. Most prevalent in young adulthood.
   iv. Linked to HLA-B27.
b. Clinical manifestations
   i. Signs and symptoms noted 2–3 weeks after initial infection.
   ii. Acute disease presents with asymmetric arthritis in knees and ankles.
      1. Three typical features are:
         (a) Diffuse swelling of fingers and toes (sausage digits).
         (b) Tenderness of the Achilles tendon.
         (c) Low back pain with sacroiliitis.
   iii. Conjunctivitis
      1. Many will develop a mild, noninfectious conjunctivitis.
   iv. Mucocutaneous lesions
      1. May note small, shallow, painless, ulcers on glans penis.
c. Diagnosis
   i. Laboratory tests reveal a leukocytosis and elevated ESR.
   ii. Synovial fluid reveals an increase in WBCs, mainly neutrophils.
   iii. X-rays reveal erosions and periosteal changes at the ischial tuberosities, greater trochanter, and Achilles tendon insertion.
      1. Sacroiliitis is also noted.

NOTES

d. Treatment
  i. NSAIDs are the primary treatment.
  ii. Sulfasalazine is second line therapy.
  iii. Antibiotics are of no use.
VIII. Rheumatoid arthritis
  a. General
   i. A chronic, systemic inflammatory disease.
   ii. More common in women of childbearing years.
   iii. Etiology is immune complex formation leading to an immune reaction.
   iv. Inflammation leads to ulceration of cartilage, ligaments, and bone.
  b. Clinical manifestations
   i. Systemic symptoms include fatigue, malaise, and pain.
   ii. Patients note prolonged morning stiffness and symptoms are made worse by movement.
   iii. Joints of the hands, wrists, elbows, shoulders, and feet are commonly affected.
     1. Joints affected include MCP and PIP.
     2. Findings include:
       (a) Ulnar deviation of fingers
       (b) Palmar subluxation of PIP joints.
       (c) Hyperextension of PIP and flexion of DIP (swan neck deformities).
       (d) Flexion of PIP and extension of DIP (boutonnière deformities).
   iv. Other physical findings include:
     1. Decreased dorsiflexion of the wrist
     2. Atrophy of the thenar eminence
     3. Neck stiffness and pain
     4. Subluxation of metatarsal heads
  c. Diagnosis
   i. Laboratory findings include anemia of chronic disease, thrombocytosis, elevated ESR, and positive for rheumatoid factor (RF).
   ii. Synovial fluid analysis reveals increased WBCs and poor mucin clot formation.
   iii. X-ray shows evidence of joint deformity, presence of cysts, loss of cartilage, and erosive changes.
     1. See Figure 4-7 for X-ray findings in rheumatoid arthritis.
  d. Treatment
   i. First-line treatment includes exercise, rest, and NSAIDs.

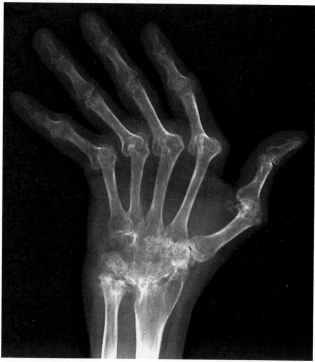

Figure 4-7 X-ray findings in rheumatoid arthritis. (From Harris ED: Kelly's Textbook of Rheumatology, 7th ed. Philadelphia, Elsevier Saunders 2005, p. 745, Fig. 51-6.)

   ii. Disease-modifying anti-rheumatic drugs (DMARDs).
     1. Hydroxychloroquine, penicillamine, gold salts, methotrexate, and azathioprine may be needed for unremitting disease.
   iii. Corticosteroid injections are used for flare-ups.
IX. Systemic lupus erythematosus (SLE)
  a. General
   i. Most common in women of reproductive age.
   ii. Acute and chronic inflammatory process with multiple organ involvement.
     1. Linked to HLA-DR2 and HLA-DR3.
   iii. May be drug-induced, secondary to hydralazine and procainamide.
  b. Clinical manifestations
   i. Systemic symptoms include fatigue, weight loss, and fever.
   ii. Affects multiple organ systems.

NOTES

1. Skin signs include facial butterfly rash and photosensitivity.
   (a) See color plate 1 for photo of typical facial rash noted in SLE.
2. Nervous system signs include seizures and psychoses.
3. Cardiac signs include pericardial effusions and myocarditis.
4. Pulmonary signs include pleural effusions and pneumonitis.
5. Renal signs include glomerulonephropathy.
6. Musculoskeletal signs include symmetrical peripheral arthralgias.

c. Diagnosis
   i. Laboratory tests reveal anemia, lymphopenia, and thrombocytopenia.
   ii. ANAs are positive.
      1. Antibodies to double-stranded DNA and anti-Sm are specific for SLE.
      2. Anti-histone is positive in drug-induced SLE.
   iii. False-positive VDRL may occur.
d. Treatment
   i. NSAIDs are useful for treatment of fever and joint pain.
   ii. Steroids are useful in cutaneous manifestations and multiple organ symptoms.
   iii. Hydroxychloroquine and chloroquine are used for the skin disease and mild systemic disease.
   iv. Severe disease may require cyclophosphamide or azathioprine.

X. Scleroderma
   a. General
      i. Multisystem disorder characterized by fibrosis of the skin, blood vessels, and visceral organs.
         1. Mechanism is overproduction and accumulation of collagen.
      ii. Two subtypes
         1. Diffuse cutaneous
            (a) Skin changes noted on extremities, face, and trunk.
            (b) Risk of visceral disease is increased early in disease.
         2. Limited cutaneous
            (a) Skin changes limited to distal extremities and face.
      iii. Typically age of onset is 20–40 years.

QUESTION

Which of the following can be used to treat acute episodes of gout?

A. Probenecid
B. Allopurinol (Zyloprim)
C. Colchicine
D. Aspirin

---

b. Clinical manifestations
   i. Raynaud's phenomenon
      1. Due to vasoconstriction of small arteries in the fingers, toes, nose, and earlobes.
   ii. Skin changes
      1. Skin becomes thick, firm, and tightly bound to underlying subcutaneous tissue.
      2. Taut skin may lead to development of contractures.
   iii. Systemic features
      1. Musculoskeletal
         (a) May develop carpal tunnel syndrome.
      2. Gastrointestinal
         (a) Dysphagia
      3. Pulmonary
         (a) Linear densities or honeycombing noted on chest X-ray.
      4. Cardiac
         (a) Pericarditis and arrhythmias
      5. Renal
         (a) Renal failure
c. Diagnosis
   i. Laboratory tests reveal an elevated ESR, anemia, and positive ANA.
      1. ANA results
   a. Anti-topoisomerase positive in diffuse cutaneous disease.
   b. Anti-centromere positive in limited cutaneous disease.
   c. Treatment
      i. Medications to control skin changes include D-penicillamine, azathioprine, and steroids.
      ii. Raynaud's can be managed by dressing warm, discontinue smoking, and use of calcium-channel blockers.

NOTES

ANSWER C EXPLANATION: *Acute episodes of gout are best treated with colchicine. Probenecid and allopurinol are used for prophylaxis and aspirin may increase the risk of developing gout.*

correct ☐   incorrect ☐

XI. Sjögren syndrome
  a. General
    i. Have inflammation and destruction of the salivary and lacrimal glands.
    ii. Etiologies
      1. Primary
      2. Secondary
        (a) Associated with RA or SLE
    iii. Typically affects women in their 50s and strongly associated with lymphoma.
  b. Clinical manifestations
    i. Patients have dry eyes, with a foreign body sensation.
    ii. Dry mouth, with an increase in dental caries, difficulty chewing, or swallowing.
    iii. May develop constipation and pancreatic insufficiency.
  c. Diagnosis
    i. Laboratory results reveal anemia of chronic disease, leukopenia, and mild eosinophilia.
    ii. ANA and RF tests are positive.
      1. Anti-La and Anti-Ro antibodies are positive.
    iii. Salivary gland biopsy will confirm the diagnosis.
  d. Treatment
    i. Artificial tears and saliva are needed.
    ii. Systemic cyclophosphamide and steroids are required in severe disease.
      1. Topical steroids in eye should be avoided due to corneal thinning.

Question 1

The Lachman's test is used to determine if an injury has occurred to which of the following ligaments?

  A. Medical collateral
  B. Posterior cruciate
  C. Lateral collateral
  D. Anterior cruciate

Question 2

A 45-year-old presents with pain in her left great toe for the past five days. Physical examination of the foot reveals a red, tender, swollen great toe. Examination of the joint fluid reveals needle-shaped, negatively birefringent crystals. Which of the following is the most likely type of crystal in the fluid?

  A. Calcium pyrophosphate
  B. Monosodium urate
  C. Cystine
  D. Tyrosine

NOTES

Question 3

A 35-year-old female presents with symmetric skin thickening of the proximal extremities, face, and trunk. The ANA is positive for anti-topoisomerase. Which of the following is the most likely diagnosis?

   A. CREST syndrome
   B. Mixed connective tissue disease
   C. Diffuse cutaneous scleroderma
   D. Systemic lupus erythematosus

Question 4

Which of the following is the initial therapy for medial epicondylitis?

   A. Surgery
   B. Antibiotics
   C. Intraarticular steroids
   D. Nonsteroidal anti-inflammatory drugs

Question 5

Which of the following is the mechanism of action of allopurinol (Zyloprim)?

   A. Inhibits renal reabsorption of uric acid
   B. Alkalinization of the urine
   C. Inhibits xanthine oxidase
   D. Activation of dihydrofolate reductase

Question 6

Osteoporosis is most commonly noted in which of the following female populations?

   A. Black
   B. Asian
   C. Caucasian
   D. Hispanic

Question 7

Which of the following is the most common type of malignant lesion to arise from bone cells?

   A. Ewing's sarcoma
   B. Chondrosarcoma
   C. Osteosarcoma
   D. Osteoid osteoma

Answer 1

ANSWER D   EXPLANATION: *The Lachman's or anterior drawer test are used to evaluate for possible anterior cruciate ligament injuries.*

Topic: Sprains/Strains

correct ☐   incorrect ☐

NOTES

Answer 2

ANSWER **B** EXPLANATION: *Gout most commonly affects middle-aged men and presents with the first metatarsophalangeal joint tender, red, swollen, and warm. Examination of the synovial fluid reveals needle-shaped, negatively birefringent crystals.*

Topic: Gout

correct ☐   incorrect ☐

Answer 3

ANSWER **C** EXPLANATION: *Scleroderma is most commonly noted in patients age 20-40 years of age and presents with thick, firm skin and Raynaud's phenomenon. Laboratory testing reveals a positive anti-topoisomerase on ANA testing.*

Topic: Scleroderma

correct ☐   incorrect ☐

Answer 4

ANSWER **D** EXPLANATION: *Medial epicondylitis presents with pain and point tenderness. Treatment consists of elimination of the activity causing symptoms, physical therapy, and nonsteroidal anti-inflammatory drugs.*

Topic: Tenosynovitis/Epicondylitis

correct ☐   incorrect ☐

Answer 5

ANSWER **C** EXPLANATION: *Allopurinol (Zyloprim) is used in the treatment of gout and lowers serum uric acid levels by inhibiting xanthine oxidase. Side effects include decreasing renal function and leukocytosis.*

Topic: Gout

correct ☐   incorrect ☐

Answer 6

ANSWER **C** EXPLANATION: *Osteoporosis is most commonly noted in Caucasian females.*

Topic: Osteoporosis

correct ☐   incorrect ☐

Answer 7

ANSWER **C** EXPLANATION: *Osteosarcoma is the most common primary malignant tumor arising from bone. More commonly noted in males ages 10-30 and is typically found in the metaphyseal areas of long bone.*

Topic: Osteosarcoma

correct ☐   incorrect ☐

NOTES

Eyes, Ears, Nose, and Throat System

5

EXAM BLUEPRINT TOPICS

Eye Disorders
Blepharitis
Blowout fracture
Cataract
Chalazion
Conjunctivitis
Corneal abrasion
Dacryoadenitis/dacryocystitis
Ectropion
Entropion
Foreign body
Glaucoma
Hordeolum
Hyphema
Macular degeneration
Orbital cellulitis
Pterygium
Retinal detachment
Retinal vascular occlusion
Retinopathy
- Diabetic
- Hypertensive

Strabismus
Ear Disorders
Acute/Chronic otitis media
Barotrauma
Cerumen impaction
Hearing impairment
Mastoiditis
Ménière's disease
Labyrinthitis
Otitis externa
Tympanic membrane perforation
Vertigo
Nose/Sinus Disorders
Acute/Chronic sinusitis
Allergic rhinitis
Epistaxis
Nasal polyps
Mouth/Throat Disorders
Acute pharyngitis
Acute tonsillitis
Aphthous ulcers
Dental abscess
Epiglottis
Laryngitis
Oral candidiasis
Oral herpes simplex
Oral leukoplakia
Peritonsillar abscess
Sialadenitis

EYE DISORDERS

I. Blepharitis
   a. General
      i. Inflammation of the eyelids.
      ii. Anterior blepharitis is a chronic bilateral inflammation of the lid margins.
         1. Two types
            (a) Staphylococcal
               (i) Due to Staphylococcus aureus or Staphylococcus epidermidis.
            (b) Seborrheic
      iii. Posterior blepharitis is inflammation of the eyelids secondary to dysfunction of the meibomian glands.
         1. Also a bilateral chronic condition.
   b. Clinical manifestations
      i. Major symptoms include irritation, burning, and itching of the eyelids.
      ii. The eyes are red-rimmed and many scales are noted on the upper and lower lashes.

NOTES

1. In staphylococcal the scales are dry and the lids red.
2. In seborrheic the scales are greasy and lid margins less red.
c. Treatment
    i. Eyelids and lid margins should be kept clean.
    ii. Staphylococcal infection is treated with antistaphylococcal antibiotics or sulfonamide eye ointment.
    iii. Posterior blepharitis is typically treated with systemic antibiotics, doxycycline or erythromycin, and a weak topical steroid.

II. Blowout fracture
    a. General
        i. Most common orbital fracture.
        ii. Occur with blunt force to the globe or orbit rim.
    b. Clinical manifestations
        i. Infraorbital anesthesia is common.
            1. Anesthesia of the maxillary teeth and upper lip is common.
        ii. Diplopia is common.
            1. If noted on upward gaze the inferior rectus muscle is entrapped.
        iii. A step-off deformity may be palpated over the intraorbital ridge.
        iv. Enophthalmos is rare.
    c. Diagnosis
        i. Plain films may note hanging teardrop sign (herniation of orbital fat into the maxillary sinus) or open bomb-bay door sign (bone fragments in the sinus).
        ii. Computed tomography (CT) scan of the orbit is needed to confirm diagnosis and determine extent of damage.
    d. Treatment
        i. Surgical repair is required if present with enophthalmos or persistent diplopia.

III. Cataract
    a. General
        i. Any opacity in the lens, with aging being the most common cause.
            1. Other causes include trauma (foreign body or blunt force), systemic disease (diabetes), smoking, congenital, and drugs (steroids, phenothiazines, or amiodarone).
            2. Cataracts are noted in 50% of patients over age 50.

ii. Due to protein that aggregates in the lens, scattering light and reducing transparency.
    1. A yellow-brown color may be noted due to these proteins.
b. Clinical manifestations
    i. Present with:
        1. Painless blurry vision or vision loss
        2. Glare
        3. Myopia
        4. Monocular double vision
        5. Absent red reflex
        6. Leukocoria
c. Diagnosis
    i. Measure visual acuity to determine impairment of vision.
    ii. Slit-lamp examination needed.
d. Treatment
    i. Surgical treatment, with or without lens implant, is the definitive treatment.

IV. Chalazion
    a. General
        i. Idiopathic, sterile chronic granulomatous inflammation of the meibomian gland.
    b. Clinical manifestations
        i. Painless, localized swelling that develops over a week.
            1. Swelling points to the conjunctival surface.
        ii. No acute inflammatory signs.
    c. Treatment
        i. Surgical excision with removal of the material is typically needed.
        ii. Intralesional steroid injections may be used in small lesions.

V. Conjunctivitis
    a. General
        i. Inflammation of the conjunctiva.
        ii. Etiologies
            1. Bacterial
                (a) *Streptococcus pneumoniae*
                (b) *Haemophilus influenzae*
                (c) *Staphylococcus aureus*
                (d) *Neisseria gonorrhoeae*
            2. Chlamydial
                (a) *Chlamydia trachomatis*
            3. Viral
                (a) Adenovirus
                (b) Herpes simplex virus types 1 and 2
                (c) Picornaviruses

NOTES

      4. Allergic
      5. Chemical
      6. Irritative
  b. Clinical manifestations
    i. Symptoms include foreign body sensation, a scratching or burning sensation, itching, and photophobia.
    ii. On physical examination note hyperemia, tearing, exudate with eyelid mattering, and pseudoptosis.
      1. Examination findings vary depending on etiology.
        (a) See Table 5-1 for comparison of signs and symptoms of conjunctivitis.
  c. Treatment
    i. Bacterial
      1. Typically self-limiting, lasting 10–14 days.
        (a) If treated will last 1–3 days.
      2. Topical broad-spectrum antibiotics (sulfonamides, tetracycline, or erythromycin) and if positive for *Neisseria* IM ceftriaxone.
    ii. Chlamydial
      1. Treat with oral tetracycline, doxycycline, erythromycin, and/or azithromycin.
      2. Topical ointments or drops can be used.
    iii. Viral
      1. No specific treatment.
      2. Herpes simplex conjunctivitis should be treated with antivirals (acyclovir) to prevent corneal involvement.

QUESTION

A 65-year-old male presents with progressive blurred vision over the past 12 months. The patient denies any pain or redness. On funduscopic examination of the eye, the retina is difficult to see secondary to the presence of an opacity. Which of the following is the most likely diagnosis?

  A. Glaucoma
  B. Cataract
  C. Amaurosis fugax
  D. Retinal artery occlusion

    iv. Allergic
      1. Topical antihistamine-vasoconstrictor agents.
      2. A short course of topical or oral steroids may be indicated.
VI. Corneal abrasion
  a. General
    i. Traumatic erosion of the corneal surface.
    ii. Secondary to trauma or contact lens wear.
  b. Clinical manifestations
    i. Present with pain, tearing, and photophobia.
    ii. A foreign body sensation is typically noted.
  c. Diagnosis
    i. Must test visual acuity.
      1. May need topical anesthetic to facilitate visual acuity testing.

Table 5-1 • Signs and Symptoms of Conjunctivitis

	Bacterial	Viral	Chlamydial	Allergic
Itching	Minimal	Minimal	Minimal	Severe
Hyperemia	Generalized: bright red	Generalized	Generalized	Generalized: milky
Tearing	Moderate	Profuse	Moderate	Moderate
Discharge	Profuse	Minimal	Profuse	Minimal
Preauricular adenopathy	Uncommon	Common	Varies	None
Sore throat and fever	Occasionally	Occasionally	Never	Never

NOTES

ANSWER **B** EXPLANATION: *Cataracts are most common in patients over age 50 and presents with progressive development of painless, blurry vision. On examination, the lens appears cloudy due to accumulation of proteins.*

correct ☐   incorrect ☐

    ii. Fluorescein staining needed to evaluate for epithelial defect.
  d. Treatment
    i. Most heal spontaneously within 48 hours.
    ii. Pain control with a cycloplegic, such as cyclopentolate or scopolamine, and oral analgesic.
    iii. Erythromycin ointment and patching may be needed.
      1. Abrasions from organic material or soft contact lenses should not be patched.
      2. Soft contact wearers are at risk of infection with *Pseudomonas* and should be treated with tobramycin or fluoroquinolone.
    iv. Follow up in 48 hours and avoid contact lenses for 1 week after healing.

VII. Dacryoadenitis/dacryocystitis
  a. General
    i. Dacryoadenitis is acute inflammation of the lacrimal gland.
      1. Rare condition seen in children, as a complication of mumps, measles, or influenzae, or in adults associated with gonorrhea.
    ii. Dacryocystitis is infection of the lacrimal gland.
      1. Occurs in infants and older women.
      2. Is unilateral and due to obstruction of the nasolacrimal duct.
      3. Common infectious agents include *H. influenzae, S. aureus,* and beta-hemolytic *Streptococcus.*
  b. Clinical manifestations
    i. Dacryoadenitis presents with severe pain, swelling, and injection over the temporal aspect of the upper eyelid.
    ii. Dacryocystitis presents with tearing and discharge. Inflammation, pain, swelling, and tenderness are noted in the tear sac area.

  c. Treatment
    i. Dacryoadenitis is observed, treated with antibiotics if needed.
      1. Surgery is rarely needed.
    ii. Dacryocystitis is treated with antibiotics and relief of the obstruction.

VIII. Ectropion
  a. General
    i. Sagging and eversion of the lower lid.
    ii. Typically bilateral and noted in the elderly.
    iii. May be caused by relaxation of the orbicularis oculi muscle.
  b. Clinical manifestations
    i. Symptoms include tearing and irritation.
    ii. On examination note sagging and eversion of the lid.
  c. Treatment
    i. Treated surgically with horizontal shortening of the lid.

IX. Entropion
  a. General
    i. Turning inward of the lower lid.
    ii. Due to laxity of the lower lid muscles.
  b. Clinical manifestations
    i. Lower lid is inverted inward.
    ii. Eyelashes may impinge on cornea and cause ulcerations.
  c. Treatment
    i. Surgery is needed to evert the lid.

X. Foreign body
  a. Clinical manifestations
    i. Surface foreign bodies present with pain and irritation that is noted with eye movement.
    ii. Intraocular foreign bodies present with discomfort or blurry vision.
      1. A history of striking metal, explosion, or projectile injury is typically present.
  b. Diagnosis
    i. Visual acuity should be determined on all patients.
    ii. With intraocular foreign bodies a slit lamp should be used to locate site of entry.
      1. CT scan or plain film X-ray should be done to identify radiopaque particles.
      2. Magnetic resonance imaging (MRI) is contraindicated.
  c. Treatment

NOTES

i. For removal of the surface foreign body a topical anesthetic and a fine-gauge needle are used to remove the foreign body.
   1. Do not use a cotton-tipped applicator.
   2. Topical anesthetic should not be used long term.
   3. Steroids should also be avoided.
ii. Intraocular foreign bodies should be removed by an ophthalmologist whenever possible.
iii. Metallic rings surrounding copper or iron fragments can be removed with a drill with a burr tip.
iv. After removal antibiotic (erythromycin) ointment should be applied and the eye pressure patched.
v. All patients should be seen within 48 hours by an ophthalmologist.

XI. Glaucoma
a. General
   i. Due to increased intraocular pressure causing optic nerve damage.
      1. Increased intraocular pressure due to impaired outflow of aqueous humor or impaired access of aqueous humor to the drainage system.
   ii. Leading cause of preventable blindness in the United States.
   iii. Classification
      1. Primary
         (a) Open-angle
            (i) Most common type of glaucoma.
            (ii) Due to inadequate drainage of aqueous humor.
         (b) Angle-closure
            (i) Restricted flow of aqueous humor.
            (ii) Acute angle-closure glaucoma is an ophthalmic emergency.
      2. Congenital
      3. Secondary
b. Clinical manifestations
   i. Primary angle-closure glaucoma presents with sudden onset of eye pain, headache, blurred vision and halos, nausea and vomiting, fixed and dilated pupil, and hyperemia.
   ii. Open angle glaucoma is asymptomatic early with gradual loss of peripheral vision, and halos around lights.
c. Diagnosis
   i. Intraocular pressure measured by tonometry.

QUESTION

A patient presents with a foreign body sensation, tearing, and pain in the right eye after hammering a nail. What is the next best step in the evaluation of this patient?

A. Orbital MRI
B. Eye culture
C. Fluorescein staining
D. Test visual acuity

   1. Goldmann applanation and Schiotz tonometry used.
   2. Normal intraocular pressure is 10–24 mm Hg.
   ii. Gonioscopy
      1. Determines if anterior chamber angle is wide (open), narrow, or closed.
   iii. Optic disk assessment
      1. Will note enlargement of optic disk, disk pallor, and increased cup-disk ratio.
   iv. Visual field defects
      1. Involves mainly the peripheral field.
d. Treatment
   i. All forms of treatment include reduction of aqueous production.
   ii. Suppression of aqueous humor production
      1. Topical beta-adrenergic blocking agents
         (a) Includes timolol maleate, betaxolol, and levobunolol.
         (b) Contraindicated in asthma and cardiac conduction defects.
         (c) Depression, confusion, and fatigue may occur.
      2. Alpha-adrenergic agonists
         (a) Includes apraclonidine and brimonidine.
         (b) High rate of allergic reactions.
      3. Topical and systemic carbonic anhydrase inhibitors
         (a) Topical medications include dorzolamide hydrochloride and brinzolamide.
            (i) Allergic reactions are common.
         (b) Systemic medications include acetazolamide.

NOTES

ANSWER **D** EXPLANATION: *Intraocular foreign bodies typically develop after the striking of metal objects. Blurry vision and pain, which worsens with eye movement, are noted. Visual acuity should be determined before any other testing is done.*

correct ☐   incorrect ☐

(i) Used in acute glaucoma.
   iii. Facilitation of aqueous outflow
      1. Parasympathomimetic agents
        (a) Includes pilocarpine and carbachol.
        (b) The irreversible anticholinesterase agents, used as parasympathomimetic agents, must be avoided during anesthesia due to potentiation of succinylcholine.
      2. Prostaglandin analogs
        (a) Includes bimatoprost, latanoprost, and travoprost.
   iv. Surgical treatment
      1. Includes peripheral iridotomy, laser trabeculoplasty, and trabeculectomy.

XII. Hordeolum
  a. General
    i. Infection of the glands of the eyelid.
    ii. Most are caused by infection with staphylococcal species.
  b. Clinical manifestations
    i. Symptoms include pain, redness, and swelling.
    ii. Internal hordeolum may point toward the skin or conjunctiva.
    iii. External hordeolum always points toward the skin.
  c. Treatment
    i. Warm compressions to area three to four times a day.
    ii. If no improvement in 48 hours, incision and drainage may be needed.
    iii. Antibiotic ointment may be helpful.

XIII. Hyphema
  a. General
    i. Traumatic forces tear vessels and bleeding into the aqueous humor.
  b. Clinical manifestations
    i. Blood may settle out into a visible layer.

  c. Treatment
    i. If more than 5% of anterior chamber filled with blood patient should rest.
    ii. Steroid drops should be started.
    iii. Avoid aspirin and nonsteroidal anti-inflammatory drugs (NSAIDs).
    iv. Will resolve by spontaneous absorption.
      1. If intraocular pressure remains elevated then surgical intervention may be required.

XIV. Macular degeneration
  a. General
    i. Age-related macular degeneration is the leading cause of permanent blindness in the elderly.
    ii. Cause is unknown.
    iii. Two types.
      1. Non-exudative
      2. Exudative
  b. Clinical manifestations
    i. In non-exudative degeneration drusen are noted ophthalmoscopically.
      1. Drusen are discrete, round, yellow-white deposits beneath the pigment epithelium and scattered throughout the macula.
      2. Visual impairment is variable.
    ii. In exudative degeneration vision loss is severe.
      1. Neovascularization may be noted on ophthalmoscopic examination.
  c. Treatment
    i. No way to prevent non-exudative degeneration.
      1. Monitor for loss of central vision with Amsler grid.
    ii. In exudative degeneration without neovascularization no medical or surgical treatment is needed.
      1. Laser photocoagulation is needed if neovascularization is present.

XV. Orbital cellulitis
  a. General
    i. Occurs most commonly in children.
    ii. May be the result of trauma or extension of sinusitis through the ethmoid sinus to the orbit.
    iii. Most common organisms are *H. influenzae* and *S. pneumoniae*.

NOTES

b. Clinical manifestations
  i. Children may present with proptosis.
  ii. Present with edema, erythema, hyperemia, and pain.
    1. Infection may spread rapidly.
  iii. Physical examination reveals chemosis, limited eye movements, reduction of vision, and erythema.
    1. Limited eye movements noted in postseptal cellulitis.
  iv. Laboratory testing reveals a leukocytosis.
c. Diagnosis
  i. CT scan or MRI needed to separate pre- from postseptal involvement.
d. Treatment
  i. Nasal decongestants and vasoconstrictors may help to drain sinuses.
  ii. IV antibiotics are required.
    1. Mild cases treated with amoxicillin and severe cases treated with ceftriaxone and vancomycin.

XVI. Pterygium
  a. General
    i. A fleshy, triangular encroachment onto the cornea.
    ii. Typically bilateral and on the nasal side.
    iii. Due to irritation secondary to ultraviolet light, drying, and wind.
  b. Clinical manifestations
    i. On physical examination note triangular lesion on the nasal side of the cornea.
  c. Treatment
    i. If large may be removed surgically.

XVII. Retinal detachment
  a. General
    i. Separation of the sensory retina from the underlying pigmented epithelium.
      1. Most common location is superior temporal area.
    ii. Caused by trauma or can be spontaneous.
    iii. Most commonly in people over age 50 and severe myopia.
  b. Clinical manifestations
    i. Patient may state that a curtain came down over their eye.
    ii. Vision is blurry and progressively worsens.
    iii. Flashes and floaters may be noted.
    iv. On funduscopic examination the retina is noted hanging in the vitreous fluid.

QUESTION

A 40-year-old presents with pain, redness, and swelling of the eye. On physical examination, swelling is noted on the upper eyelid. Visual acuity is normal. Which of the following is the most likely diagnosis?

A. Retinal detachment
B. Hyphema
C. Hordeolum
D. Dacryoadenitis

  c. Treatment
    i. Immediate ophthalmologic referral needed.
    ii. Patient should keep head position so that gravity helps the detached portion of the retina fall back into place.
    iii. Photocoagulation or cryotherapy may be needed to correct the tear.

XVIII. Retinal vascular occlusion
  a. General
    i. Typically present with painless vision loss.
    ii. Central vein occlusion is noted in patients over age 50 and associated with cardiovascular disease.
  b. Clinical manifestations
    i. Central retinal artery occlusion presents with painless monocular vision loss.
      1. Often proceeded by amaurosis fugax.
      2. On funduscopic examination a cherry-red spot is noted on the macula.
    ii. Branch retinal artery occlusion presents with sudden loss of visual field and reduced visual acuity.
      1. On funduscopic examination cotton-wool spots are noted in the area of the retina supplied by the artery.
    iii. Central retinal vein occlusion presents with sudden painless vision loss.
      1. Funduscopic examination varies from small retinal hemorrhages to cotton-wool spots to deep and superficial retinal hemorrhages

NOTES

ANSWER C EXPLANATION: *Hordeolum is an infection of the glands of the eyelid. Symptoms include pain, redness, and swelling. Visual acuity is no affected.*

correct ☐   incorrect ☐

c. Treatment
  i. Referral to an ophthalmologist is required.
  ii. In central retinal artery occlusion IV acetazolamide is used to decrease intra-ocular pressure and thrombolytic agent is infused into the artery. This can result in return of vision if given within 8 hours.
    1. Ocular massage can also decrease intraocular pressure.
  iii. Central vein occlusion is treated with laser photocoagulation if neovascularization is present.
    1. Aspirin may be helpful.

XIX. Retinopathy
  a. Diabetic
    i. General
      1. Changes in retinal vessels lead to microaneurysms, neovascularizations, hemorrhages, and edema.
      2. Occur faster in diabetes type II than type I.
      3. Classified as either proliferative or nonproliferative.
    ii. Clinical manifestations
      1. Varies with classification.
        (a) Proliferative
          (i) Neovascularization
          (ii) Hemorrhage in the vitreous body.
          (iii) May lead to retinal detachment.
        (b) Nonproliferative
          (i) Venous dilatation
          (ii) Microaneurysms
          (iii) Retinal hemorrhages
          (iv) Edema
          (v) Hard exudates
      2. See color plate 2 for funduscopic exam in diabetic retinopathy.

    iii. Diagnosis
      1. Based on history and funduscopic examination.
    iv. Treatment
      1. Management of blood sugar and blood pressure is vital.
      2. Yearly ophthalmoscopic examination is needed for patients with diabetes.
      3. Neovascularization is treated with laser photocoagulation.
      4. Laser surgery for macular edema.
  b. Hypertensive
    i. General
      1. Due to systemic hypertension.
    ii. Clinical manifestations
      1. Vision is impaired.
      2. On funduscopic examination note:
        (a) Silver or copper wiring
        (b) Arteriovenous (AV) nicking
        (c) Flame-shaped hemorrhages
        (d) Cotton-wool spots
        (e) Retinal edema
        (f) Retinal pigmentation
    iii. Diagnosis
      1. Based on history and physical examination findings.
    iv. Treatment
      1. Will have improvement with blood pressure control.

XX. Strabismus
  a. General
    i. Defined as any deviation from perfect ocular alignment.
    ii. Misalignment may be in any direction.
      1. Esotropia is convergent strabismus (crossed eyes).
        (a) The most common type of strabismus.
      2. Exotropia is divergent strabismus.
    iii. Present in 4%–5% of children.
      1. Stable ocular alignment not present until age 2 months.
  b. Clinical manifestations
    i. Children present with diplopia, scotoma, and amblyopia.
    ii. On physical examination the strabismus may be noted on inspection.
    iii. Convergence testing is used to test for disjunctive movements.

NOTES

c. Diagnosis
   i. Angle of strabismus determined by the cover-uncover test.
   ii. Hirschberg test is used to determine eye position by evaluating for centering of light reflection in both eyes.
d. Treatment
   i. Treatment should be started as soon as possible.
   ii. Nonsurgical treatment.
      1. Occlusion therapy is used to treat amblyopia.
         (a) The sound eye is covered to stimulate the amblyopic eye.
      2. Spectacles are used to treat strabismus and prisms are used to treat diplopia.
   iii. Surgical treatment
      1. Resection and recession are used to strengthen and weaken the appropriate muscles.

EAR DISORDERS

I. Acute otitis media
   a. General
      i. Due to inflammation that results in fluid collection in the middle ear.
      ii. Risk factors include:
         1. Daycare attendance
         2. Sibling with acute otitis media
         3. Parental smoking
         4. Drinking from a bottle while lying flat
      iii. Etiology
         1. Most cases are viral (respiratory syncytial virus, rhinovirus, influenzae, and enterovirus).
         2. Bacterial causes include:
            (a) *S. pneumoniae*
            (b) *H. influenzae*
            (c) *Moraxella catarrhalis*
            (d) *S. aureus*
            (e) Group A *Streptococcus*
   b. Clinical manifestations
      i. Children present with irritability, crying, lethargy, and pulling at their ears.
      ii. Older children and adults present with earache and ear drainage.

QUESTION

A 60-year-old male presents with sudden, painless loss of vision in the right eye. On examination, a pale retina with a cherry-red spot at the macula is noted. What is the most likely diagnosis?

A. Amaurosis fugax
B. Retinal detachment
C. Vitreous hemorrhage
D. Central retinal artery occlusion

---

      iii. Physical examination reveals an erythematosus tympanic membrane (TM).
         1. TM may be bulging, retracted, or perforated.
         2. An air-fluid level may be noted behind the TM and mobility of the TM is diminished.
         3. Hearing may be decreased.
   c. Diagnosis
      i. Based on history and physical examination.
      ii. Culture, via tympanocentesis, is rarely done, unless patient appears toxic or has recurrent infection.
   d. Treatment
      i. Symptomatic treatment, mainly pain control, is required.
      ii. Antibiotic treatment includes:
         1. Amoxicillin
         2. Erythromycin/sulfisoxazole
         3. Amoxicillin/clavulanate
         4. Cefpodoxime
         5. Trimethoprim/sulfamethoxazole
      iii. Most patients start to respond in 48–72 hours.
      iv. Complications include chronic otitis media, mastoiditis, and intracranial extension.
      v. Recurrent disease may require placement of tympanostomy tubes or tonsillectomy/adenoidectomy.
II. Chronic otitis media
   a. General
      i. Complication of acute otitis media.
   b. Clinical manifestations
      i. Present with persistent or recurrent purulent otorrhea with TM perforation.

NOTES

ANSWER **D** EXPLANATION: *Sudden, painless loss of vision is noted in central retinal artery occlusion. On examination, a cherry-red spot is noted on the macula is noted.*

correct ☐   incorrect ☐

    ii. Typically have some degree of conductive hearing loss without pain.

    iii. May develop a cholesteatoma.

      1. A mass of squamous epithelium debris that forms at the site of invasion.

      2. This mass can invade surrounding bone and lead to meningitis and brain abscess.

  c. Treatment

    i. Treatment is very difficult and consists of surgery.

      1. Includes mastoidectomy, myringoplasty, and tympanoplasty.

    ii. Systemic antibiotics may also be needed.

III. Barotrauma

  a. General

    i. Injury caused by barometric pressure change.

    ii. Usually results from water diving, ascending into the atmosphere, or mechanical respiratory support.

    iii. Injury can occur in the ears, sinuses, or lungs.

  b. Clinical manifestations

    i. External ear barotrauma

      1. Patients experience pain and bloody discharge.

      2. May note petechiae, hemorrhagic blebs, or rupture of the TM on physical examination.

    ii. Middle ear barotrauma

      1. Due to impaired eustachian tube functioning, secondary to upper respiratory infection (URI), allergy, or trauma.

      2. Noted in patients with URI and flying in a plane.

        (a) Pain and fullness noted on descent if patient fails to "pop" ears.

    iii. Decompression sickness ("the bends")

      1. Occurs most often after divers descend and remain deeper than 10 meters.

      2. Due to nitrogen becoming insoluble and forming bubbles in the blood and tissue.

      3. Present with steady, throbbing pain in the joints, pruritus, headache, seizures, hemiplegia, and visual disturbances.

      4. Pulmonary effects include substernal pain, dyspnea, and cough.

  c. Treatment

    i. Treatment of ear barotrauma consists of keeping ear dry, pain control, decongestants, or antihistamines.

      1. Prevent with use of decongestants prior to flying.

    ii. Treatment of decompression sickness consists of recompression therapy in a compression chamber.

IV. Cerumen impaction

  a. General

    i. Precipitated by use of cotton-tipped applicators to clean ears.

    ii. Foreign bodies in the external ear canal may also be present.

  b. Clinical manifestations

    i. Present with decreased hearing (conduction type), pressure or fullness in the ear, dizziness, tinnitus, or pain.

    ii. On physical examination the TM may not be visualized and the external auditory canal may be occluded with cerumen.

  c. Treatment

    i. Cerumen softeners are used and then a cerumen spoon or loop is used to remove the cerumen.

      1. Softening of the cerumen can occur with half strength hydrogen peroxide, mineral oil, or over-the-counter preparations.

    ii. Irrigation of the ear may also be needed.

V. Hearing impairment

  a. General

    i. Almost 10% of the adult population has some hearing loss.

    ii. Two types of hearing loss:

      1. Conductive

        (a) Lesion in the auricle, external auditory canal, or middle ear.

      2. Sensorineural

        (a) Lesion in the inner ear or eighth cranial nerve.

NOTES

b. Etiologies
  i. Conductive
    1. Obstruction of external auditory canal due to cerumen, foreign body, swelling, neoplasm, or TM perforation.
    2. Cholesteatoma
      (a) A benign, slow-growing lesion that destroys bone and normal ear tissue.
      (b) On examination note perforated TM with white debris.
    3. Otosclerosis
      (a) Due to fixation of the ossicular bones and results in a low-frequency conductive hearing loss.
  ii. Sensorineural
    1. Presbycusis
      (a) Most common cause of sensorineural hearing loss and is age-associated.
      (b) High-frequency hearing loss.
    2. Ménière's disease
      (a) See VII V below.
    3. Drug-induced
      (a) Mechanism is damage to hair cells in the organ of Corti.
      (b) Common medications include salicylates, quinine, aminoglycosides, cisplatin, and loop diuretics.
c. Diagnosis
  i. Differentiate conductive and sensorineural hearing losses with the Weber and Rinne tests.
    1. Weber
      (a) Vibrating tuning fork placed on the head in the midline.
      (b) With unilateral conductive hearing loss the tone is perceived in the affected ear.
      (c) With unilateral sensorineural hearing loss the tone is perceived in the unaffected ear.
    2. Rinne
      (a) Vibrating tuning fork placed near opening of auditory canal (air conduction) and then placed on mastoid process (bone conduction).
      (b) Normally and with sensorineural hearing loss the air conduction is greater than bone conduction.
      (c) With conductive hearing loss the bone conduction is greater than air conduction.
  ii. Audiologic assessment
    1. Used to determine level of hearing loss.
d. Treatment
  i. Conductive hearing loss can be treated with surgical intervention and correction.
  ii. Sensorineural hearing loss is permanent and corrected with hearing aids.

VI. Mastoiditis
  a. General
    i. A rare complication of otitis media.
      1. Caused by same microorganisms as otitis media.
    ii. Infection of the mastoid air cells.
  b. Clinical manifestations
    i. Present with pain, swelling, tenderness, and redness behind the ear in the area of the mastoid bone.
    ii. On physical examination the mastoid area is red and tender and the pinna may be displaced.
  c. Diagnosis
    i. X-ray of the mastoid bone may show soft-tissue swelling, loss of mastoid bone mass, and lytic lesions.
  d. Treatment
    i. Treatment the same as otitis media but must treat for 3–4 weeks.
    ii. Mastoidectomy may be needed in severe disease.
    iii. Complications include brain abscess and septic lateral sinus thrombosis.
VII. Ménière's disease
  a. General
    i. Results from malfunction of the endolymphatic sac in the inner ear.
  b. Clinical manifestations
    i. Present with debilitating vertigo, progressive sensorineural hearing loss, and tinnitus.
      1. Onset of vertigo is sudden and lasts minutes to hours.
        (a) Rarely lasts longer than 24–48 hours.
    ii. May also note a fullness or pressure in the affected ear.
    iii. Physical examination is typically normal.

NOTES

c. Diagnosis
    i. Based on history and physical examination.
    ii. Electronystagmography with warm and cold calorics can be used to differentiate central from peripheral causes of vertigo.
d. Treatment
    i. May be pharmacologic or surgical.
    ii. Pharmacologic treatment consists of:
        1. Diazepam for acute disease
        2. Trimethobenzamide hydrochloride
        3. Meclizine
        4. Dimenhydrinate
        5. Hydrochlorothiazide
        6. Triamterene
    iii. Surgical drainage of the endolymphatic system or ablation of the eighth cranial nerve or labyrinth may be needed in severe cases.
    iv. Patients should also be instructed to avoid caffeine, alcohol, and smoking.

VIII. Labyrinthitis (Vestibular neuronitis)
a. General
    i. Acute unilateral infection or inflammation of the vestibular system.
        1. Typically due to viral infection.
        2. A history of recent URI.
    ii. May last 7–10 days and typically is self-limited.
b. Clinical manifestations
    i. Present with rotational vertigo, nystagmus, nausea, and vomiting.
        1. Nystagmus is horizontal-rotatory away from affected side.
        2. No tinnitus or hearing loss.
    ii. On physical examination the vertigo remains whether the patient opens or closes the eyes.
c. Diagnosis
    i. CT scan may be needed to rule out central causes of dizziness.
d. Treatment
    i. Typically self-limiting and may require symptomatic treatment.
        1. Pharmacologic management includes:
            (a) Diazepam
            (b) Meclizine
            (c) Dimenhydrinate
        2. Side effects include drowsiness and sedation.

    ii. Complications are uncommon.
IX. Otitis externa
a. General
    i. Defined as infection and inflammation of the external auditory canal.
    ii. Four different categories.
        1. Acute localized
        2. Acute diffuse (swimmer's ear)
        3. Chronic
        4. Malignant
    iii. Etiology includes:
        1. *S. aureus*
        2. Group A *Streptococcus*
        3. *Pseudomonas aeruginosa*
        4. *Aspergillus*
b. Clinical manifestations
    i. Acute localized infection present with pain and tenderness,
        1. On physical examination the canal is erythematosus and tenderness is noted over the tragus.
        2. Preauricular lymphadenopathy may be noted.
    ii. Acute diffuse disease presents with pain and itching.
        1. On physical examination the canal is erythematosus, swollen, and hemorrhagic.
    iii. Chronic disease presents with drainage and itching.
    iv. Malignant disease presents with a severe, necrotizing infection.
        1. Associated with elderly diabetic patients and infection due to *P. aeruginosa*.
c. Diagnosis
    i. Based on history and physical examination.
d. Treatment
    i. Treatment is started with gentle cleaning with saline or alcohol and acetic acid mixture.
    ii. Topical neomycin, polymyxin, and quinolone are also started.
    iii. IV anti-pseudomonal antibiotics, such as ceftazidime or piperacillin, plus aminoglycosides or fluoroquinolones, are required for the treatment of malignant otitis externa.
X. Tympanic membrane perforation
a. General

NOTES

    i. Occur as a result of penetrating or noise trauma.

    ii. Occurs typically in the pars tensa, anteriorly or inferiorly.

  b. Clinical manifestations

    i. Present with acute onset of pain, hearing loss, and with or without bloody otorrhea.

    ii. May also have tinnitus and vertigo.

  c. Diagnosis

    i. Perforation is noted on otoscopic examination.

  d. Treatment

    i. Most perforated tympanic membranes will heal spontaneously.

    ii. A follow-up hearing test is needed to confirm that hearing has returned to baseline.

    iii. Patient should be instructed not to get any water in the ear.

XI. Vertigo

  a. General

    i. Vertigo described as a dizziness, spinning, imbalance, lightheadedness, or sensation of ground moving.

    ii. Due to a disturbance in the vestibular system.

    iii. Physiologic vertigo

      1. Etiologies include:

        (a) Due to mismatch in sensory systems.

        (b) Patient subjected to unfamiliar head movements.

        (c) Unusual head or neck positions.

        (d) Spinning

    iv. Pathologic vertigo

      1. Etiologies include:

        (a) Peripheral

          (i) Severe vertigo with sudden onset.

          (ii) Nystagmus is horizontal or rotatory.

          (iii) Other symptoms include tinnitus, hearing loss, nausea, and vomiting.

          (iv) Etiologies include:

            (1) Benign paroxysmal positional vertigo

            (2) Labyrinthitis

            (3) Acoustic neuroma

            (4) Ototoxic drugs

        (b) Central

          (i) Less severe and vague vertigo.

QUESTION

Which of the following medications can lead to irreversible hearing loss?

A. Penicillin

B. Thorazine

C. Salicylates

D. Hydrochlorothiazide

          (ii) Nystagmus is vertical or bidirectional.

          (iii) Etiologies include:

            (1) Multiple sclerosis

            (2) Vertebrobasilar insufficiency

  (c) See Table 5-2 for comparison of peripheral and central vertigo.

Table 5-2 • Peripheral and Central Vertigo

Sign/Symptom	Peripheral	Central
Severity of vertigo	Marked, spontaneous	Mild, gradual
Tinnitus/deafness	Often present	Usually absent
Vertical nystagmus	Never	Occasionally
Horizontal nystagmus	Uncommon	Common
Duration	Finite, intermittent	Variable, chronic
Central nervous system signs	None	Common
Etiologies	Infection	Vascular
	Ménière's	Neoplasm
	Trauma	
	Toxin	

ANSWER C EXPLANATION: *The most common medications causing sensorineural hearing loss include salicylates, quinine, aminoglycoside, cisplatin, and loop diuretics.*

correct ☐   incorrect ☐

b. Diagnosis
  i. Dix-Hallpike maneuver is used to assist in the diagnosis of benign paroxysmal positional vertigo.
  ii. Electronystagmography (calorics), warm and cold, to test vestibular function.
c. Treatment
  i. Treatment of acute vertigo consists of bed rest and medications.
    1. Medications include:
      (a) Antihistamines such as meclizine and dimenhydrinate.
      (b) Tranquilizers such as diazepam and clonazepam.
      (c) Phenothiazine such as prochlorperazine.
      (d) Glucocorticoids

NOSE/SINUS DISORDERS

I. Acute sinusitis
  a. General
    i. Defined as a sinusitis for less than 4 weeks duration.
    ii. Typically occur as a result of a preceding viral upper respiratory tract infection.
    iii. Mechanism includes obstruction of the sinus ostia or impaired ciliary clearance.
    iv. Etiologies include allergic rhinitis, barotrauma, chemical irritants, and infectious.
      1. Infectious agents include bacterial, viral, and fungal.
        (a) Bacterial
          (i) *S. pneumoniae*
          (ii) *H. influenzae* (nontypeable)
          (iii) *M. catarrhalis*
          (iv) Anaerobes
          (v) *P. aeruginosa*
          (vi) *S. aureus*
        (b) Viral
          (i) Rhinovirus
          (ii) Parainfluenzae
          (iii) Influenzae
        (c) Fungal
          (i) *Rhizopus*
          (ii) *Rhizomucor*
          (iii) *Mucor*
          (iv) *Aspergillus*
  b. Clinical manifestations
    i. Present with fever, nasal drainage and congestion, facial pain or pressure, and headache.
      1. Upper molar tooth pain and halitosis is associated with bacterial sinusitis.
    ii. Sinus pressure or pain is localized over infected sinus.
      1. Maxillary sinus is most frequently infected, followed by ethmoid, frontal, and sphenoid.
    iii. Physical examination tenderness with palpation is noted over the infected sinus.
      1. Decreased transillumination may be noted.
    iv. Laboratory testing reveals a leukocytosis.
  c. Diagnosis
    i. Signs and symptoms should be present for greater than 7 days.
    ii. CT scan or sinus X-ray may reveal air-fluid levels, opacification, and mucosal thickening.
      1. See Figure 5-1 for X-ray of sinus infection.
  d. Treatment
    i. For symptoms present for less than 7 days, decongestants and nasal saline lavage may be helpful.
    ii. For symptoms present greater than 7 days or more severe symptoms, antibiotics are indicated.
      1. Amoxicillin, trimethoprim-sulfamethoxazole, cefuroxime, clarithromycin, and azithromycin are indicated.
II. Chronic sinusitis
  a. General
    i. Defined by signs and symptoms lasting greater than 12 weeks.

NOTES

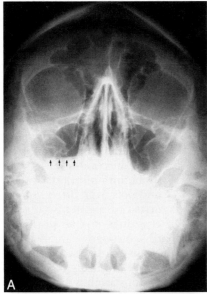

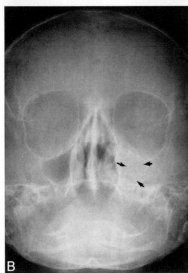

Figure 5-1 Sinus infection X-ray. Note air-fluid levels. (From Mettler FA: Essentials of Radiology, 2nd ed. Philadelphia, Elsevier Saunders, 2005, p. 37, Fig. 2-27a.)

 ii. Associated with infection by bacteria or fungi.
 iii. Mechanism is based on impaired mucociliary clearance from repeated infections.
  1. Certain conditions, such as cystic fibrosis, can predispose patients to chronic bacterial sinusitis.

QUESTION

A 3-year-old presents with irritability and lethargy. On physical examination, a fluid level is noted behind the right TM and the TM mobility is decreased. Which of the following is the most likely diagnosis?

 A. Barotrauma
 B. Otitis externa
 C. TM perforation
 D. Acute otitis media

 b. Clinical manifestations
  i. Present with headaches, fatigue, irritability, low-grade fever, facial pressure, and postnasal discharge.
 c. Diagnosis
  i. CT scan is used to determine extent of disease and response to therapy.
 d. Treatment
  i. Includes repeated courses of antibiotics or antifungals, intranasal glucocorticoids, and irrigation of the sinus.
  ii. Surgery may be needed to remove impacted mucus.
III. Allergic rhinitis
 a. General
  i. One of the most common allergic diseases in the United States.
  ii. May have onset at any age, but incidence of onset is greatest during adolescence and peak prevalence during ages 20–30.
  iii. A type 1 hypersensitivity reaction mediates the allergic response.
   1. Involves the excess production of IgE.
   2. Two phases:
    (a) Early phase
     (i) Due to degranulation of mast cells, evokes an inflammatory response and release of histamine, leukotrienes, cytokines, and prostaglandins.
     (ii) Occurs within 10–15 minutes of exposure.

NOTES

ANSWER **D** EXPLANATION: *Acute otitis media is common in young children who present with irritability, crying, and lethargy. On examination, the TM is red, swollen, a fluid level may be present, and TM mobility is decreased.*

correct ☐   incorrect ☐

    (iii) Symptoms include sneezing, rhinorrhea, itching, and increased vascular permeability.
  (b) Late phase
    (i) Release of cytokines and leukotrienes cause an influx of inflammatory cells (eosinophils).
    (ii) Can begin 4–6 hours after initial exposure.
    (iii) Symptoms include nasal congestion and postnasal drip.
  iv. Etiologies
    1. Seasonal
      (a) Occur during certain seasons and typically due to tree pollen in the spring, grasses in the late spring and summer, and weeds in the fall.
    2. Perennial
      (a) Symptoms are usually constant and typically due to indoor allergens, such as dust mites, animal dander, cockroaches, and mold spores.
  b. Clinical manifestations
    i. Seasonal allergic rhinitis presents with sneezing, watery rhinorrhea, itching of the nose, eyes, and throat, red and watery eyes, and nasal congestion.
      1. Symptoms are worse in the morning and aggravated by dry, windy conditions.
      2. Physical examination of the nose reveals blue, pale, boggy turbinates; wet, swollen mucosa; and nasal congestion.
    ii. Perennial allergic rhinitis presents with nasal congestion and postnasal drip.
      1. Physical examination may be normal or just reveal nasal congestion.
    iii. In children may note allergic shiners, mouth breathing, and the nasal salute.

  c. Diagnosis
    i. Allergy testing is done to establish the presence of atopic disease.
    ii. Other tests include skin testing (skin prick test and intradermal testing) and in vitro testing (RAST test).
  d. Treatment
    i. Are three major options:
      1. Avoidance and environmental control
        (a) Consists of avoidance of outdoor allergens, keeping windows closed, using air conditioning, decreasing home humidity, removal of carpets and pets from often-used living areas, encase items in hypoallergenic coverings, and air purifiers.
      2. Pharmacotherapy
        (a) Done through a variety of medications.
        (b) Antihistamines are most effective on early phase symptoms and have little effect on nasal congestion.
        (c) Intranasal corticosteroids are the most effective medication for overall control of allergic rhinitis.
          (i) May take 1–2 weeks for maximum effect.
          (ii) Act on the late phase symptoms.
          (iii) No systemic side effects compared to oral corticosteroids.
        (d) Decongestants improve nasal congestion, but have no effect on sneezing, rhinorrhea, or pruritus.
        (e) Anticholinergics control only rhinorrhea.
        (f) Intranasal cromolyn must be used prior to onset of symptoms.
        (g) See Table 5-3 for medications used in allergic rhinitis.
      3. Immunotherapy
        (a) Attempts to increase the threshold level for the appearance of symptoms.
        (b) Done through the gradual increase in dose of antigen until a reaction occurs.
IV. Epistaxis
  a. General
    i. Common etiologies of epistaxis.
      1. Infection
      2. Trauma
      3. Allergic rhinitis

NOTES

4. Atrophic rhinitis
5. Hypertension
6. Tumors
   ii. Divided into two groups.
      1. Anterior
         (a) Make up 90% of nosebleeds and most
             originate from Kiesselbach plexus.
      2. Posterior
         (a) More common in the elderly and
             due to arteriosclerosis.
b. Clinical manifestations
   i. Anterior bleeds are typically unilateral and
      without sensation of blood in the posterior
      pharynx.

QUESTION

A patient presents with a 2-week history of upper molar and facial pain on the right side. On exam tenderness and decreased transillumination is noted below the right eye. Which of the following is the most likely diagnosis?

A. Allergic rhinitis
B. Acute sinusitis
C. Mastoiditis
D. Otitis externa

Table 5-3 • Medications for Allergic Rhinitis

Class	Medication	Mechanism of Action	Side Effects
Antihistamines	**First generation:** Diphenhydramine Hydroxyzine Chlorpheniramine **Second generation:** Fexofenadine Loratadine Cetirizine Azelastine	Antagonize the H1 receptor-mediated effects of histamine.	First-generation side effects include sedation and anticholinergic effects. Second generation have little sedation and no anticholinergic effects.
Decongestants	Oxymetazoline	Act on alpha-adrenergic receptors of the mucosa of the respiratory tract	May have rebound nasal congestion.
Corticosteroids (intranasal and oral)	**Nasal:** Triamcinolone Budesonide Fluticasone Mometasone	Act at a wide variety of steps, cell types, and mediators suppressing inflammatory response.	Nasal corticosteroids have no systemic side effects. Oral corticosteroids may suppress the HPA axis.
Mast-cell stabilizers	Cromolyn	Inhibit the release of mediators, such as histamine, from mast cells.	
Anticholinergic agents	Ipratropium bromide	Antagonize the action of acetylcholine at muscarinic receptors.	
Leukotriene modifiers	Montelukast	Antagonize the action of leukotriene receptors or inhibit the formation or leukotrienes.	

HPA, Hypothalamic-pituitary-adrenal.

NOTES

ANSWER **B** EXPLANATION: *Acute sinusitis, symptoms of less than four weeks in duration, presents with upper molars and facial pain, fever, and nasal drainage. On examination, tenderness and decreased transillumination is noted over the infected sinus.*

correct ☐   incorrect ☐

ii. Posterior bleeds are typically profuse and blood is noted draining down posterior pharynx.
c. Treatment
    i. Anterior nosebleeds are treated with the following:
      1. Direct pressure
        (a) Compress elastic area of nose for 10–15 minutes.
      2. Vasoconstrictive agents
        (a) Agents include phenylephrine, oxymetazoline, or epinephrine.
      3. Nasal packing
        (a) Perform when direct pressure or vasoconstrictors are not successful.
        (b) Consider prophylactic treatment against toxic shock syndrome.
          (i) Includes cephalexin, clindamycin, or amoxicillin/clavulanate.
      4. Cautery
        (a) Done with silver nitrate or electrocautery.
    ii. Posterior nosebleeds are treated with the following:
      1. Posterior nasal packing
        (a) Carry a significant morbidity, includes difficulty swallowing, otitis media, sinusitis, and hypoxia.
      2. Embolization
      3. Ligation
V. Nasal polyps
  a. General
    i. Two types:
      1. Eosinophilic
        (a) Most common type.
        (b) Associated with intrinsic asthma and aspirin sensitivity.

      2. Neutrophilic
        (a) Associated with cystic fibrosis, sinusitis, and immune deficiency.
  b. Clinical manifestations
    i. May cause severe obstruction and anosmia.
    ii. Type of nasal secretion varies with type of polyp.
      1. Eosinophilic type presents with seromucous secretion.
      2. Neutrophilic type presents with purulent secretions.
    iii. On physical examination polyps will be noted.
    iv. Nasal cytology reveals increased eosinophils, with or without increased number of basophils, in eosinophilic type and increased neutrophils, with or without bacteria, in neutrophilic type.
  c. Treatment
    i. Eosinophilic type treated with intranasal or oral corticosteroids.
    ii. Neutrophilic type treated with antibiotics.

MOUTH/THROAT DISORDERS

I. Acute pharyngitis/Tonsillitis
  a. General
    i. Acute infection of the pharyngeal mucosa
    ii. Etiologies include:
      1. *Streptococcus pyogenes*
      2. Adenovirus
      3. Rhinovirus
      4. Enterovirus
      5. Influenzae A and B
      6. Epstein-Barr virus
      7. Respiratory syncytial virus
  b. Clinical manifestations
    i. Presents with mild sore throat to severe pain with swallowing or talking, with or without fever.
    ii. On physical examination the pharynx is erythematosus with or without exudates and cervical lymphadenopathy is noted.
    iii. Symptoms and physical examination findings vary with etiology.
      1. Rhinorrhea suggests viral etiology.
      2. Pharyngeal exudates suggest streptococcal or Epstein-Barr.

NOTES

3. Vesicles or ulcers suggest herpes simplex.
4. Conjunctival congestion suggests adenovirus.
   c. Diagnosis
   i. Diagnosis of *S. pyogenes* can be made with rapid strep screen or throat culture.
   d. Treatment
   i. Complications include rheumatic fever and acute glomerulonephritis.
   ii. If bacterial treatment consists of penicillin, amoxicillin, erythromycin, clarithromycin, or azithromycin.
   iii. Symptomatic treatment consists of fluids, warm saline gargles, and NSAIDs.

II. Aphthous ulcers
   a. General
   i. One of the most common oral lesions.
   ii. Etiology is unknown, but may be linked to human herpesvirus 6.
   iii. Three factors known to predispose to ulcer formations.
      1. Immune imbalance
      2. Defect in mucosal barrier
      3. Allergic response
   iv. Involve the nonkeratinized epithelium and begin as an erythematosus macule that ulcerates and forms a central fibropurulent eschar.
   b. Clinical manifestations
   i. Present with multiple, painful ulcers that measure from 2–3 mm to several cm in diameter.
   ii. Mainly involve the labial or buccal mucosa.
   iii. Disease may be more severe in immunocompromised patients.
   c. Treatment
   i. Treatment consists of topical corticosteroids, such as dexamethasone or fluocinonide.

III. Dental abscess
   a. General
   i. Periodontal abscess may be focal or diffuse.
   ii. Due to entrapment of plaque and debris in the periodontal pocket.
   iii. Periodontal disease is the most common cause of tooth loss.
   iv. Gingivitis is the acute and chronic inflammation of the gingiva.

QUESTION

Which of the following medications is a mast cell stabilizer?

A. Montelukast (Singulair)
B. Oxymetazoline (Afrin)
C. Ipratropium bromide (Atrovent)
D. Cromolyn sodium (Intal)

1. Due to local irritation and microbial invasion.
2. Gums are bluish-red, swollen, and bleed easily.
3. Local débridement is needed and possibly oral antibiotics, such as penicillin or metronidazole.
   b. Clinical manifestations
   i. Present with a painful, red, fluctuant swelling of the gingiva.
   ii. Gingiva is very tender to palpation.
   iii. Pus can be expelled from the periodontal pocket after probing of the pocket.
   c. Treatment
   i. Small abscesses can be treated with warm saline rinses and oral antibiotics penicillin or erythromycin.
   ii. Large abscesses require incision and drainage.

IV. Epiglottis
   a. General
   i. A respiratory emergency.
   ii. More common in children ages 2–6 and adults.
   iii. Caused by:
      1. *H. influenzae* type b
      2. *S. pneumoniae*
      3. *S. pyogenes*
      4. *S. aureus*
   b. Clinical manifestations
   i. Present with a short, rapidly progressive febrile illness.
   ii. Also have sore throat, pain with swallowing, and shortness of breath.
   iii. On physical examination the patient appears toxic, assumes a forward leaning

NOTES

ANSWER **D** EXPLANATION: *Cromolyn sodium is a mast cell stabilizer.*

correct ☐   incorrect ☐

position, neck-extended position, and with drooling of secretions.
1. A child may also present with stridor and tachypnea.
iv. Indirect laryngoscopy demonstrates a cherry-red epiglottis.
v. Examination of the pharynx should be attempted only if intubation is available.
c. Diagnosis
i. Laboratory tests reveal a leukocytosis and blood cultures are typically positive.
ii. X-ray of the neck shows an enlarged edematous epiglottis (thumbprint sign) and normal subglottic space.
1. See Figure 5-2.

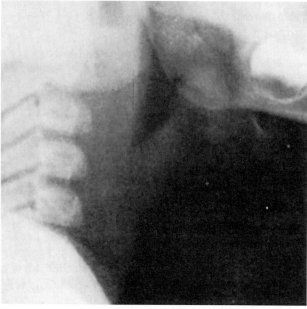

Figure 5-2 Soft-tissue X-ray of lateral neck showing an edematous epiglottis space (thumbprint sign). (From Behrman RE: Nelson's Textbook of Pediatrics, 17th ed. Philadelphia, Elsevier Saunders 2004, p. 1406, Fig. 371-2.)

d. Treatment
i. Maintaining a patent airway is most important.
ii. Antibiotic treatment consists of:
1. Cefotaxime
2. Ceftriaxone
3. Ampicillin/sulbactam
4. Chloramphenicol
iii. Secondary attacks can be decreased with the prophylactic use of rifampin.
iv. Incidence of disease has decreased with mass vaccination for *H. influenzae* type b.
V. Laryngitis
a. General
i. Defined as inflammation of the larynx caused by a variety of infectious agents.
1. Most frequent noninfectious cause is voice abuse.
ii. Most commonly due to viral agents, such as rhinovirus, influenzae, adenovirus, respiratory syncytial virus, or parainfluenzae.
1. Bacterial cause less common and typically due to *S. pyogenes* or *M. catarrhalis*.
b. Clinical manifestations
i. Symptoms include hoarseness, aphonia, rhinitis, and pharyngitis.
ii. On physical examination the larynx is hyperemic, edematous, and with or without ulcerations.
c. Treatment
i. Treatment is typically supportive with voice rest, warm saline gargles, and increased humidity
VI. Oral candidiasis
a. General
i. Most cases due to infection with the fungal organism *Candida albicans*, which can infect any mucosal surface in the body.
ii. *Candida* is normal flora in many areas of the body and only causes disease when normal host defenses are altered.
b. Clinical manifestations
i. Presents with multiple white patches on the tongue, palate, and other areas of the oral mucosa.
ii. The patches are easily removed by scraping with a tongue blade to reveal a red, irritated mucosa.

NOTES

c. Diagnosis
  i. Budding yeast and hyphae can be seen on KOH prep or Gram stain of the scrapings.
d. Treatment
  i. Topical antifungal agents, such as nystatin or clotrimazole, are effective.
  ii. If systemic treatment is required then fluconazole or itraconazole are effective.
  iii. Dentures must be removed and properly cleaned.

VII. Oral herpes simplex
a. General
  i. Typically due to herpes simplex type 1 (HSV-1), but herpes simplex type 2 can also cause infection.
  ii. Present with an acute infection, the virus lies dormant and is then reactivated to cause latent infections.
    1. Reactivation may occur secondary to trauma, fever, stress, or exposure to ultraviolet light.
b. Clinical manifestations
  i. Appear as a group or single vesicular lesion that becomes pustular to form single or multiple ulcers.
  ii. May present with a burning pain prior to vesicle formation.
  iii. Lesions can be very painful and last 5–10 days.
  iv. Fever and lymphadenopathy can also be noted, and may occur prior to the appearance of the vesicles.
c. Diagnosis
  i. Giemsa stain may reveal giant multinucleated cells (Tzanck smear).
  ii. Immunofluorescence or antigen-detection testing can be used in oral herpes infections to assist in diagnosis.
  iii. Viral culture can be used.
d. Treatment
  i. Treatment consists of the antivirals acyclovir, valacyclovir, or famciclovir.
    1. Can be given orally or used topically.
  ii. Avoiding contact with infected patients can reduce the risk of transmission.
  iii. Suppression therapy with antivirals can be used if history of frequent recurrences.

QUESTION

A 5-year-old child presents looking acutely ill and with a temperature of 103°F. The patient prefers to sit up and lean forward. He is drooling and can barely speak. The mother states that the patient was fine 24 hours ago. Which of the following is the most likely diagnosis?

  A. Croup
  B. Epiglottitis
  C. Bronchiectasis
  D. Foreign body aspiration

VIII. Oral leukoplakia
a. General
  i. Leukoplakia appears as white patches in the oral cavity that cannot be removed with scraping.
    1. Noted in smokers and thought to be premalignant.
  ii. Oral hairy leukoplakia is a white lesion found on the sides of the tongue or soft palate.
    1. Is not malignant or premalignant.
    2. Maybe noted in patients with human immunodeficiency virus (HIV), posttransplant, or on steroids.
b. Clinical manifestations
  i. Appear as white patches that cannot be removed with scraping.
c. Diagnosis
  i. Biopsy is required to evaluate for malignant conditions.
d. Treatment
  i. Acyclovir can be used, but lesions will recur when medication stopped.

IX. Peritonsillar abscess
a. General
  i. A complication of adenotonsillitis and typically due to infection with a mixture of aerobic and anaerobic bacterial organisms.
  ii. Develops when a bacterial infection extends beyond the tonsillar capsule and into surrounding tissues.

NOTES

ANSWER **B** EXPLANATION: *Epiglottis, most common in children age 2-6, is a rapidly progressive disease that presents with sore throat, dysphagia, and shortness of breath. On examination, the child appears toxic, is leaning forward, and drooling. Examination of the pharynx should be avoided unless intubation is available.*

correct ☐   incorrect ☐

1. Abscess develops between the capsule wall and the pharyngeal muscles.
   b. Clinical manifestations
      i. Present with severe odynophagia.
      ii. On physical examination the infected tonsil is displaced to the midline or beyond.
   c. Diagnosis
      i. Needle aspiration confirms the diagnosis.
   d. Treatment
      i. Needle aspiration or incision and drainage may be required.
      ii. Systemic antibiotics, such as penicillin or clindamycin, are required.

X. Sialadenitis
   a. General
      i. Inflammation resulting from decreased saliva production or alterations in saliva flow.
      ii. There may or may not be an obstruction.
         1. A sialolithiasis (stone in the salivary duct) may be the cause.
      iii. Typically noted only in adults.
   b. Clinical manifestations
      i. Present with painful swelling of the salivary gland, especially with eating.
      ii. If a stone is present it may be palpated.
   c. Diagnosis
      i. CT scan may be needed to rule out a malignant tumor.
      ii. Sialography may be helpful in finding an obstruction.
   d. Treatment
      i. Conservative therapy and surgical gland excision are the most successful treatment.
         1. Conservative treatment consists of oral hygiene, increased hydration, massage of affected gland, and use of sialagogues.

Question 1

Which of the following is a clinical finding of bacterial conjunctivitis?

A. Conjunctival itching
B. Bright red hyperemia
C. Profuse discharge
D. Periauricular adenopathy

Question 2

Which of the following is the first step in the evaluation of the patient with a foreign body in the eye?

A. Visual acuity
B. Schiotz tonometry
C. Fluorescein staining
D. MRI scanning

NOTES

Question 3

A patient presents with vertigo after a recent URI. The patient denies tinnitus or hearing loss. On physical examination the vertigo is present with the patient's eyes open or closed. Which of the following is the most likely diagnosis?

    A. Vestibular neuronitis
    B. Ménière's disease
    C. Acoustic neuroma
    D. Multiple sclerosis

Question 4

A 75-year-old presents with epistaxis. The bleeding is brisk and blood is noted in the posterior pharynx. Which of the following is the most appropriate intervention?

    A. Anterior nasal packing
    B. Silver nitrate
    C. Vasoconstrictors
    D. Embolization

Question 5

A 30-year-old presents with odynophagia. On physical examination the uvula is noted to be to the left of midline. Which of the following is the treatment of choice?

    A. Erythromycin
    B. Cefazolin
    C. Vancomycin
    D. Clindamycin

Question 6

Which of the following is a risk factor for malignant otitis externa?

    A. Smoking
    B. Diabetes
    C. Neomycin use
    D. Perforated tympanic membrane

Question 7

Which of the following type of hypersensitivity immune response is noted in allergic rhinitis?

    A. Type I
    B. Type II
    C. Type III
    D. Type IV

Answer 1

ANSWER C EXPLANATION: *Bacterial conjunctivitis presents with bright red hyperemia, moderate tearing, and profuse discharge. Preauricular adenopathy is more common in viral conjunctivitis.*

Topic: Conjunctivitis

correct ☐   **incorrect** ☐

NOTES

Answer 2

ANSWER **A** EXPLANATION: *Visual acuity should be determined before the evaluation of any patient with possible ocular foreign body.*

Topic: Foreign body-ocular

correct ☐   incorrect ☐

Answer 3

ANSWER **A** EXPLANATION: *Vestibular neuronitis (labyrinthitis) typically develops after a viral infection and presents with vertigo (present with eyes open or closed), nystagmus, nausea, and vomiting. No tinnitus or hearing loss is noted.*

Topic: Labyrinthitis

correct ☐   incorrect ☐

Answer 4

ANSWER **D** EXPLANATION: *Epistaxis that is profuse and with blood present in the posterior pharynx is typical of posterior epistaxis. Posterior epistaxis is most commonly treated with posterior nasal packing and possibly embolization or ligation.*

Topic: Epistaxis

correct ☐   incorrect ☐

Answer 5

ANSWER **D** EXPLANATION: *Odynophagia and displacement of the uvula or tonsil past midline is the typical presentation of peritonsillar abscess. Peritonsillar abscess is typically treated with systemic antibiotics such as penicillin or clindamycin.*

Topic: Peritonsillar abscess

correct ☐   incorrect ☐

Answer 6

ANSWER **B** EXPLANATION: *Malignant otitis externa is most commonly noted in elderly diabetic patients and typically due to infection with Pseudomonas aeruginosa.*

Topic: Otitis externa

correct ☐   incorrect ☐

Answer 7

CORRECT ANSWER **A** EXPLANATION: *Type I hypersensitivity reaction, with increase production of IgE, mediates the immune response in allergic rhinitis.*

Topic: Allergic rhinitis

correct ☐   incorrect ☐

NOTES

Reproductive System

6

EXAM BLUEPRINT TOPICS

Uterus
Dysfunctional uterine bleeding
Endometrial cancer
Endometriosis/Adenomyosis
Leiomyoma
Metritis
Prolapse
Ovary
Cysts
Neoplasms
Cervix
Carcinoma
Cervicitis
Dysplasia
Incompetent
Vagina/Vulva
Cystocele
Neoplasm
Rectocele
Vaginitis
Menstrual Disorders
Amenorrhea
Dysmenorrhea
Premenstrual syndrome
Menopause
Breast
Abscess
Carcinoma
Fibroadenoma
Fibrocystic disease
Mastitis
Pelvic Inflammatory Disease
Contraceptive Methods
Infertility
Uncomplicated Pregnancy
Prenatal diagnosis/care
Normal labor/delivery
Complicated Pregnancy

Abortion
Abruptio placentae
Dystocia
Ectopic pregnancy
Gestational diabetes
Gestational trophoblastic disease
Molar pregnancy
Multiple gestation
Placenta previa
Postpartum hemorrhage
Pregnancy-induced hypertension
Premature rupture of membranes
Rh incompatibility

I. Menstrual Cycle
   a. Menarche
      i. Average age of onset is between ages 12 and 13.
      ii. The menstrual cycle is typically irregular, due to anovulatory cycles, for the first 6 months to 1 year after menarche.
   b. Menstrual cycle (see Figure 6-1)
      i. Two phases: follicular and luteal phases.
      ii. Follicular phase
         1. Release of follicle-stimulating hormone (FSH) from the pituitary results in development of primary ovarian follicle.
         2. Ovarian follicle produces estrogen, which causes the uterine lining to proliferate.
         3. At mid-cycle, day 14, luteinizing hormone (LH) spikes in response to the estrogen surge. This stimulates release of the ovum from the follicle.
      iii. Luteal phase
         1. Begins after release of the ovum.
         2. Follicle remnants in the ovary develop into the corpus luteum and secrete progesterone.

NOTES

3. Progesterone maintains the uterine lining in preparation for implantation of the fertilized ovum.
   (a) If fertilization occurs the developing trophoblast synthesizes human chorionic gonadotropin (hCG) that maintains the corpus luteum until the placenta develops.
4. If no fertilization the corpus luteum degenerates and progesterone levels fall.
5. Without progesterone the endometrial lining is sloughed off.
6. The withdrawal of estrogen and progesterone leads to gradual increase in FSH.
7. Release of FSH results in development of primary ovarian follicles and the start of the follicular phase.

II. Tanner staging (see Table 6-1)

III. Uterus
   a. Dysfunctional bleeding
      i. General
         1. A diagnosis of exclusion. If no pathologic cause of menorrhagia, metrorrhagia, or menometrorrhagia the diagnosis is made.
         2. May be secondary to anovulation with a disruption of the hypothalamic-pituitary-gonadal that causes continuous estrogen stimulation of the endometrium that overgrows and sloughs off at irregular times and varying amounts.
         3. Typically occurs near menarche and menopause.
      ii. Diagnosis
         1. A careful workup including history and physical to rule out other causes before the diagnosis is made.
         2. Endometrial sampling is the gold standard to determine if ovulation is occurring.

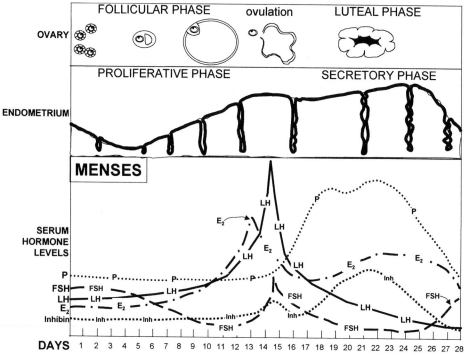

Figure 6-1 The normal menstrual cycle. (From Larsen PR: Williams Textbook of Endocrinology, 10th ed. Philadelphia, Elsevier Saunders 2003, p. 607, Fig. 16-22.)

NOTES

Table 6-1 • Tanner Staging

		Breast Development
	Average Age (years)	Description
Stage 1		Preadolescent, elevation of papilla only
Stage 2	10.1–12.3	Breast bud stage, elevation of breast and papilla, areolar enlargement
Stage 3	11.0–13.2	Further enlargement of breast and areola without separation of contour
Stage 4	11.9–14.3	Projection of areola and papilla to form the secondary mound
Stage 5	13.6–17.1	Mature stage, projection of papilla only as areola recedes to breast contour
		Pubic Hair (Male and Female)
	Average Age (years)	Description
Stage 1		Preadolescent, no pubic hair
Stage 2	M 12.4–14.5 F 10.5–12.9	Sparse growth of long, slightly pigmented downy hair, mainly at base of penis or along labia
Stage 3	M 12.9–14.9 F 11.3–12.9	Darker, coarser, curled hair spread sparsely over junction of pubes
Stage 4	M 13.3–15.4 F 11.9–14.0	Hair resembles adult in type, distribution smaller than adult, no spread to medial surface of thighs
Stage 5	M 14.1–16.3 F 13.3–15.5	Adult in quantity and type of distribution of the horizontal pattern
		Genital Development (Male)
	Average Age (years)	Description
Stage 1		Preadolescent, testes, scrotum, and penis same size and proportion as early childhood
Stage 2	10.6–12.7	Enlargement of scrotum and testes, skin of scrotum darkens and changes texture, penis little or no change
Stage 3	11.8–13.9	Enlargement of penis, first in length, testes and scrotum grow further
Stage 4	12.8–14.8	Increased size of penis, growth in breadth and development of glans, darkening of scrotal skin and enlargement of testes and scrotum
Stage 5	13.8–16.0	Adult size and shape

NOTES

iii. Treatment
1. Oral contraceptives are used to regulate menstrual cycle if patient not hemorrhaging and is stable.
2. If excessive bleeding, use conjugated estrogens.
3. With ovulatory dysfunctional uterine bleeding, nonsteroidal anti-inflammatory drugs (NSAIDs) can decrease menstrual blood loss.
4. If no response to medical therapy may use surgical intervention.
  (a) Dilation and curettage is the first treatment of choice.
  (b) Hysterectomy is the definitive surgery and used for refractory cases.

b. Endometrial cancer
i. General
1. Most common gynecologic cancer in the United States.
  (a) Median age at diagnosis is 60 years.
2. Most common type is adenocarcinoma, followed by mucinous, clear cell, and squamous cell.
3. Prognostic factors include:
  (a) Histologic grade
  (b) Myometrial invasion
  (c) Histologic type
ii. Risk factors
1. Nulliparity
2. Late menopause
3. Diabetes mellitus
4. Obesity
5. Unopposed estrogen therapy
6. Tamoxifen use
iii. Clinical manifestations
1. Most common symptom is irregular bleeding, including prolonged heavy periods or spotting.
2. Typically have a normal pelvic examination.
iv. Diagnosis
1. Endometrial biopsy is the test of choice.
2. Pelvic ultrasound needed to rule out fibroids, polyps, and endometrial hyperplasia.
v. Treatment
1. Depends on staging.

2. Treatment includes surgical staging, total abdominal hysterectomy and bilateral salpingo-oophorectomy, and postoperative radiation therapy.
3. High-dose progestins are the first-line treatment for advanced and recurrent disease.

c. Endometriosis
i. General
1. Presence of endometrial tissue outside the endometrial cavity.
  (a) Most common sites are ovary, pelvic peritoneum, round ligament, fallopian tubes, and sigmoid colon.
2. Found in women of reproductive age.
ii. Clinical manifestations
1. Symptoms include dysmenorrhea, dyspareunia, infertility, abnormal bleeding, and chronic pelvic pain.
  (a) Symptoms vary with area involved.
2. Physical examination findings are subtle early in the disease.
  (a) When disease more disseminated may note uterosacral nodularity or a fixed or retroverted uterus.
  (b) If an ovary is involved a tender, fixed adnexal mass may be noted.
iii. Diagnosis
1. Direct visualization with laparoscopy is required to make the diagnosis.
iv. Treatment
1. Treatment aimed at suppression and atrophy of endometrial tissue.
2. Options include:
  (a) Oral contraceptives or medroxyprogesterone
    (i) Suppresses ovulation and menstruation, avoiding dysmenorrhea.
    (ii) Conception not possible.
  (b) Danazol, an androgen derivative, or gonadotropin-releasing hormone
    (i) Suppress FSH and LH, which results in diminished estrogen production and decrease in endometriosis.
    (ii) Side effects of danazol include acne, weight gain, edema, and hirsutism.

NOTES

(iii) Side effects of gonadotropin-releasing hormone include hot flashes and decreased bone density.

(c) Surgical treatment
  (i) Conservation options include ablation, electrocauterization, or excision of visible endometriosis.
  (ii) Definitive therapy includes abdominal hysterectomy and bilateral salpingo-oophorectomy, lysis of adhesions, and removal of endometriosis lesions.

d. Adenomyosis
  i. General
     1. Extension of endometrial glands and stroma into the uterine musculature.
     2. Cause is unknown.
     3. Typically develops in parous women in their late 30s or early 40s.
     4. Increased risk of endometriosis and leiomyoma.
  ii. Clinical manifestations
     1. Patients may be asymptomatic.
     2. Most common symptoms are secondary dysmenorrhea, menorrhagia, or both.
     3. On physical examination may note an enlarged uterus with a soft consistency.
  iii. Diagnosis
     1. Definitive diagnosis made via hysterectomy.
     2. Magnetic resonance imaging (MRI) may identify adenomyosis.
  iv. Treatment
     1. Analgesics may be used in mild disease.
     2. Hysterectomy is the only definitive treatment.

e. Leiomyoma
  i. General
     1. Also called fibroids.
     2. Due to local proliferation of smooth muscle cells of the uterus.
        (a) Etiology is unknown.
     3. Typically occur in women of childbearing age and regress during menopause.
     4. More common in African-American women.
  ii. Clinical manifestations
     1. Most women have no clinical symptoms.

QUESTION

Which of the following stimulates release of the ovum from the follicle on day 14 of the menstrual cycle?

A. Inhibin
B. Progesterone
C. Luteinizing hormone
D. Follicle-stimulating hormone

     2. Most common symptom is abnormal uterine bleeding.
     3. Symptoms also include pressure-related symptoms (pelvic pressure, fullness, or heaviness) and infertility.
     4. Physical examination reveals masses noted on bimanual or abdominal exam.
        (a) Mass is a nontender, irregular, enlarged uterus.
  iii. Diagnosis
     1. Pelvic ultrasound reveals hypoechogenic areas among normal myometrial material.
  iv. Treatment
     1. Treatment is typically not required.
     2. Treatment needed if severe pain, infertility, or evidence of growth.
        (a) Medical treatment to shrink the fibroids includes medroxyprogesterone, danazol, and gonadotropin-releasing hormone agonists.
        (b) Surgical treatment includes myomectomy and hysterectomy.

f. Metritis
  i. General
     1. Endometritis is infection of the uterine endometrium.
     2. Endomyometritis is infection invading into the myometrium.
     3. Infection preceded by instrumentation or disruption of the intrauterine cavity.
        (a) Most common after cesarean section, vaginal deliveries, dilation and evacuation or curettage, and intrauterine device (IUD) placement.

NOTES

ANSWER C Explanation: *At mid-cycle, day 14, luteinizing hormone spikes to stimulate release of the ovum from the follicle.*

correct ☐   incorrect ☐

    ii. Clinical manifestations
        1. Patients typically have fever.
        2. Bimanual examination reveals uterine tenderness.
        3. Lab tests reveal a leukocytosis.
    iii. Diagnosis
        1. Based on clinical history and presence of uterine tenderness, fever, and elevated white blood cell (WBC) count.
    iv. Treatment
        1. Treatment of severe disease is IV clindamycin or gentamicin.
        2. Mild disease is treated with cephalosporins.
        3. Chronic disease is treated with doxycycline.
  g. Prolapse
    i. General
        1. Abnormal protrusion of the uterus through the pelvic floor aperture.
        2. Due to injury or stretching of the cardinal ligaments.
        3. Occurs most commonly in multiparous women.
        4. Most commonly secondary to childbirth injury, but also noted with pelvic tumors, sacral nerve disorders, systemic disorders (obesity and asthma), and local conditions (ascites).
    ii. Clinical manifestations
        1. Present with a firm mass in the lower vagina, cervix projecting through the introitus, and vaginal inversion with cervix and uterus projecting between the legs.
        2. Physical examination reveals descent of the cervix to the lower third of the vagina or through the introitus with bearing down or straining.
    iii. Diagnosis
        1. Based on physical examination findings.

    iv. Treatment
        1. Kegel exercises can be used for prevention.
        2. Medical treatment includes a vaginal pessary and use of estrogens to improve tissue tone.
        3. Surgical treatment to improve vaginal support may be needed.
IV. Ovaries
  a. Cysts
    i. General
        1. Functional cysts result from normal physiologic functioning of the ovaries.
        2. Two types of functional cysts: follicular and corpus luteum cysts.
        3. Most commonly occur between puberty and menopause.
        4. Smoking increases risk of functional cysts.
    ii. Clinical manifestations
        1. Follicular cysts are typically asymptomatic, but large cysts can cause pelvic pain, dyspareunia, and lead to ovarian torsion.
          (a) Tend to be less than 8 cm in size.
        2. Lutein cysts may cause pelvic pain and amenorrhea or delayed menses.
          (a) Tend to be larger than follicular cysts and more firm or solid on palpation.
        3. Physical examination varies with type of cyst.
        4. A torsed or ruptured cyst will cause pain on palpation, acute abdominal pain, and rebound tenderness.
        5. Polycystic ovarian disease
          (a) Present with anovulation, oligomenorrhea, amenorrhea, hirsutism, obesity, and enlarged ovaries.
    iii. Diagnosis
        1. Pelvic ultrasound is the test of choice for the workup of ovarian cysts.
    iv. Treatment
        1. Treatment varies with age and size of cyst.
          (a) Premenarchal with cyst greater than 2 cm: treated with exploratory laparotomy.

NOTES

(b) Reproductive age and cyst less than 6 cm: observed for 6 weeks.
(c) Reproductive age and cyst greater than 8 cm: treated with exploratory laparotomy.
(d) Postmenopausal age and palpable cyst: treated with exploratory laparotomy.
   2. Polycystic ovarian disease
      (a) Treatment depends on symptoms and desire for fertility.
         (i) If desiring fertility start clomiphene citrate.
b. Neoplasms
   i. General
      1. Third most common cancer of the female genital tract.
      2. Ovarian carcinoma primarily spreads by direct exfoliation of malignant cells.
      3. Cause is unknown but may be due to malignant transformation of ovarian tissue after long period of chronic uninterrupted ovulation.
      4. Increased risk with positive family history, history of uninterrupted ovulation, and breast cancer.
         (a) Oral contraceptives may have a protective effect.

QUESTION

A 36-year-old female presents with a 4-year history of infertility, severe dysmenorrhea, and increasing dyspareunia. Pelvic exam reveals a 5-cm right ovarian mass. Nodules are palpated along the uterosacral ligament. Which of the following is the most likely diagnosis?

   A. Ectopic pregnancy
   B. Endometriosis
   C. Sertoli-Leydig cell tumor
   D. Follicular cyst

      5. See Table 6-2 for summary of ovarian carcinoma.
   ii. Clinical manifestations
      1. Patients are often asymptomatic until disease is advanced.
      2. May present with vague lower abdominal pain and abdominal enlargement.
      3. Physical examination reveals a solid, fixed pelvic mass and possible ascites.
         (a) Malignant tumors tend to be fixed, solid, bilateral, and nodular.

Table 6-2 • Summary of Ovarian Carcinoma

	Epithelial Tumors	Germ Cell	Sex Cord Stroma
Frequency	65%–70%	15%–20%	5%–10%
Age group	50s	1–25	All ages
Clinical	Elevated CA-125	Rapidly enlarging mass	Have hormone production
Treatment	Surgery Cisplatin-based chemotherapy	Surgery Multidrug chemotherapy	Surgery
Cell types	Serous Mucinous Endometrioid Clear cell	Teratoma Choriocarcinoma Dysgerminoma	Sertoli-Leydig cell Fibroma Granulosa-theca cell
5-year survival	Less than 20%	60–85%	90%

NOTES

ANSWER **B** EXPLANATION: *Endometriosis presents with infertility, dysmenorrhea, dyspareunia, and chronic pelvic pain. On examination, an ovarian or adnexal mass be noted.*

correct ☐   incorrect ☐

   iii. Diagnosis
      1. Pelvic ultrasound is the test of choice.
        (a) Malignant masses tend to be greater than 8 cm in size, solid, multilocular, and bilateral.
      2. Tumor markers such as CA-125, alpha-fetoprotein, and hCGs.
   iv. Treatment
      1. Varies with cell type.
V. Cervix
  a. Carcinoma
    i. General
      1. Cervical cancer and premalignant cervical dysplasia are correlated with onset of sexual activity at an early age and increased number of sexual partners.
      2. Human papillomavirus is the primary causative agent.
        (a) Serotypes 16, 18, and 31 are correlated with cervical cancer.
      3. Most common cell type is squamous cell carcinoma followed by adenocarcinoma.
        (a) Clear cell carcinoma, a type of adenocarcinoma, is linked to exposure in utero of diethylstilbestrol (DES) exposure.
    ii. Clinical manifestations
      1. Classic presentation is postcoital bleeding.
        (a) Other symptoms may include abnormal vaginal bleeding, watery discharge, or pelvic pain.
      2. On bimanual examination a mass within the cervix may be palpated.
    iii. Diagnosis
      1. Screen for disease with Pap smear.
        (a) Recommendation for annual Pap smear in anyone until 3 years after

onset of sexual activity or age 21, whatever is first.
      2. With any abnormal Pap smear the cervix should be biopsied colposcopically.
    iv. Treatment
      1. With microinvasion carcinoma a cone biopsy should be performed if fertility wishes to be maintained.
      2. With invasive cervical carcinoma radical hysterectomy is indicated, if not spread beyond the cervix, uterine corpus, and vagina.
      3. Curative or palliative radiation therapy can also be used.
      4. Cisplatin-based chemotherapy with radiation therapy has been found to be effective against bulky stage disease.
  b. Cervicitis
    i. General
      1. Most common infectious agents include:
        (a) *Chlamydia trachomatis*
        (b) *Neisseria gonorrhoeae*
        (c) Herpes simplex virus
        (d) *Candida albicans*
        (e) *Trichomonas vaginalis*
        (f) *Gardnerella vaginalis*
    ii. Clinical manifestations
      1. Acute cervicitis
        (a) Primary symptom is purulent vaginal discharge.
          (i) Gonorrhea: thick and creamy
          (ii) Gardnerella: thin and gray discharge
          (iii) Candidiasis: white and curd-like discharge
          (iv) Chlamydia: purulent discharge
          (v) Trichomonas: foamy and greenish-white
        (b) Other symptoms include leukorrhea (caused by endocervical inflammation), infertility, pelvic discomfort, and dyspareunia.
        (c) On physical examination note acutely inflamed, edematous cervix with purulent discharge.
      2. Chronic cervicitis
        (a) Leukorrhea is the major symptom.

NOTES

 iii. Diagnosis
  1. Diagnosis made through various smears.
   (a) Wet mount: motile flagellated *T. vaginalis* may be noted.
   (b) In candidiasis KOH prep may reveal spores or hyphae.
   (c) Clue cells noted in *G. vaginalis* infection.
   (d) Gram stain reveals Gram-negative, intracellular diplococci in gonorrhea.
 iv. Treatment
  1. Treat based on specific organism.
   (a) *T. vaginalis*: metronidazole
   (b) Candidiasis: nystatin, miconazole or clotrimazole.
   (c) *G. vaginalis*: metronidazole
   (d) Gonorrhea: ceftriaxone or azithromycin.
   (e) Chlamydia: doxycycline or azithromycin.
  2. See infectious disease chapter for more information on treatment for the specific organisms.
c. Dysplasia
 i. General
  1. Thought to be a precursor to cervical cancer.
  2. Cervical intraepithelial neoplasia I (CIN I) takes 7 years to become cervical cancer; it takes 4 years for CIN II to become cervical cancer.
 ii. Clinical manifestations
  1. No clinical signs or symptoms.
 iii. Diagnosis
  1. Diagnosis made by Pap smear and confirmed by biopsy.
 iv. Treatment
  1. CIN I followed with colposcopy every 3–4 months.
  2. CIN II or III treated with destruction or excision of the lesions.
   (a) Cryotherapy or laser therapy can be used.
   (b) Loop electrosurgical excision procedure (LEEP) is used to remove endocervical lesions.

QUESTION

CA-125 is elevated in which of the following?

 A. Leiomyoma
 B. Endometriosis
 C. Ovarian cancer
 D. Cervical cancer

 d. Incompetent cervix
  i. General
   1. With an incompetent cervix fetal membranes are exposed to vaginal flora and risk of increased trauma.
   2. Infection, vaginal discharge, and premature rupture of membranes are common in patients with incompetent cervix.
   3. Increased risk of incompetent cervix with surgery or cervical trauma.
  ii. Clinical manifestations
   1. Patients present with painless dilation and effacement of the cervix, often during the second trimester of pregnancy.
   2. May also note bleeding, vaginal discharge, or rupture of membranes.
  iii. Diagnosis
   1. Diagnosis based on physical examination.
  iv. Treatment
   1. Strict bed rest.
   2. Placement of a cerclage, a suture placed vaginally to close the cervix.
VI. Vagina/Vulva
 a. Cystocele
  i. General
   1. Descent of a portion of the posterior bladder wall and trigone into the vagina.
   2. Typically due to the trauma of parturition.
  ii. Clinical manifestations
   1. A small cystocele causes no significant symptoms.
   2. If large the patient may complain of vaginal pressure or a protruding mass.
   3. Symptoms are aggravated with prolonged standing, coughing, or straining.

NOTES

ANSWER **C** EXPLANATION: *The tumor marker CA-125 is elevated in ovarian cancer. May also be elevated in pregnancy, menstruation, and endometriosis.*

correct ☐   incorrect ☐

4. Urinary incontinence is also noted.
5. On physical examination a relaxed vaginal outlet with a thin-walled, smooth bulging mass involving the anterior vaginal wall.
   (a) With straining the mass may project through the vaginal introitus.
iii. Treatment
   1. Kegel exercises may assist in prevention.
   2. Medical measures include a vaginal pessary, Kegel exercises, or estrogens.
   3. Surgery seldom indicated unless cystocele is large.
      (a) An anterior vaginal colporrhaphy is most effective in patients with a large cystocele.
b. Neoplasm
   i. Vaginal
   1. General
      (a) Peak incidence in women in their 50s.
      (b) Most common type is epithelial.
         (i) Increased risk of clear cell adenocarcinoma of the vagina with exposure to DES.
   2. Clinical manifestations
      (a) Many are asymptomatic or may present with vaginal discharge, bleeding, and vaginal pruritus.
   3. Diagnosis
      (a) Disease is screened for with the Pap smear and colposcopy.
      (b) Diagnosis is confirmed by biopsy.
   4. Treatment
      (a) Surgical resection and radiation therapy are used to treat vaginal carcinoma.
      (b) 5-year survival varies with clinical stage.

   ii. Vulva
   1. General
      (a) More common in older patients with peak incidence in women in their 60s.
   2. Clinical manifestations
      (a) Symptoms include vulvar pruritus and vulvodynia.
      (b) May also present with vulvar bleeding or mass.
   3. Diagnosis
      (a) Confirmed with biopsy.
   4. Treatment
      (a) Wide local excision with regional lymphadenectomy is the treatment of choice.
      (b) If metastatic disease is noted pelvic radiation is indicated.
c. Rectocele
   i. General
   1. Herniation of the rectum into the vaginal vault.
   2. Due to injury of the endopelvic fascia of the rectovaginal septum.
   ii. Clinical manifestations
   1. Small rectoceles are typically asymptomatic.
   2. With larger rectoceles vaginal pressure, rectal fullness, and incomplete evacuation are noted.
   3. On physical examination a soft, thin-walled rectovaginal septum projecting into the vagina.
   iii. Diagnosis
   1. Based on history and physical examination findings.
   iv. Treatment
   1. Medical measures include increasing fluids and laxatives.
   2. Surgical measures include posterior colpoperineorrhaphy.
d. Vaginitis
   i. Yeast infection
   1. General
      (a) Most commonly caused by *C. albicans*.
      (b) Predisposing factors include use of antibiotics, diabetes mellitus, and decreased cellular immunity.
      (c) Make up 20%–25% of all causes of vaginitis.

NOTES

2. Clinical manifestations
   (a) Symptoms include vulvar and vaginal pruritus, burning, dysuria, dyspareunia, and vaginal discharge.
   (b) On physical examination there is vulvar edema and erythema with a thick white vaginal discharge.
3. Diagnosis
   (a) Branching hyphae and spores noted on KOH prep.
   (b) Gram stain and culture are also used in diagnosis.
4. Treatment
   (a) Consists of azole agents via topical application.
   (b) Oral fluconazole is also effective.
ii. *Trichomonas vaginalis*
   1. General
      (a) A sexually transmitted disease (STD) caused by a unicellular flagellated protozoan.
      (b) Make up 15%–20% of all causes of vaginitis.

2. Clinical manifestations
   (a) Present with a profuse unpleasant smelling discharge.
   (b) The discharge may be yellow or green in color and frothy in appearance.
   (c) May also note vulvar erythema, edema, and pruritus.
   (d) On physical examination may note erythematosus, punctate epithelial papillae, or a strawberry appearance of the cervix.
3. Diagnosis
   (a) Wet prep reveals motile protozoan.
   (b) See Figure 6-2.
4. Treatment
   (a) Treatment consists of metronidazole for 7 days.
iii. *Gardnerella vaginalis*
   1. General
      (a) Risk factors include low socioeconomic status, IUD usage, multiple sexual partners, and smoking.

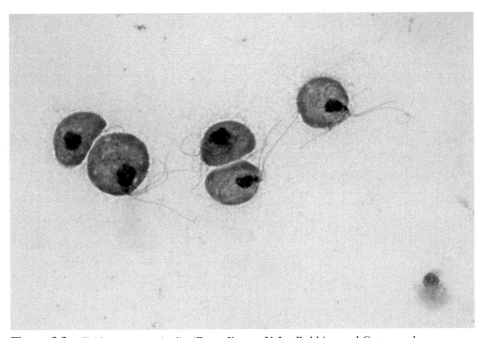

Figure 6-2   *Trichomonas vaginalis.* (From Kumar V. In: Robbins and Cotran, eds.: Pathologic Basis of Disease, 7th ed. Philadelphia, Elsevier Saunders 2005, p. 1064, Fig. 22-4.)

NOTES

(b) Make up 40%–50% of all causes of vaginitis.

2. Clinical manifestations

(a) Patients may be asymptomatic.

(b) Symptomatic patients note a profuse nonirritating discharge with a fishy odor.

3. Diagnosis

(a) On wet prep note epithelial cells covered by bacteria (clue cells).

(i) Clue cells are vaginal squamous epithelial cells covered with *G. vaginalis*, giving the cells a granular appearance.

(ii) See Figure 6-3.

(b) The fish odor can be enhanced with addition of KOH to the vaginal prep (Whiff test).

4. Treatment

(a) Consists of metronidazole or clindamycin.

VII. Menstrual disorders

a. Amenorrhea

i. General

1. Amenorrhea is the absence of menses.

(a) Primary amenorrhea is absence of menses in a woman who has not undergone menarche by age 16.

(i) See Table 6-3 for etiologies.

(b) Secondary amenorrhea is the absence of menses for 3 menstrual cycles or 6 months in a woman who previously had normal menses.

(i) Leading cause of secondary amenorrhea is pregnancy.

(ii) See Table 6-4 for etiologies.

ii. Clinical manifestations

1. Primary

(a) Workup based on phenotypic picture.

(i) Based on presence or absence of uterus and breasts.

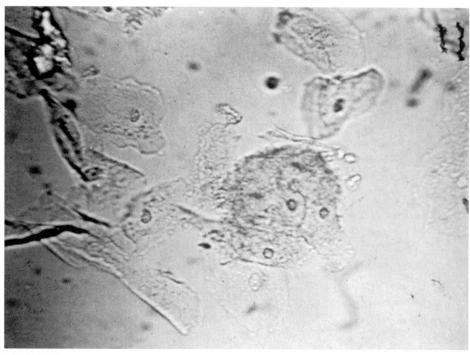

Figure 6-3 Clue cells seen in bacterial vaginosis. (From Ferri FF: Ferri's Clinical Advisor: Instant Diagnosis and Treatment. Philadelphia, Elsevier Saunders 2005, p. 876, Fig. 1-290.)

NOTES

Table 6-3 • Causes of Primary Amenorrhea

Outflow Obstruction	End-organ Disease	Central Regulatory Disease
Imperforate hymen	Ovarian failure	Hypothalamic disorder
Transverse vaginal septum	Gonadal agenesis	Pituitary disorder
Vaginal agenesis		
Testicular feminization		

QUESTION

A multiparous female presents with complaint of vaginal pressure and rectal fullness. She states she has to use laxatives to have a bowel movement. On examination, a soft, reducible mass bulging into the lower half of the vaginal wall is noted. Which of the following is the most likely diagnosis?

A. Irritable bowel syndrome
B. Intussusception
C. Rectocele
D. Cystocele

Table 6-4 • Causes of Secondary Amenorrhea

Anatomic	Ovarian Dysfunction	Hyperprolactinemia	Hypothalamic Disorders
Asherman syndrome	Premature ovarian failure	Primary hypothyroidism	Stress
Cervical stenosis	Polycystic ovarian disease	Medications Dopamine antagonists TCA MAO inhibitors Pituitary tumor	Exercise Anorexia nervosa Weight loss

TCA, Tricyclic antidepressants; MOA, Monoamine oxidase.

(b) Workup of a phenotypic female with absence of either uterus or breasts must include karyotype studies, testosterone level, and FSH level.

iii. Diagnosis
  1. See Table 6-5 for diagnostic features of primary amenorrhea.
  2. Diagnosis of secondary amenorrhea
    (a) Begins with a pregnancy test.
    (b) Thyroid-stimulating hormone (TSH) and prolactin levels should be checked to evaluate for hypothyroidism and hyperprolactinemia.
    (c) If prolactin is normal a progesterone challenge test should be done.
      (i) If patient has withdrawal bleeding this indicates that estrogen levels

are adequate and outflow tract is patent.

iv. Treatment
  1. Primary
    (a) Patients with a functional uterus and congenital abnormalities can be treated with surgery to allow menses flow.
    (b) Patients without a uterus are treated with estrogen replacement to effect breast development and prevent osteoporosis.
  2. Secondary
    (a) Treat underlying cause.
    (b) Patients with a positive progesterone challenge test should be treated with oral contraceptives to prevent endometrial hyperplasia.

NOTES

ANSWER C EXPLANATION: *Rectocele, herniation of the rectum into the vaginal vault, is due to injury to the rectovaginal septum. Symptoms include vaginal pressure and rectal fullness. On examination, a soft, thin-walled rectovaginal septum is noted in the vaginal vault.*

correct ☐   incorrect ☐

b. Dysmenorrhea
   i. General
      1. Pain and cramping during the menstrual cycle that interferes with normal daily activities.
      2. Classified as primary or secondary.
      3. Etiology
         (a) Primary dysmenorrhea has no obvious cause.
            (i) May be due to high levels of prostaglandins.
         (b) Secondary dysmenorrhea is due to endometriosis, fibroids, cervical stenosis, or pelvic adhesions.
   ii. Clinical manifestations
      1. Primary dysmenorrhea
         (a) Pain typically occurs on the first or second day of menstruation.
         (b) Associated symptoms may include headache, nausea, and vomiting.
         (c) On physical examination no abnormalities are typically noted except generalized tenderness in the lower abdomen/pelvis.
      2. Secondary dysmenorrhea
         (a) Patients with cervical stenosis present with scant menses and severe cramping pain that is relieved with increased menstrual flow.
            (i) Physical examination reveals scarring of the external os.
         (b) Patients with pelvic adhesions typically have a history of pelvic infections or prior pelvic surgery.
   iii. Diagnosis
      1. Primary dysmenorrhea is diagnosed based on history and lack of organic cause.
   iv. Treatment
      1. Primary dysmenorrhea is treated with NSAIDs and oral contraceptive pills.
      2. Treatment of secondary dysmenorrhea is based on the cause.
         (a) Endometriosis is treated with oral contraceptives, medroxyprogesterone, danazol, or surgery.
         (b) Cervical stenosis is treated with cervical dilation.
         (c) Pelvic adhesions are treated with NSAIDs and oral contraceptive pills. If no relief, surgery can be used to lyse the adhesions.
c. Premenstrual syndrome (PMS)
   i. General
      1. Occurs during the second half of the menstrual cycle.
      2. Etiology is unknown.
   ii. Clinical manifestations
      1. Symptoms include somatic, emotional, and behavioral complaints.

Table 6-5 • Diagnosis of Primary Amenorrhea		
	Uterus Present	**Uterus Absent**
Breasts present	Testicular feminization Müllerian agenesis	Congenital abnormalities
Breasts absent	Gonadal agenesis Enzyme deficiency in testosterone synthesis	Gonadal failure/agenesis Hypothalamic-pituitary axis dysfunction Hypothalamic, pituitary, or ovarian dysfunction

NOTES

(a) Somatic complaints include breast swelling and tenderness, bloating, headache, fatigue, and constipation.
(b) Emotional complaints include irritability, depression, anxiety, and libido changes.
(c) Behavioral complaints include food cravings, poor concentration, and sensitivity to noise.

   iii. Diagnosis
1. Based on history and physical examination.
2. To confirm diagnosis the patient must have a symptom-free follicular phase, for about 1 week.

   iv. Treatment
1. NSAIDs and oral contraceptive pills bring symptomatic relief.
2. Antidepressant drugs may be needed in some cases.

VIII. Menopause
  a. General
    i. Denotes the final menstruation and marks the end of reproductive capabilities.
    ii. In the United States occurs between the ages of 48–52.
      1. If menopause occurs before age 40 it is considered premature.
    iii. Due to diminished estrogen production that leads to increased levels of FSH and LH.
    iv. With menopause women lose the benefits of estrogen on lipid profile and vascular endothelium.
      1. Leads to increased risk of coronary artery disease.
      2. Also have loss of bone resorption that leads to osteopenia and osteoporosis.
  b. Clinical manifestations
    i. Symptoms include vasomotor flushing, sweats, mood changes, and depression.
      1. Due to fall in estradiol levels.
    ii. Physical examination may reveal decreasing breast size, and vaginal, urethral, and cervical atrophy.

QUESTION

Which of the following is the most common cause of secondary amenorrhea?

A. Obesity
B. Pregnancy
C. Turner's syndrome
D. Testicular feminization

---

    iii. Laboratory tests reveal an elevated FSH.
  c. Diagnosis
    i. Based on history and physical examination.
  d. Treatment
    i. Hormone replacement therapy may be considered.
      1. Benefits include stroke and myocardial infarction protection, decreased osteopenia and decreased number of hip fractures, and improvement of symptoms noted during menopause.
      2. Risk factors include cholestatic hepatic dysfunction, increased incidence of estrogen dependent neoplasm, increased risk of thromboembolic events, or undiagnosed vaginal bleeding.
      3. Progesterone is used in combination with estrogen therapy to decrease risk of endometrial hyperplasia and cancer.

IX. Breast
  a. Abscess
    i. General
      1. An acute inflammatory process that results in the formation of a collection of pus.
      2. Many breast abscesses are lactational.
      3. May also develop in patients with acute mastitis.
      4. Lactational breast abscess typically due to *Staphylococcus aureus.*
      5. Subareolar breast abscess is typically due to a mixed infection, including anaerobes, staphylococci, and streptococci.

NOTES

ANSWER **B** EXPLANATION: *Secondary amenorrhea, the absence of menstrual periods for six months in a women who had previously been regular, is most commonly due to pregnancy.*

correct ☐   incorrect ☐

---

    ii. Clinical manifestations
      1. May present with a painful, erythematosus mass in the breast with occasional drainage through the skin or nipple duct.
    iii. Diagnosis
      1. Based on physical examination findings.
    iv. Treatment
      1. Incision and drainage required.
      2. Carcinoma should be excluded by performing a biopsy.
      3. Antibiotics are needed.
        (a) Lactational abscess can be treated with nafcillin, cefazolin, or vancomycin.
        (b) Subareolar abscess requires broad-spectrum antibiotics.
      4. Complications
        (a) Fistula may develop in subareolar abscess.
  b. Carcinoma
    i. General
      1. One in nine American women will develop breast cancer during their lifetime.
        (a) Most cases diagnosed after age 40.
      2. Risk factors
        (a) Increasing age
        (b) Family history of gynecologic malignancies
        (c) First-degree relative with breast cancer
        (d) Personal history of breast cancer
        (e) Exposure to ionizing radiation before age 30
        (f) Significant alcohol use
      3. Prevention
        (a) Early pregnancy
        (b) Prolonged lactation

        (c) Chemical or surgical sterilization
        (d) Exercise
        (e) Low-fat diet
    ii. Clinical manifestations
      1. Present with masses, skin changes, nipple discharge, or symptoms of metastatic disease.
        (a) Breast pain is rarely a symptom of breast cancer.
      2. Mass most often detected by patient on self-breast examination.
        (a) Mass is typically nontender, irregular, firm, and immobile.
        (b) Half occur in the upper outer quadrant of the breast.
        (c) Monthly self-breast examinations 5 days after menses are recommended for all patients over age 20.
      3. Skin dimpling, tissue edema, "peau d'orange" appearance, and nipple retraction or discharge may be noted.
      4. May also have nonspecific symptoms such as anorexia, weight loss, fatigue, dyspnea, and bone pain.
    iii. Diagnosis
      1. Mammogram used to detect early lesions.
        (a) Screening guidelines:
          (i) Baseline mammogram at age 30–35.
          (ii) Mammogram every 1–2 years between ages 40–50.
          (iii) Annual mammogram after age 50.
        (b) Findings suggestive of carcinoma:
          (i) Spiculated mass
          (ii) Asymmetric local fibrosis
          (iii) Microcalcifications with a linear, branched pattern
        (c) See Figure 6-4 for mammogram results of breast cancer.
      2. Ultrasound also used to separate fluid-filled cysts from solid masses.
      3. Needle biopsy, fine-needle aspiration, or excisional biopsy needed to diagnosis.
        (a) If fine-needle aspiration is negative an excisional biopsy should be done.

NOTES

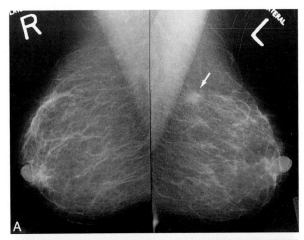

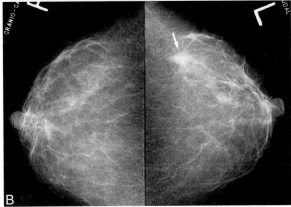

Figure 6-4 Mammogram of breast cancer. (From Mettler FA: Essentials of Radiology, 2nd ed. Philadelphia, Elsevier Saunders, 2005, p. 118, Fig. 4-2.)

QUESTION

A 23-year-old female presents with profuse, green foul smelling, vaginal discharge. KOH prep and whiff are negative. Which of the following is the most appropriate treatment?

    A. Metronidazole (Flagyl)

    B. Fluconazole (Diflucan)

    C. Clindamycin (Cleocin)

    D. Penicillin

    4. Types of invasive breast cancer:
        (a) Infiltrating ductal carcinoma
        (b) Invasive lobular carcinoma
        (c) Paget's disease of the nipple
        (d) Inflammatory breast carcinoma
        (e) See Table 6-6 for summary of noninvasive breast cancer.
  iv. Treatment
    1. Surgical treatment options:
        (a) Wide local excision or lumpectomy
            (i) This is a breast-conserving treatment option.
            (ii) Can be used if tumor less than 4 cm and tumor not fixed to underlying tissue.
        (b) Simple mastectomy
            (i) Includes removal of breast tissue, nipple-areolar complex, and skin.

Table 6-6 • Types of Noninvasive Breast Cancer

Type	Age	Mammogram Results	Diagnosis	Treatment
Ductal carcinoma in situ	50s	Clustered microcalcifications	Needle or excisional biopsy	Surgical excision
Lobular carcinoma in situ	40s	Not seen on mammogram	Diagnosed incidentally on biopsy for other condition	Local excision

NOTES

ANSWER A EXPLANATION: *Trichomonas presents with profuse, green, fouling smelling vaginal discharge. Wet mount is positive for the presence of motile protozoan. First line treatment is metronidazole.*

correct ❏   incorrect ❏

(ii) This is no axillary node dissection.
(c) Modified radical mastectomy
  (i) Includes removal of breast tissue, nipple-areolar complex, skin, pectoralis fascia, and axillary lymph nodes.
(d) Radical mastectomy
  (i) Includes removal of breast tissue, nipple-areolar complex, skin, axillary lymph nodes, and pectoralis major and minor.
2. Medical treatment options:
(a) Include chemotherapy and hormone (anti-estrogen) therapy.
(b) Are used to control micrometastases.
(c) Are indicated in lymph node–positive patients or high-risk lymph node–negative patients.
(d) Chemotherapy typically includes cyclophosphamide, methotrexate, and 5-fluorouracil (CMF).
(e) The most common hormone therapy is tamoxifen.
3. Prognosis
(a) Overall 5-year disease-free survival rate is 94%.
  (i) Survival rate varies with stage of cancer.
(b) Patients with positive estrogen and progesterone receptor have a more favorable prognosis.
c. Fibroadenoma
  i. General
    1. Benign tumors most commonly noted in women under the age of 40.
  ii. Clinical manifestations

1. On physical examination are palpated as round, well-circumscribed, rubbery, nontender, mobile firm lesion.
  (a) Lesions may change during menstrual cycle or pregnancy.
2. Most are 1–5 cm in diameter.
3. No axillary involvement or nipple discharge.
iii. Diagnosis
  1. Diagnosis based on physical examination and biopsy results.
iv. Treatment
  1. If no family history of breast cancer and the patient is stable, she can be followed clinically.
  2. If suspicious for cancer a fine-needle aspiration should be done.
  3. Large fibroadenoma can be removed by excisional biopsy.
d. Fibrocystic disease
  i. General
    1. Very common benign breast condition.
    2. Common in women between the ages of 30–40.
    3. Due to exaggerated stromal response to hormones.
  ii. Clinical manifestations
    1. Present with breast swelling, pain, and tenderness.
    2. Are typically multiple, well demarcated, and mobile.
    3. May involve both breasts and vary through menstrual cycle.
    4. No axillary lymph node involvement or nipple discharge.
  iii. Diagnosis
    1. Biopsy needed to diagnosis possible carcinoma.
  iv. Treatment
    1. Decreasing intake of nicotine and caffeine may reduce symptoms.
    2. If symptoms are severe danazol, an androgen, can be used.
e. Mastitis
  i. General
    1. Regional infection of the breast.

NOTES

2. Typically seen in lactating women and caused by patient's skin flora or oral flora of infant.
3. Organism enters through erosion or crack in the nipple.

  ii. Clinical manifestations
1. Present with fever, chills, and malaise.
2. On physical examination the area is tender, red, and warm to the touch.
3. Laboratory tests may reveal an elevated WBC count.

  iii. Diagnosis
1. Diagnosis made based on physical exam findings.

  iv. Treatment
1. Treated with dicloxacillin.
2. Complications include development of breast abscess.
3. Patients should be instructed to continue to breast-feed or use a breast pump to prevent accumulation of infected material.

X. Pelvic inflammatory disease (PID)
  a. General
    i. A serious complication of STDs.
      1. Infectious agents include *N. gonorrhoeae*, *C. trachomatis*, and anaerobic organisms.
    ii. Increased risk of infertility and ectopic pregnancy with PID.
    iii. Incidence highest in the 15–19-year-old age group.
    iv. Risk factors: nonwhite ethnicity, being unmarried, cigarette smoking, and use of IUDs.
    v. Barrier contraceptives decrease the risk of PID.
  b. Clinical manifestations
    i. Major symptom is abdominal or pelvic pain.
      1. Pain can be bilateral or unilateral and described as a burning, cramping, or stabbing pain.
    ii. May also note increased vaginal discharge, abnormal bleeding, dyspareunia, and gastrointestinal or urinary tract symptoms.
    iii. Fever may be noted.
    iv. On physical examination note lower abdominal tenderness, cervical motion tenderness (Chandelier's sign), and purulent cervical discharge.
    v. Laboratory tests reveal an elevated WBC count.
  c. Diagnosis
    i. Ultrasound is not helpful in making the diagnosis.
    ii. Definitive diagnosis is made by laparoscopy.
    iii. Cultures are obtained to identify the causative agent.
  d. Treatment
    i. Patients often need to be hospitalized.
    ii. Antibiotics include broad-spectrum cephalosporins, such as cefoxitin or cefotetan, and doxycycline.
    iii. Clindamycin and gentamicin can be used if patient allergic to cephalosporins.

XI. Contraceptive methods
  a. Natural methods
    i. Periodic abstinence (rhythm method)
      1. Method
        (a) Requires abstinence shortly before and after the predicted ovulation period.
        (b) Ovulation assessment methods include basal temperature, menstrual cycle tracking, evaluation of cervical mucus, and monitoring for premenstrual or ovulatory symptoms.
      2. Effectiveness
        (a) Failure rate is high at 20%–40%.
      3. Advantages/disadvantages
        (a) No use of chemicals or barriers.
        (b) May require long periods of abstinence.

QUESTION

Which of the following is a risk factor for the development of breast cancer?

A. Significant alcohol intake
B. Surgical sterilization
C. Early pregnancy
D. Low-fat diet

NOTES

ANSWER **A** EXPLANATION: *Risk factors for breast cancer include positive family history of breast or gynecologic cancer, exposure to ionizing radiation, and excessive alcohol intake. Prevention is seen with low-fat diet, early pregnancy, and surgical sterilization.*

correct ☐   incorrect ☐

    (c) Must be motivated to monitor and use ovulation assessment methods.
  ii. Coitus interruptus
    1. Method
      (a) Requires withdrawal of penis from vagina before ejaculation.
    2. Effectiveness
      (a) Failure rate is high at 15%–25%.
    3. Advantages/disadvantages
      (a) Must have sufficient self-control to withdraw before ejaculation.
  iii. Lactational amenorrhea
    1. Method
      (a) After delivery ovulation is delayed due to hypothalamic suppression of ovulation secondary to nursing and lactation.
      (b) Should be used for a maximum of 6 months after delivery.
    2. Effectiveness
      (a) Failure rate is high at 15%–55%.
      (b) Failure rate can be decreased to 2% if method not used for longer than 6 months and breast-feeding is the only form of nutrition for the infant.
  iv. Natural methods are physiologically based, do not use barriers, and are the least effective method of contraception.
b. Barrier methods
  i. Male/female condom
    1. Method
      (a) Male condom is placed over the penis and prevents the ejaculate from entering the female reproductive tract.
      (b) Female condom has two flexible rings; one is placed into the vagina and the other stays outside near the introitus.
    2. Effectiveness
      (a) Male condom has a failure rate of 10%–15%.
        (i) Decreases to 2% if used properly.
      (b) Female condom has a failure rate of 15%–20%.
    3. Advantages/disadvantages
      (a) Male condoms are widely available and prevent the transmission of STDs.
        (i) Only method of contraception that protects against human immunodeficiency virus (HIV).
      (b) Female condom protects against STDs; but is more costly than male condoms.
  ii. Diaphragm
    1. Method
      (a) A domed sheet of rubber or latex that is placed in the vagina so that it covers the cervix.
      (b) Must be placed before intercourse and left in place for 6–8 hours after intercourse.
      (c) Spermicide must also be used.
    2. Effectiveness
      (a) Failure rate is 5%–20%.
    3. Advantages/disadvantages
      (a) May lead to bladder irritation and cystitis.
      (b) If diaphragm left in place too long the patient could become colonized with *S. aureus* and develop toxic shock syndrome.
      (c) Diaphragm must be fitted and replaced every 5 years or when a patient gains or loses more than 10 pounds.
  iii. Cervical cap
    1. Method
      (a) Small, soft cap that fits over the cervix and held in place by suction.
    2. Effectiveness
      (a) Failure rate is 5%–20% and mostly due to movement of the cap.

NOTES

3. Advantages/disadvantages
  (a) Can be left in place for 1–2 days.
  (b) Must be fitted and requires use of spermicide.
  iv. Contraceptive sponge
    1. Method
      (a) A soft, polyurethane sponge embedded with nonoxynol-9, a spermicide.
      (b) Placed in the vagina in front of the cervix.
    2. Effectiveness
      (a) Failure rate is 6%–18% in nulliparous women and 10%–30% in parous women.
    3. Advantages/disadvantages
      (a) No longer available in the United States, but is available in Canada.
      (b) Effective for 24 hours.
      (c) Increase risk of toxic shock syndrome.
c. Spermicides
  i. Method
    1. Disrupt the cell membrane of sperm and act as a mechanical barrier to sperm in the cervical canal.
    2. Must be placed in the vagina 30 minutes before intercourse.
    3. May be used alone but more effective if used with condoms, diaphragms, or cervical caps.
  ii. Effectiveness
    1. Failure rate is 3%–20%.
  iii. Advantages/disadvantages
    1. Widely available in a variety of forms, vaginal creams, jellies, suppositories, and foam.
    2. Can cause vaginal irritation.
    3. Can protect against STDs.
d. Intrauterine devices (IUDs)
  i. Method
    1. Plastic or metal device that is placed in the endometrial cavity.
    2. May elicit a spermicidal inflammatory response resulting in the sperm being destroyed.
    3. Have no effect on ovulation.
  ii. Effectiveness
    1. Very low failure rate of 1%–3%.
  iii. Advantages/disadvantages
    1. Contraindications to use of IUD

QUESTION

Which of the following physical examination finding is noted in pelvic inflammatory disease?

A. Adnexal mass
B. Uterine prolapse
C. Cherry red cervix
D. Cervical motion tenderness

      (a) Absolute
        (i) Current pregnancy
        (ii) Abnormal vaginal bleeding
        (iii) Gynecologic cancer
        (iv) Acute cervical or uterine infection
        (v) History of PID
      (b) Relative
        (i) Nulliparity
        (ii) Prior ectopic pregnancy
        (iii) History of STD
        (iv) Moderate to severe dysmenorrhea
    2. Must be prescribed, inserted, and removed by a health care provider.
    3. Decreases risk of ectopic pregnancy.
e. Hormonal
  i. Oral contraceptive/Contraceptive patch
    1. Method
      (a) Composed of progesterone or progesterone and estrogen.
      (b) Interfere with the pulsatile release of FSH and LH and suppress ovulation.
      (c) Also change the endometrium to not allow for implantation.
    2. Effectiveness
      (a) Very effective with a theoretic failure rate of less than 1%. Actual failure rate is about 3%.
        (i) May have decreased effectiveness due to interaction with other medications.
          (1) Effectiveness decreased with concurrent use of many antibiotics, including penicillins, tetracycline,

NOTES

ANSWER **D** EXPLANATION: *On examination, pelvic inflammatory disease presents with lower abdominal tenderness, cervical motion tenderness, and vaginal discharge.*

correct ☐   incorrect ☐

sulfonamides, rifampin, phenytoin, and barbiturates.
3. Advantages/disadvantages
   (a) Complications include increased coagulability and increased risk of pulmonary embolism, thromboembolism, stroke, and myocardial infarction.
      (i) Increased risk with increased doses of estrogen.
   (b) Oral contraceptive pills are contraindicated in women over age 35 who smoke.
      (i) See Table 6-7 for contraindications.
   (c) Oral contraceptive pills decrease risk of ovarian and endometrial cancer, ectopic pregnancy, anemia, and PID.

Table 6-7 • Contraindication to Use of Oral Contraceptive Pills

Absolute	Relative
Thromboembolism	Uterine fibroids
Pulmonary embolism	Lactation
Myocardial infarction	Diabetes mellitus
Stroke	Hypertension
Breast/endometrial cancer	
Hepatic tumor or abnormal liver function	

ii. Norplant
   1. Method
      (a) Sustained release of levonorgestrel, a progestin.
      (b) Placed in the subcutaneous tissue and slowly released over 5 years.
      (c) Mechanism of action is via suppression of ovulation, thickening cervical mucus, and making endometrium unsuitable for implantation.
   2. Effectiveness
      (a) Very low failure rate of 0.09%–0.2%.
   3. Advantages/disadvantages
      (a) May lead to irregular vaginal bleeding, headaches, weight gain, and mood changes.
      (b) No delay in fertility when discontinued.
iii. Depo-Provera
   1. Method
      (a) Progestin that is injected IM and slowly released over 3 months.
      (b) Mechanism of action is via suppression of ovulation, thickening cervical mucus, and making endometrium unsuitable for implantation.
   2. Effectiveness
      (a) Very low failure rate of 0.3%.
   3. Advantages/disadvantages
      (a) May lead to irregular vaginal bleeding, depression, breast tenderness, and weight gain.
      (b) Long-term use may lead to loss of bone mineral density, osteoporosis, and osteoporotic fracture.
      (c) After discontinuing may have a significant delay, up to 18 months, in return of normal ovulation.
f. Sterilization
   i. Tubal sterilization
      1. Method
         (a) Pregnancy by surgically blocking both fallopian tubes and preventing sperm and ovum from meeting.

NOTES

(b) Can be done by clipping, banding, or coagulation of the tubes.
(c) Performed under general anesthesia.
2. Effectiveness
(a) Failure rate of only 0.2%–0.4%.
3. Advantages/disadvantages
(a) Very low rate of ectopic pregnancy.
(b) May be reversed but success rates vary from 40%–80%.
ii. Vasectomy
1. Method
(a) Sterilization via ligation of vas deferens.
(b) Can be performed under local anesthesia.
(c) Due to possibility of viable sperm being present in the proximal collecting system another form of contraception should be used for 4–6 weeks until azoospermia can be confirmed.
2. Effectiveness
(a) Failure rate is less than 1%.
3. Advantages/disadvantages
(a) Complications are rare and include bleeding and infection after the procedure.
(b) Success rate of re-anastomosis is 60%–70%.
g. Emergency contraception
i. Method
1. Thought to be due to inhibition or delay in ovulation and insufficient corpus luteum function.
2. Products contain ethinyl estradiol and/or levonorgestrel.
ii. Effectiveness
1. Failure rate of 15%–25%.
2. Most effective when used within 72 hours of unprotected intercourse.
iii. Advantages/disadvantages
1. Should not be used in patients with a known or suspected pregnancy.
2. If pregnancy does occur emergency contraception has no effect on fetal development.

QUESTION

Which of the following is an absolute contraindication to the use of oral contraceptives?

A. Thromboembolic disorder
B. Diabetes mellitus
C. Hypertension
D. Cholestasis

XII. Infertility
a. General
i. Infertility is defined as the inability to conceive after 1 year of unprotected intercourse.
ii. Male factors are attributed to 40% of cases of infertility, female factors to 40%, and unidentifiable factors in 20%.
b. Male infertility
i. Etiology
1. May be due to endocrine causes, anatomic defects, abnormal sperm production or motility, and sexual dysfunction.
2. Risk factors include exposure to chemicals, radiation, and excessive heat.
3. See Table 6-8.

Table 6-8 • Etiologies of Male Infertility		
Endocrine	**Abnormal Spermatogenesis**	**Sexual Dysfunction**
Hypothalamic dysfunction	Mumps orchitis	Retrograde ejaculation
Pituitary failure	Varicocele	Impotence
Anabolic steroids	Cryptorchidism	
Thyroid disease		
Hyperprolactinemia		

ANSWER A EXPLANATION: *Absolute contraindications to the use of oral contraceptions include thromboembolism, pulmonary embolism, myocardial infarction, stroke, breast/endometrial cancer, and hepatic tumor or elevated liver function tests.*

correct ☐   incorrect ☐

ii. Diagnosis
   1. Review for history of previous pregnancies fathered by patient, chemical or toxin exposure, and history of STDs, mumps, or trauma to the genitals.
   2. Physical examination should include signs of testosterone deficiency, varicocele, and patency of urethral meatus.
   3. Laboratory evaluation includes semen analysis.
      (a) Analysis includes sperm count, volume, motility, morphology, pH, and WBC count.
      (b) If abnormal, evaluation should continue with thyroid testing and serum testosterone, prolactin, and FSH level.
iii. Treatment
   1. Avoid tight underwear, hot tubs, and environmental exposures.

2. Reproductive techniques such as intracytoplasmic sperm injection.
   (a) Sperm are retrieved and a single sperm is injected directly into an egg and then implanted.
c. Female infertility
   i. Etiology
      1. May be due to ovulatory, cervical, uterine, tubal, or peritoneal causes.
      2. Ovulatory factors disrupt the hypothalamic pituitary ovarian axis and lead to infertility by impairing follicle formation, ovulation, or endometrial development.
      3. See Table 6-9.
   ii. Diagnosis
      1. May require laparoscopic evaluation, evaluation for evidence of ovulation, endometrial biopsy, progestin challenge, FSH, LH, prolactin and thyroid function tests, and pelvic examination.
   iii. Treatment
      1. Varies with etiology.
      2. Ovulation can be induced with clomiphene citrate.
         (a) Clomiphene stimulates release of gonadotropin-releasing hormone which stimulates FSH and LH release and follicular development.
         (b) Major side effect is multiple-gestation pregnancy.

Table 6-9 • Etiologies of Female Infertility

Cervical	Uterine	Tubal	Peritoneal	Ovulatory
Cervical stenosis	Malformations	Pelvic inflammatory disease	Adhesions	Pituitary insufficiency
Cervicitis	Leiomyoma Asherman syndrome	Tubal ligation Endometriosis	Endometriosis	Hyperprolactinemia Polycystic ovarian disease Ovarian tumor Thyroid disease Obesity

NOTES

3. Techniques such as intrauterine insemination (IUI), in vitro fertilization (IVF), and gamete intrafallopian transfer (GIFT) can also be used.

XIII. Uncomplicated pregnancy
  a. Prenatal diagnosis/care
    i. Pregnancy diagnosis
      1. In the patient with normal menstrual periods a delay of more than a few days may suggest pregnancy.
      2. Diagnosis can be made by serum or urine assay for beta-human chorionic gonadotropin (beta-hCG).
        (a) May detect pregnancy as early as 4–7 days after the first missed menstrual cycle.
      3. Ultrasound can also be used to confirm or detect a pregnancy as early as 5 weeks by detecting the gestational sac or the fetal heart at 6 weeks.
      4. Pregnancy dating
        (a) Nägele's rule
          (i) Estimated date of confinement (EDC) is date of last menstrual period minus 3 months plus 7 days.
        (b) Ultrasound
          (i) Uses fetal crown-to-rump length, at 5–12 weeks, to determine gestational age.
          (ii) Can also use femur length.
        (c) Other landmarks
          (i) Fetal quickening at 16–20 weeks
          (ii) Fetal heart tones
            (1) 10 weeks by Doppler ultrasound
            (2) 20 weeks by non-electrical fetoscope
      5. Signs and symptoms of pregnancy
        (a) Chadwick's sign
          (i) Bluish discoloration of the vagina and the cervix.
        (b) Goodell's sign
          (i) Softening and cyanosis of the cervix after 4 weeks.
        (c) Breast swelling and tenderness
        (d) Development of the lines of nigra from the umbilicus to the pubis.
        (e) Palmar erythema

        (f) Symptoms include amenorrhea, nausea and vomiting, breast pain, and quickening.
      6. Time frames
        (a) First trimester
          (i) Lasts until 14 weeks gestational age.
        (b) Second trimester
          (i) Lasts from 14–28 weeks gestation.
        (c) Third trimester
          (i) Lasts from 28 weeks gestation to delivery.
    ii. Prenatal care
      1. Initial visit
        (a) Complete history, including history of prior pregnancies, and physical examination are required.
          (i) Exam with Pap smear and cultures for gonorrhea and chlamydia are required.
        (b) Initial laboratory tests include complete blood count, blood type and antibody screen, rapid plasma reagin (RPR), rubella titer, hepatitis B surface antigen, and urinalysis.
          (i) HIV counseling and testing should be offered.
      2. Follow-up visits
        (a) With each return visit the patient should have weight and blood pressure checked, urinalysis, measurement of fundal height, and evaluation of fetal heart tones.
          (i) Fundal height varies with gestational age.

NOTES

ANSWER **A** EXPLANATION: *Dysfunctional uterine bleeding is best diagnosed with an endometrial biopsy, to determine if ovulation has occurred.*

correct ☐   incorrect ☐

    (1) 12 weeks: above pubic symphysis
    (2) 14–16 weeks: midway between pubic symphysis and umbilicus
    (3) 20–22 weeks: level of umbilicus
    (4) 22–38 weeks: height equal to gestational age (weeks)
    (5) 38–40 weeks: 203 cm below xiphoid process
  (b) Genetic and congenital screening
    (i) Typically occurs during the second trimester.
    (ii) Between weeks 15–18 evaluate with the triple screen.
      (1) Tests include maternal serum alpha-fetoprotein, beta-hCG, and estriol.
      (2) Elevated alpha-fetoprotein correlated with increased risk of neural tube defect and Down syndrome.
    (iii) Screening ultrasound
      (1) Offered between weeks 18–20.
      (2) Provides a fetal anatomic survey.
  (c) Oral glucose tolerance testing (OGTT)
    (i) Completed during second trimester if screening tests are positive for diabetes.
    (ii) Fasting result greater than 95–100 mg/dL or 1-hour result greater than 170–190 mg/dL significant for gestational diabetes on OGTT.

b. Normal labor/delivery
  i. General
    1. Defined as contractions that cause change in cervical effacement or dilation.
  ii. Examination
    1. Obstetric
     (a) Includes determining fetal presentation and lie.
      (i) Determined by using the Leopold maneuvers that involve palpating the maternal abdomen.
      (ii) Fetal lie evident if the infant is transverse or longitudinal in the uterus.
      (iii) Fetal presentation is if the infant is breech or vertex.
     (b) If fetal position or lie is difficult to determine an ultrasound can be used.
    2. Cervical
     (a) Cervical examination assists with determining phase of labor and labor progression.
     (b) Based on five items:
      (i) Dilation
       (1) Determines how open the cervix is at the internal os.
       (2) Ranges from closed to 10 cm.
      (ii) Effacement
       (1) Determines how thin the cervix is between internal and external os.
       (2) Is typically 3–5 cm in length and measured in percent effacement.
      (iii) Station
       (1) Determined by relationship of the fetal head to the ischial spines of the pelvis.
       (2) Zero station is when the presenting part is at the level of the ischial spines.
       (3) Ranges from −3 to +3 or −5 to +5, with negative stations being above the ischial spines and positive stations being below the ischial spines.

NOTES

(iv) Cervical position
  (1) Determines if cervical position is posterior, mid, or anterior.
(v) Cervical consistency
  (1) Determines if the cervix is firm, soft, or in between.
(c) Bishop scoring system used to determine if cervix is favorable to spontaneous delivery.
  (i) A score of greater than 8 is favorable.

iii. Induction and augmentation
1. General
  (a) Induction of labor is an attempt to begin labor in a nonlaboring patient.
    (i) Indications for induction include postterm pregnancy, preeclampsia, premature rupture of membranes, or fetal distress or growth retardation.
  (b) Augmentation of labor is the process of increasing already present labor.
2. Induction preparation
  (a) Success of induction is related to Bishop score. A score of less than 5 leads to increased number of failed inductions.
  (b) Can prepare a patient for induction by use of prostaglandins to ripen the cervix.
    (i) Contraindications to the use of prostaglandins include maternal asthma or glaucoma, more than one prior cesarean section, or unstable fetal status.
3. Induction
  (a) Can be performed with amniotomy or Pitocin.
  (b) Pitocin, given by continuous IV infusion, stimulates uterine contraction.
  (c) Amniotomy is the rupture of the amniotic sac with the use of an amniotic hook.

> # QUESTION
>
> What is the gestational age if the fundal height is at the level of the umbilicus?
>
> A. 12 weeks
> B. 16 weeks
> C. 20 weeks
> D. 24 weeks

4. Augmentation
  (a) Pitocin and amniotomy can also be used to augment labor in those with inadequate labor.
iv. Fetal monitoring
1. Contraction monitoring
  (a) External tocometer is used to obtain record of the contractions.
  (b) Used to monitor frequency of contractions and to compare to fetal heart monitoring record.
2. Fetal heart monitoring
  (a) Continuous monitoring is done after determining baseline to monitor for fetal distress.
  (b) Baseline fetal heart rate is between 110–160 beats/minute.
    (i) With rates above 160 the fetal distress may be secondary to infection, hypoxia, or anemia.
  (c) Fetal heart tracing should show variability between heartbeats.
  (d) Decelerations can be noted on fetal heart monitoring.
    (i) Early decelerations
      (1) Begin and end at the same time as the contraction.
      (2) A result of increased vagal tone due to head compression during the contraction.
    (ii) Variable decelerations
      (1) Occur at any time and drop more than early or late decelerations.

NOTES

---

(2) A result of umbilical cord compression.
(iii) Late decelerations
(1) Begin at peak of a contraction and slowly return to baseline after the contraction is complete.
(2) A result of uteroplacental compromise.
3. Fetal scalp electrode
(a) Used to sense depolarizations of the fetal heart.
(b) Used in the fetus with repetitive decelerations or difficult to monitor externally.
(c) Contraindications include fetal thrombocytopenia, maternal hepatitis or HIV.
4. Fetal scalp pH
(a) If fetal heart tracings are abnormal fetal scalp pH can be obtained to evaluate for fetal hypoxia and acidosis.
(b) pH greater than 7.25 is normal and less than 7.20 is abnormal.
5. Intrauterine pressure catheter
(a) Used to determine timing and strength of contractions.
(b) Used in those patients difficult to monitor externally or when absolute values of contraction strength are needed.
v. Labor progression
1. Cardinal movements of labor
(a) Engagement
(i) When the fetal presenting part enters the pelvis.
(b) Flexion
(i) Head flexes to allow the smallest diameter to present to the pelvis.

(c) Descent
(i) Passage of the head into the pelvis.
(d) Internal rotation
(i) Fetal vertex moves from occiput transverse position to a position where the sagittal suture is parallel to the anteroposterior diameter of the pelvis.
(e) Extension
(i) Vertex extends as it passes beneath the pubic symphysis.
(f) External rotation
(i) Fetus externally rotates after head is delivered so that the shoulders can be delivered.
2. Stages of labor
(a) Stage 1
(i) Begins with the onset of labor to complete dilation and effacement of the cervix.
(ii) Average duration is 10–12 hours in nulliparous and 6–8 hours in multiparous patients.
(iii) Divided into two phases:
(1) Latent phase from onset of labor until 3–4 cm of dilation.
(2) Active phase ranges until greater than 9 cm of dilation.
(iv) Transit time affected by three things.
(1) Power: the strength and frequency of contractions.
(2) Passenger: size and position of the fetus.
(3) Pelvis: size and shape of the pelvis.
(b) Stage 2
(i) From the time of full dilation and effacement to delivery of the infant.
(ii) Normal time frame is less than 2 hours in nulliparous and less than 1 hour in multiparous patients.

NOTES

(iii) Once fetal head is delivered the mouth and upper airway should be suctioned.

(iv) If stage two is prolonged an operative vaginal delivery may be needed.

   (1) Means use of forceps or vacuum extraction.

(v) Episiotomy may be needed to speed up delivery, minimize risk of laceration, or assist with shoulder dystocia.

   (1) Two common types: midline and mediolateral.

   (2) Lacerations

(a) First-degree: involves mucosa and skin.

(b) Second-degree: extends into perineal body but not the anal sphincter.

(c) Third-degree: extends into or through the anal sphincter.

(d) Fourth-degree: anal mucosa is entered.

(c) Stage 3

(i) From delivery of the infant to delivery of the placenta.

(ii) Normal time frame is less than 30 minutes.

(iii) Three signs of placental separation:

   (1) Cord lengthening

   (2) Rush of blood

   (3) Uterine fundal rebound

(iv) Retained placenta

   (1) Diagnosis made when placenta has not been delivered in 30 minutes

   (2) May be removed by manual extraction.

XIV. Complicated pregnancy

  a. Abortion

    i. General

      1. Spontaneous abortion is a pregnancy that ends before week 20 of gestation.

      (a) Between 60%–80% of all spontaneous abortions occur during the first trimester.

QUESTION

A 25-year-old female who is G_1P_0 and known to be 12 weeks pregnant presents with painless spotting since this AM. Pelvic examination reveals blood in the vagina with a closed cervical os. The uterus is non-tender to palpation and consistent in size with 12 weeks gestation. Which of the following is the most likely diagnosis?

  A. Inevitable abortion

  B. Threatened abortion

  C. Incomplete abortion

  D. Complete abortion

2. Most first-trimester abortions are associated with abnormal chromosomes, while second-trimester abortions are associated with infection, uterus/cervix abnormalities, exposure to toxins, and trauma.

3. Many different definitions:

  (a) Complete: complete expulsion of all products of conception before 20 weeks gestation.

  (b) Incomplete: partial expulsion of some but not all products of conception before 20 weeks gestation.

  (c) Inevitable: no expulsion of products, but bleeding and dilation of the cervix evidence that a viable pregnancy is not likely.

  (d) Threatened: any intrauterine bleeding before 20 weeks gestation, without dilation or expulsion of products of conception.

  (e) Missed: death of the fetus before 20 weeks gestation with complete retention of the products of conception.

  ii. Diagnosis

    1. Present with vaginal bleeding, abdominal cramping, abdominal pain, and decreased symptoms of pregnancy.

    2. Serial beta-hCG levels should be obtained and doubling should occur

NOTES

ANSWER **B** EXPLANATION: *A threatened abortion is defined as any intrauterine bleeding before 20 weeks gestation, without dilation or expulsion of products of conception.*

correct ☐   incorrect ☐

    every 48 hours early in pregnancy in a viable pregnancy.
    3. Ultrasound should be obtained to detect fetal heart activity.
  iii. Treatment
    1. Incomplete or missed abortions should be allowed to finish.
    2. Dilation and evacuation may be required to remove all products of conception.
    3. Patients with threatened abortions should be placed on pelvic rest and monitored for continued bleeding.
    4. All Rh-negative patients should receive RhoGAM with any vaginal bleeding.
b. Abruptio placentae
  i. General
    1. The premature separation of the placenta from the uterine wall.
    2. Most occur after 30 weeks gestation and before labor.
    3. May result in premature delivery, uterine tetany, disseminated intravascular coagulation (DIC), and shock.
    4. Cause is unknown, but risk factors include maternal hypertension, prior history of abruptio placentae, maternal trauma, advanced age, multiparity, smoking, and alcohol use.
  ii. Clinical manifestations
    1. Present with third-trimester vaginal bleeding and severe abdominal pain.
    2. On physical examination will note vaginal bleeding and a firm, tender uterus.
  iii. Diagnosis
    1. Diagnosis based on clinical findings.
    2. Confirmed by inspection of the placenta at time of delivery.
  iv. Treatment
    1. First step is to stabilize the patient and prepare for more hemorrhage.

    2. Prepare for delivery and monitor for complications such as DIC and shock.
c. Dystocia: Shoulder
  i. General
    1. Impaction of the anterior shoulder against the pubic symphysis after delivery of the head.
    2. Rate is 1 in 300 live births.
     (a) Increased risk in newborns with macrosomia.
  ii. Clinical manifestations
    1. On examination the fetal head may appear to retract toward the maternal perineum.
  iii. Diagnosis
    1. Warning signs include prolonged second stage of labor and the use of forceps or vacuum with delivery.
  iv. Treatment
    1. McRoberts maneuver used to disimpact the shoulder.
     (a) Maternal thighs flexed onto the abdomen increases inlet diameter and removes sacral prominence as a possible obstruction.
     (b) Suprapubic pressure can also be used with this maneuver to disimpact the shoulder.
    2. Complications
     (a) Maternal complications include soft-tissue injury.
     (b) Fetal complications are more severe and include brachial plexus injury including Erb's palsy, clavicle fracture, and fetal hypoxia.
d. Ectopic pregnancy
  i. General
    1. Implantation of the egg occurs outside of the uterus, most commonly in the fallopian tubes.
    2. Occurs in approximately 1 in 100 pregnancies.
    3. Risk factors for ectopic pregnancy include history of STD or PID, prior ectopic pregnancy, previous abdominal or tubal surgery, endometriosis, or use of IUD.
  ii. Clinical manifestations
    1. Symptoms include unilateral pelvic pain and vaginal bleeding.

NOTES

2. On physical examination may note a tender adnexal mass, uterus small for gestational age, and cervical bleeding.
3. Laboratory results reveal beta-hCG levels low for gestational age and a level that does not double every 48 hours early in the pregnancy.

iii. Diagnosis
1. Based on symptoms, physical examination, and laboratory findings.
2. Ultrasound may reveal an adnexal mass or extrauterine pregnancy.
3. If no mass on physical exam or ultrasound follow patient with serial beta-hCG levels to evaluate for possible ectopic pregnancy.

iv. Treatment
1. Patient should be stabilized if the ectopic pregnancy has ruptured and then an exploratory laparotomy should be performed.
2. Methotrexate can be used in uncomplicated, stable ectopic pregnancies.

e. Gestational diabetes
i. General
1. Impaired carbohydrate metabolism that first manifests during pregnancy.
2. Risk factors for the development of diabetes during pregnancy include age over 25 years, obesity, positive family history, history of macrosomia, and previous miscarriage.
3. Patients who develop gestational diabetes are at an increased risk of developing gestational diabetes in later pregnancies and overt diabetes within 5 years

ii. Clinical manifestations
1. If patient has one or more risk factors screen for diabetes at first prenatal visit.
2. Screening typically done at end of second trimester.
3. Screening is done by measuring glucose 1-hour after a 50-g glucose load.
   (a) Normal fasting glucose is less than 105 mg/dL and normal 1-hour glucose post 50-g glucose load is less than 140 mg/dL.

iii. Diagnosis
1. Oral glucose tolerance test (OGTT) done if screening test is positive.

QUESTION

What is the most common site of implantation of an ectopic pregnancy?

A. Fallopian tube
B. Uterus
C. Cervix
D. Vagina

Table 6-10 • Complications of Diabetes during Pregnancy

Maternal	Fetal
Preeclampsia	Macrosomia
Miscarriage	Traumatic delivery
Infection	Shoulder dystocia
Postpartum hemorrhage	Delayed organ maturity
Vascular or end-organ involvement	Congenital abnormalities
Neuropathy	Intrauterine growth retardation

2. OGTT involves a 100-g glucose dose and measuring fasting, and 1-, 2-, 3-hour postglucose load blood glucose levels.
3. Gestational diabetes is diagnosed if two or more of the levels are elevated.

iv. Treatment
1. Strict glucose control is vital to the well-being of the mother and infant.
2. Diet control with an American Dietetic Association (ADA) diet is indicated.
3. Insulin may be needed if control with diet is inadequate.
4. Oral hypoglycemic agents are not indicated due to crossing the placenta and possible teratogenic effects.

NOTES

ANSWER **A** EXPLANATION: *The most common site of an ectopic pregnancy is the fallopian tube.*

correct ☐   incorrect ☐

f. Gestational trophoblastic disease
  i. General
    1. Wide group of interrelated disease resulting in abnormal proliferation of trophoblastic tissue.
    2. Four major groups:
      (a) Molar pregnancy: benign
      (b) Invasive mole
        (i) A malignant disorder in which the molar villi and trophoblasts penetrate the myometrium.
      (c) Choriocarcinoma: malignant
      (d) Placental site trophoblastic tumor: malignant
  ii. Clinical manifestations
    1. Irregular or heavy vaginal bleeding early in the pregnancy.
    2. All are able to produce hCG.
  iii. Diagnosis
    1. hCG serves as a tumor marker for this disease.
    2. Ultrasound can be used to aid in diagnosis.
  iv. Treatment
    1. Varies with type of disease.
    2. Malignant types are very sensitive to chemotherapy.
g. Molar pregnancy (hydatidiform moles)
  i. General
    1. Two types:
      (a) Complete
        (i) Results from fertilization of an empty ovum by a normal sperm.
        (ii) Have trophoblastic development and the absence of fetal parts.
      (b) Incomplete
        (i) Results when two sperm fertilize a normal ovum at the same time.
    2. Incidence 1 in 1000 pregnancies; occurs most commonly in women under age 20 or over age 40.
  ii. Clinical manifestations

    1. Present with painless, irregular, or heavy vaginal bleeding early in pregnancy.
    2. May also note severe nausea and vomiting.
    3. Physical examination may reveal molar clusters (grape-like) protruding into the vagina and blood in the cervical os in complete molar pregnancy.
      (a) Physical exam normal in incomplete molar pregnancy.
    4. Laboratory results reveal a markedly elevated beta-hCG, relative to that of a normal pregnancy.
    5. Ultrasound reveals no fetal heart tones.
  iii. Diagnosis
    1. Based on laboratory and ultrasound results.
  iv. Treatment
    1. Immediate removal of uterine contents.
    2. Monitor beta-hCG levels for 1 year to identify invasive moles.
    3. Pregnancy should also be avoided during this 1-year follow-up.
h. Multiple gestation
  i. General
    1. Monozygotic, or identical, twins result when a fertilized ovum divides into two separate ova.
    2. Dizygotic, or nonidentical, twins result when two ova are released and fertilized.
    3. 1 in 80 pregnancies result in twins.
    4. Triplets occur in 1 in 8000 pregnancies.
      (a) Increased risk with ovulation-enhancing drugs.
  ii. Complications
    1. Increased risk of preterm labor, umbilical cord prolapse, postpartum hemorrhage, gestational diabetes, preeclampsia, and placenta previa.
  iii. Diagnosis
    1. Possible diagnosis indicated by rapid uterine growth, excessive maternal weight gain, and elevated beta-hCG.
    2. Diagnosed by ultrasound.
  iv. Treatment
    1. Because of increased risk of complications multiple gestations should be managed as a high-risk pregnancy.
i. Placenta previa
  i. General

NOTES

1. Abnormal implantation of the placenta over the internal cervical os.
   (a) Complete previa occurs when the placenta completely covers the internal os.
   (b) Partial previa occurs when the placenta covers part of the internal os.
   (c) Marginal previa occurs when the edge of the placenta reaches the margin of the os.
2. Major cause of antepartum bleeding.
3. Bleeding is due to disruptions in placental attachment during normal development and thinning of the cervix during the third trimester.
4. May be complicated by placenta accreta in which there is abnormal invasion of the placenta into the uterine wall.
   (a) Placenta accreta does not allow the placenta to separate from the uterine wall after delivery.
   (b) Results in severe hemorrhage and treated with hysterectomy.

ii. Clinical manifestations
1. Presents with sudden and profuse, painless vaginal bleeding after week 28 gestation.
2. Vaginal examination is contraindicated in placenta previa.

iii. Diagnosis
1. Diagnosis is made by ultrasound.

iv. Treatment
1. If placenta previa is suspected stabilize patient, prepare for bleeding, and delivery via cesarean section.
2. If signs of fetal distress or severe hemorrhaging, emergency cesarean section is indicated.

j. Postpartum hemorrhage
   i. General
   1. Defined as blood loss greater than 500 cc in a vaginal delivery and greater than 1000 cc in a cesarean section.
   2. See Table 6-11 for etiologies of postpartum hemorrhage.

   ii. Diagnosis
   1. Uterine atony is the major cause of postpartum bleeding.
      (a) On physical examination the uterus will be soft, enlarged, and boggy.

QUESTION

A 30-year-old female, in her 37th week of pregnancy, presents with sudden onset of painless, profuse vaginal bleeding. Vitals are as pulse 106/minute, respirations 20/min, blood pressure 106/64 mm Hg, and temperature 98.6°F. Which of the following is the most likely diagnosis?

A. Cervical laceration
B. Abruptio placentae
C. Uterine rupture
D. Placenta previa

Table 6-11 • Etiology of Postpartum Bleeding	
Vaginal	**Cesarean**
Vaginal and cervical lacerations	Uterine atony
Uterine atony	Surgery
Placenta accreta	Placenta accreta
Retained products of conception	Uterine rupture
Uterine inversion or rupture	

(b) Treated with IV oxytocin and uterine massage.

iii. Treatment
1. Fluid resuscitation should be started and monitor for signs of DIC.

k. Pregnancy-induced hypertension
   i. General
   1. In the obstetric patient hypertension is defined as a blood pressure greater than 140/90 mm Hg.
   2. Four defined hypertensive states in pregnancy:
      (a) Preeclampsia and eclampsia
      (b) Chronic hypertension
         (i) Defined as hypertension present before conception, before 20 weeks gestations, or continuing more than 6 weeks postpartum.

NOTES

ANSWER D EXPLANATION: *Placenta previa, a major cause of antepartum bleeding, presents with sudden, painless, profuse bleeding after 28 weeks gestation.*

correct ☐   incorrect ☐

(c) Chronic hypertension with superimposed preeclampsia
   (i) Defined as worsening hypertension or worsening proteinuria in the last half of pregnancy.
(d) Transient hypertension
   (i) Hypertension that develops between midpregnancy and 48 hours after delivery.
ii. Preeclampsia
   1. General
      (a) Presence of edema, proteinuria, and hypertension.
         (i) May develop any time after 20 weeks gestation, but typically seen in the third trimester.
      (b) Involves generalized arteriolar vasoconstriction and intravascular depletion.

(c) Maternal complications are related to the arteriolar vasoconstriction and include renal failure, oliguria, edema, thrombocytopenia, and DIC.
(d) Fetal complications are related to prematurity and include intrauterine growth restriction, placental abruption, fetal distress, and stillbirth.
2. Clinical manifestations (see Table 6-12 for clinical manifestations).
3. Diagnosis
   (a) Based on physical examination and laboratory findings.
4. Treatment
   (a) Delivery is the ultimate treatment.
   (b) Magnesium sulfate is started to decrease risk of seizures.
   (c) In severe disease hydralazine can be used to control blood pressure.
iii. Eclampsia
   1. General
      (a) Defined as the development of seizures in a preeclamptic patient not attributed to any other cause.
   2. Clinical manifestations
      (a) Seizures are tonic-clonic.
   3. Diagnosis

Table 6-12 • Clinical Manifestations of Preeclampsia

Severity	Blood Pressure (mm Hg)	Proteinuria	Edema	Other
Mild	140/90 to 160/110 or ≥30 increase in systolic BP ≥15 increase in diastolic BP	>300 mg/24 hr or 1–2+ on dipstick	Hands and/or face	
Severe	>160/110	>5 g/24 hr or 3–4+ on dipstick	Hands and/or face	Altered consciousness Headache Abdominal pain Elevated liver function tests Oliguria Pulmonary edema Thrombocytopenia

NOTES

(a) Based on findings of elevated blood pressure, proteinuria, edema, and seizures.
   (i) Not all patients will have proteinuria.
4. Treatment
   (a) Seizure control and prophylaxis with magnesium sulfate.
   (b) Blood pressure control with hydralazine.
   (c) Once patient is stable delivery should be started.

iv. **HELLP** syndrome
1. General
   (a) Subcategory of severe preeclampsia.
   (b) Uncommon, but has a high rate of stillbirth and neonatal death.
2. Clinical manifestations
   (a) Patients present with the following:
      (i) **H**emolytic anemia
      (ii) **E**levated **L**iver function tests
      (iii) **L**ow **P**latelets
   (b) Physical examination may reveal epigastric pain due to liver capsule distention and progressive nausea and vomiting.
3. Diagnosis
   (a) Based on laboratory
4. Treatment
   (a) Delivery is the definitive treatment.

l. Premature rupture of membranes
i. General
1. Defined as rupture of membranes at least 1 hour before the onset of labor.
2. Preterm rupture of membranes is rupture that occurs before 37 weeks gestation.
3. Prolonged premature rupture of membranes is rupture more than 18 hours before onset of labor.
ii. Clinical manifestations
1. Suspected with a history of leaking amniotic fluid from the vagina.
iii. Diagnosis
1. Nitrazine or fern test confirms diagnosis.
   (a) Nitrazine test detects the pH of the fluid that is alkaline if amniotic fluid.
   (b) Fern test detects crystallization of salts in the amniotic fluid.
iv. Treatment
1. Evaluate for signs of infection, chorioamnionitis.
   (a) Chorioamnionitis is infection of the amniotic fluid.
      (i) Commonly caused by group B *Streptococcus* and treated with IV antibiotics.

m. Rh incompatibility
i. General
1. If a woman is Rh-negative and the fetus is Rh-positive she may become sensitized to Rh antigen and develop antibodies.
2. Antibodies may cross the placenta and cause hemolysis of the fetal red blood cells.
ii. Diagnosis
1. In a patient who has a positive antibody screen for Rh a titer should be checked and monitored throughout the pregnancy.
   (a) If titer increases then amniocentesis should be performed and the amniotic fluid tested for bilirubin.
   (b) Bilirubin levels used to predict severity of disease.
   (c) Ultrasound is used to evaluate for signs of fetal hydrops and a fetal hemoglobin is obtained.
2. If placenta abruption or any antepartum bleeding occurs a Kleihauer-Bethke test is needed to test for the amount of fetal blood cells in the maternal circulation.
   (a) RhoGAM dose may need to be increased based on test results.
iii. Treatment
1. If patient is Rh-negative and has a negative antibody screen the goal is to keep the patient from becoming sensitized.
   (a) With any exposure to fetal blood the patient should be given RhoGAM, anti-D immunoglobulin.
   (b) RhoGAM is given at 28 weeks gestation and then again postpartum if neonate is Rh-positive.
2. In the sensitized Rh-negative patient with severe disease fetal transfusion may be needed.

NOTES

Question 1

Which of the following physical examination findings is typically seen in fibroadenoma of the breast?

A. Rubbery mass
B. Dimpling
C. Retraction
D. Nipple flattening

Question 2

What is the average doubling time during the first trimester of pregnancy for beta-HCG?

A. 2 days
B. 4 days
C. 6 days
D. 8 days

Question 3

A 23-year-old female presents with pain in the abdominal and sacral region. The pain is worse during menses and during intercourse. On examination the patient's uterus is fixed and painful with movement and there are palpable nodular areas that are tender to palpation. Her ovaries are also enlarged. Which of the following is the most likely diagnosis?

A. Ectopic pregnancy
B. Uterine leiomyoma
C. Pelvic inflammatory disease
D. Endometriosis

Question 4

A 30-year-old female presents with a non-tender mass in the right breast. No nipple discharge is noted. Which of the following is the next best step in the evaluation of this patient?

A. Simple mastectomy
B. Excisional biopsy
C. Fine needle aspiration
D. Mammography

Question 5

Which of the following is the treatment of choice for Trichomonas?

A. Podophyllin
B. Doxycycline
C. Metronidazole
D. Nystatin

Question 6

Which of the following is a contraindication to estrogen hormone replacement therapy?

A. Thromboembolic disease
B. Melanoma of the skin
C. Osteoporosis
D. Ulcerative colitis

NOTES

Question 7

Release of which of the following hormones results in development of the primary ovarian follicle?

- A. Estrogen
- B. Progesterone
- C. Luteinizing hormone
- D. Follicle stimulating hormone

Answer 3

ANSWER **D** EXPLANATION: *Endometriosis, presence of endometrial tissue outside the endometrial cavity, presents with dysmenorrhea and dyspareunia. On physical examination the ovaries may be enlarged and the uterus is fixed and painful with any movement of the uterus.*

Topic: Endometriosis

correct ☐   incorrect ☐

Answer 1

ANSWER **A** EXPLANATION: *Dimpling, retraction, and nipple flattening or discharge are more commonly noted in breast cancer. Fibroadenoma presents with well-circumscribed, rubbery, non-tender, mobile, firm mass.*

Topic: Fibroadenoma

correct ☐   incorrect ☐

Answer 4

ANSWER **C** EXPLANATION: *The evaluation of the patient with a breast mass includes a fine needle aspiration followed by excisional biopsy if aspirate is negative.*

Topic: Breast carcinoma

correct ☐   incorrect ☐

Answer 2

ANSWER **A** EXPLANATION: *During the first trimester of a normal pregnancy the beta-HCG will double every two days. In ectopic pregnancy the beta-HCG does not double as expected.*

Topic: Ectopic pregnancy

correct ☐   incorrect ☐

Answer 5

ANSWER **C** EXPLANATION: *Trichomonas vaginalis presents with foul smelling, green vaginal discharge and is treated with metronidazole (Flagyl).*

Topic: Vaginitis

correct ☐   incorrect ☐

NOTES

Answer 6

ANSWER **A** EXPLANATION: *Estrogen replacement therapy may be considered in patients with menopause, but is contraindicated in patients with hepatic dysfunction and history of thromboembolic events.*

Topic: Menopause

correct ☐   incorrect ☐

Answer 7

ANSWER **D** EXPLANATION: *release of FSH from the pituitary results in development of primary ovarian follicles. The ovarian follicle produces estrogen which causes the uterine lining to proliferate.*

Topic: Menstrual cycle

correct ☐   incorrect ☐

NOTES

Endocrine System

7

EXAM BLUEPRINT TOPICS

Diseases of the Thyroid Gland
Hyperparathyroidism
Hypoparathyroidism
Hyperthyroidism

- Graves' disease
- Thyroid storm

Hypothyroidism
Thyroiditis
Neoplastic disease
Diseases of the Adrenal Gland
Cushing syndrome
Acute/Chronic corticoadrenal insufficiency
Glucocorticoids
Primary hyperaldosteronism
Diseases of the Pituitary Gland
Acromegaly/Gigantism
Dwarfism/Short stature
Diabetes insipidus
Hyperprolactinemia
Diabetes Mellitus
Type 1
Type 2
Hypoglycemia
Lipid Disorders
Hypercholesterolemia
Hypertriglyceridemia

GENERAL

I. Information
  a. If have excess hormone, order a suppression test.
  b. If have decreased levels of hormone, order a stimulation test.
  c. Primary disease means malfunction of the target organ.
  d. Secondary disease means malfunction of hypothalamus and pituitary gland.
II. Hypothalamic function
  a. There are a number of releasing factors.
    i. Gonadotropin-releasing hormone (GnRH) stimulates release of follicle-stimulating hormone (FSH) and luteinizing hormone (LH).
    ii. Thyrotropin-releasing hormone (TRH) stimulates release of thyroid-stimulating hormone (TSH).
    iii. Corticotropin-releasing factor (CRF) stimulates release of adrenocorticotropic hormone (ACTH).
III. Feedback loops
  a. Central basis of endocrine system.
  b. With positive feedback, production of a hormone causes increased release of the stimulating hormone.
  c. With negative feedback, production of a hormone causes decreased release of the stimulating hormone.
    i. See Figure 7-1.

DISEASES OF THE THYROID GLAND

I. Hyperparathyroidism
  a. General
    i. More common in females than males and patients over age 50.
    ii. Caused by hypersecretion of parathyroid hormone.
      1. Due to parathyroid adenoma, hyperplasia, or carcinoma.
    iii. Causes excessive excretion of calcium and phosphate by the kidney.
    iv. Primary hyperparathyroidism due to excessive parathyroid hormone and

NOTES

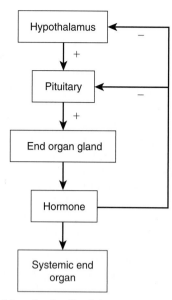

Figure 7-1 Negative feedback loop.

multiple endocrine neoplasia and secondary hyperparathyroidism due to renal failure, metastatic bone disease, osteomalacia, and multiple myeloma.
  b. Clinical manifestations
    i. Most patients are asymptomatic.
    ii. If symptomatic have "bones, stones, abdominal groans, psychic moans, and fatigue overtones."
      1. Skeletal changes include loss of cortical bone and gain of trabecular bone, bone pain, and arthralgias.
      2. Urinary complaints include polyuria, polydipsia, and kidney stones.
      3. Hypercalcemia may cause constipation, fatigue, anemia, weight loss, and hypertension in mild cases and increased thirst, anorexia, nausea, and, vomiting in severe cases.
  c. Diagnosis
    i. Laboratory results reveal hypercalcemia, low phosphate, and increased alkaline phosphatase (if bone disease is present).
      1. Diagnosis confirmed with presence of elevated levels of parathyroid hormone.

    ii. Must rule out malignant tumors, multiple myeloma, and sarcoidosis as a cause of hypercalcemia.
  d. Treatment
    i. Parathyroidectomy is recommended in patients with symptomatic disease.
      1. Postsurgical complications include hypocalcemia paresthesias and possibly tetany.
    ii. Medical treatment for hypercalcemia includes large fluid intake and bisphosphonates.
    iii. Complications include pathologic fractures, urinary tract infections, and renal failure.
II. Hypoparathyroidism
  a. General
    i. Most commonly noted after thyroidectomy, surgical removal of parathyroid adenoma, or autoimmune, congenital, familial.
    ii. Pseudohypoparathyroidism is due to renal resistance to parathyroid hormone.
  b. Clinical manifestations
    i. Acute disease causes circumoral tingling, tetany, muscle cramps, irritability, and seizures.
    ii. Chronic disease symptoms include lethargy, personality changes, blurry vision, and mental retardation.
    iii. Chvostek's sign and Trousseau's phenomenon are positive.
    iv. Nails may be brittle and skin dry.
    v. Deep tendon reflexes may be hyperactive.
  c. Diagnosis
    i. Laboratory tests reveal low-serum calcium, high-serum phosphate, low-urine calcium, and alkaline phosphatase is normal.
    ii. Parathyroid hormone levels are low.
  d. Treatment
    i. Treatment of acute attack includes IV calcium gluconate, vitamin D supplement, and magnesium supplement if levels are low.
    ii. Maintenance therapy includes calcium and vitamin D supplements.
      1. Monitor serum calcium every 3 months.
III. Hyperthyroidism
  a. General
    i. Etiologies include:
      1. Graves' disease

NOTES

2. Toxic nodules of the thyroid
   (a) Typically noted in the elderly.
   (b) No eye or skin changes as seen in Graves' disease.
3. Subacute thyroiditis
4. Hashimoto's thyroiditis
5. Pregnancy/Trophoblastic tumors
6. Use of amiodarone (hypothyroidism more common)

b. Graves' disease
   i. General
      1. The most common cause of hyperthyroidism.
      2. Have diffuse enlargement and hyperactivity of the thyroid gland and presence of antibodies against the gland.
         (a) Have formation of autoantibodies to TSH receptors and stimulates the gland to hyperfunction.
      3. More common in females and onset typically between ages 20–40.
      4. Associated with other autoimmune diseases.
   ii. Clinical manifestations
      1. Present with signs and symptoms of hyperthyroidism (see Table 7-1).
      2. Physical examination presents with pretibial myxedema, exophthalmos, lid lag, and hyperreflexia.
      3. Goiter, often with a bruit, is noted.
      4. Patients may present with atrial fibrillation.
   iii. Diagnosis
      1. Serum triiodothyronine (T_3), thyroxine (T_4), and free T_4 are increased with a decreased TSH.
      2. Elevated antimicrosomal and antithyroglobulin antibodies titers.
   iv. Treatment
      1. Propranolol is used for treatment of symptoms until hyperthyroidism is resolved.
         (a) Symptoms include tachycardia, tremor, diaphoresis, anxiety, and palpitations.
      2. Thiourea drugs, methimazole and propylthiouracil, are used to inhibit hormone synthesis.

QUESTION

Which of the following laboratory abnormality is noted in hyperparathyroidism?

A. Hypermagnesemia
B. Hyperphosphatemia
C. Hyperkalemia
D. Hypercalcemia

   (a) Safe to use in pregnancy.
3. Radioactive iodine is used to destroy an overactive thyroid.
   (a) Avoid in pregnant patients.
4. Thyroid surgery, while not used widely, is usually preferred for pregnant patients.

c. Thyroid storm
   i. General
      1. Rare, severe form of thyrotoxicosis.
      2. May occur with stressful illness, thyroid surgery, or radioactive iodine.
      3. Very high mortality rate.
   ii. Clinical manifestations
      1. Present with marked delirium, severe tachycardia, vomiting, diarrhea, dehydration, and high fever.
   iii. Diagnosis

Table 7-1 • Signs and Symptoms of Hyperthyroidism

Appetite change	Nervousness
Exertional shortness of breath	Palpitations
Diarrhea	Sleep disturbances
Headache	Sweating
Fatigue	Tremor
Heat intolerance	Weakness
Irritability	Weight loss
Menstrual disturbances	Hyperactivity

NOTES

ANSWER D EXPLANATION: *Laboratory abnormalities in hyperparathyroidism include hypercalcemia, low phosphorus, and elevated alkaline phosphatase (if bone disease present).*

correct ☐   incorrect ☐

1. Elevated free T_4 and decreased TSH.
   iv. Treatment
      1. Treatment consists of thiourea drug, iodide, propranolol, and steroids.
         (a) Avoid propranolol in patients with heart failure.
      2. Avoid aspirin, as it will raise free T_4 levels by displacement of thyroid hormone from carrier proteins.
      3. Treatment with radioactive iodide or surgery is undertaken when patient is euthyroid.
IV. Hypothyroidism
   a. General
      i. Etiologies include:
         1. Autoimmune thyroiditis (Hashimoto's)
            (a) Most common cause of hypothyroidism.
            (b) More common in females.
         2. Post-ablative hypothyroidism
         3. Drug-induced: lithium, sulfonamides, amiodarone
         4. Iodine deficiency
      ii. Myxedema coma
         1. Hypothyroidism precipitated by an acute illness or trauma.
            (a) Very high mortality rate.
         2. Present with signs and symptoms of hypothyroidism, hypothermia, and impaired mentation.
         3. Patients present with hyponatremia and hypoglycemia.
         4. Treatment is IV levothyroxine.
   b. Clinical manifestations
      i. Signs and symptoms of hypothyroidism (see Table 7-2).
      ii. Physical examination reveals thin, brittle nails, thinning hair and lateral half of eyebrows, bradycardia, and delayed return of deep tendon reflexes.

Table 7-2 • Signs and Symptoms of Hypothyroidism

Arthralgias	Fatigue
Cold intolerance	Lethargy
Constipation	Menstrual disturbances
Decreased appetite	Muscle cramps
Decreased memory	Paresthesias
Decreased perspiration	Sleepiness
Depression	Weight gain
Dry skin	

c. Diagnosis
   i. Laboratory findings include low free T_4 and increased TSH in primary hypothyroidism.
   ii. Patients with Hashimoto's thyroiditis have high titers for antibodies to thyroperoxidase and thyroglobulin.
   iii. See Table 7-3 for interpretation of thyroid function tests.

Table 7-3 • Thyroid Function Test Interpretation

	TSH Level	Thyroid Hormone Level
Overt hyperthyroidism	Low or undetectable	Elevated FT_4 or FT_3
Subclinical hyperthyroidism	Low or undetectable	Normal FT_4 or FT_3
Overt hypothyroidism	>5 mIU/L	Low FT_4
Subclinical hypothyroidism	>5 mIU/L	Normal FT_4

FT_4, free thyroxine; FT_3, free triiodothyronine

d. Treatment
   i. Thyroid supplement with levothyroxine.
      1. Smaller starting doses should be started in the elderly and patients with coronary artery disease.
V. Thyroiditis
   a. General
      i. Classified as:
         1. Chronic lymphocytic (Hashimoto's) thyroiditis
            (a) More common in females than males and tends to be familial.
            (b) Associated with other autoimmune diseases such as diabetes, Addison's disease, etc.
         2. Subacute thyroiditis
            (a) More common in young and middle-aged females.
            (b) Viral infection suggested as the cause.
         3. Suppurative thyroiditis
            (a) Rare disorder caused by pyogenic bacteria.
         4. Riedel's thyroiditis
            (a) Very rare and more commonly noted in middle-aged and elderly females.
   b. Clinical manifestations
      i. Chronic lymphocytic presents with fatigue, dry mouth and eyes, and a diffusely enlarged, firm nodular thyroid.
      ii. Subacute thyroiditis presents with a painful, enlarged thyroid.
      iii. Suppurative thyroiditis presents with a very painful, tender, red thyroid gland.
      iv. Riedel's thyroiditis presents with a stoney hard thyroid gland and signs of dysphagia, dyspnea, pain, and hoarseness.
   c. Diagnosis
      i. Thyroid antibodies present in chronic lymphocytic (Hashimoto's) thyroiditis.
      ii. Radioactive iodide uptake is low in subacute thyroiditis.
   d. Treatment
      i. Chronic lymphocytic is treated with levothyroxine.
      ii. Subacute thyroiditis is treated with aspirin for pain and inflammation.
      iii. Suppurative thyroiditis is treated with antibiotics and surgical drainage if needed.

QUESTION

A 30-year-old female presents with fatigue, loss of hair, weight gain, and prolonged menstrual periods. Which of the following lab results would the physician assistant except to see?

A. Low T_4, low T_3, low TSH
B. Low T_4, low T_3, high TSH
C. High T_4, normal T_3, low TSH
D. Normal T_4, low T_3, normal TSH

   iv. Riedel's thyroiditis is treated with short-term steroid therapy and long-term treatment with tamoxifen.
VI. Neoplastic disease
   a. General
      i. Almost always manifests as a palpable thyroid nodule.
      ii. Cause of thyroid cancer is unknown.
      iii. Risk factors include radiation to the head and neck and genetic causes.
      iv. Twice as common in females than males, but males have a worse prognosis.
      v. Papillary carcinoma is the most common type and is the least aggressive.
   b. Clinical manifestations
      i. Present with a single, hard nodule that is showing rapid, painless growth.
         1. Cancer more likely etiology of a thyroid nodule in a child or a patient over age 60.
   c. Diagnosis
      i. Thyroid hormone levels are typically normal.
      ii. An iodine-123 (^{123}I) scan will reveal a thyroid nodule that is cold.
      iii. Diagnosis is based on cytology findings of a fine-needle aspiration of the thyroid.
      iv. Thyroid ultrasound can also be helpful to determine if nodule is cystic or fluid-filled.
   d. Treatment
      i. Thyroid surgery, a lobectomy or near-total thyroidectomy, is indicated.
      ii. ^{131}I ablation is used in patients who have undergone a near-total thyroidectomy to destroy the remainder of the thyroid gland,

NOTES

ANSWER **B** EXPLANATION: *Hypothyroidism presents with fatigue, hair loss, weigh gain, cold tolerance, depression, and decreased appetite. Laboratory tests reveal an elevated TSH and low T3 and T4.*

correct ☐   incorrect ☐

DISEASES OF THE ADRENAL GLAND

I. General
   a. Location/function
      i. Located on top of the kidneys.
      ii. Each gland is composed of a cortex and medulla.
         1. Cortex
            (a) Composed of three zones that produce different steroid hormones.
            (b) See Table 7-4.
         2. Medulla
            (a) A sympathetic ganglion produces catecholamines.
   b. Tests of adrenocortical function:
      i. Urine free cortisol
         1. Used for adrenal hyperfunctioning not adrenal insufficiency.
      ii. Plasma cortisol
         1. There is a diurnal variation in cortisol levels.
         2. Normal range 5–20 µg/dL.
      iii. Plasma ACTH levels
         1. Normal range is up to 100 pg/mL.
      iv. Provocative tests
         1. ACTH stimulation test
            (a) Screening test for adrenal hypofunction.
         2. Corticotropin-releasing hormone
            (a) Used to separate ACTH-dependent from ACTH-independent hypercortisolism.
         3. Dexamethasone suppression test
            (a) Used to screen for adrenal hyperfunction.

II. Cushing syndrome
   a. General
      i. Caused by glucocorticoid excess.
      ii. Causes of Cushing syndrome
         1. ACTH-dependent
            (a) ACTH-secreting pituitary tumor (Cushing's disease)
               (i) Most common cause
            (b) Nonpituitary ACTH-secreting neoplasm
               (i) Small cell carcinoma of the lung
               (ii) Endocrine tumors of foregut origin
               (iii) Pheochromocytoma
               (iv) Ovarian tumors
         2. ACTH-independent
            (a) Adrenal adenoma
            (b) Adrenal carcinoma
            (c) Glucocorticoid administration
   b. Clinical manifestations
      i. Classically present with the following:
         1. Weight gain
            (a) Mainly centripetal with deposits in the dorsocervical fat pad (buffalo hump) and supraclavicular fossa.
         2. Plethora
            (a) Present with a ruddy complexion.

Table 7-4 • Adrenal Gland Cortex

Zone	Hormone Produced	Hormone Function	Hormone Controlling Release
Zona glomerulosa	Aldosterone	Regulates sodium balance	Renin
Zona fasciculate	Cortisol	Maintains physiologic integrity	ACTH
Zona reticularis	Androgen and estrogen precursors	Production of androgens and estrogens	Androgen-stimulating hormone

ACTH, adrenocorticotropic hormone

NOTES

3. Striae
   (a) Violaceous and occurring in thin skin.
4. Hypertension
5. Proximal muscle weakness
   (a) Test patient's ability to rise unassisted from a squatting position.
6. Oligomenorrhea or amenorrhea
   ii. Laboratory findings
      1. May see hyperglycemia, hypokalemia, and a leukocytosis.
c. Diagnosis
   i. Lab tests reveal an elevated cortisol level.
      1. Best tested for with the urine free cortisol level.
   ii. Dexamethasone screening test (dexamethasone given at night with cortisol measured in the morning) with a low AM cortisol level excludes Cushing syndrome.
   iii. The corticotrophin-releasing hormone test, with the measurement of ACTH levels, is used to separate ACTH-dependent from ACTH-independent disease.
d. Treatment
   i. Surgical removal of tumor is indicated followed by hormone replacement therapy.
   ii. Adrenal inhibitors include metyrapone and ketoconazole.

III. Acute corticoadrenal insufficiency (adrenal crisis)
a. General
   i. Due to insufficient cortisol.
   ii. Most commonly seen in patients with primary adrenal insufficiency (Addison's disease).
   iii. Adrenal crisis may occur after the following:
      1. Following stress such as trauma, surgery, or infection.
      2. Sudden withdrawal of adrenocortical hormone.
      3. Bilateral adrenalectomy
      4. Following injury to both adrenals
b. Clinical manifestations
   i. Patients complain of headache, nausea and vomiting, abdominal pain, and diarrhea.
   ii. Confusion or coma may be present.

QUESTION

Which of the following causes Cushing's syndrome?

A. Glucocorticoid deficiency
B. Glucocorticoid excess
C. Aldosterone deficiency
D. Aldosterone excess

---

   iii. On physical examination the patient is hypotensive and signs of cyanosis, dehydration, and hyperpigmentation of the skin may be present.
   iv. Laboratory results reveal the following:
      1. Eosinophilia
      2. Hyponatremia
      3. Hyperkalemia
      4. Hypoglycemia
c. Diagnosis
   i. Evaluate patient for possible cause such as infection.
   ii. Diagnosis made by simplified cosyntropin stimulation test.
      1. A cortisol level below 20 µg/dL is a positive test.
   iii. Plasma ACTH levels will be elevated if patient has primary adrenal disease.
d. Treatment
   i. Acute
      1. Antibiotics for possible bacterial infection.
      2. IV saline and hydrocortisone must be given immediately.
   ii. Convalescent
      1. Continue with hydrocortisone and, as dosage decreases, may need to add mineralocorticoid to the treatment.

IV. Chronic corticoadrenal insufficiency
a. General
   i. Caused by destruction or dysfunction of the adrenal cortex.
   ii. Etiology
      1. Autoimmune destruction
         (a) Most common.
      2. Tuberculosis
      3. Bilateral adrenal hemorrhage

NOTES

4. Adrenoleukodystrophy
   (a) X-linked disorder with accumulation of long chain fatty acids in the adrenal cortex, testes, and brain.
   b. Clinical manifestations
   i. Symptoms include weakness, fatigability, weight loss, myalgias, arthralgias, fever, anorexia, anxiety, and nausea and vomiting.
   ii. On physical examination hypotension with orthostatics and hyperpigmentation is noted
      1. Pigmentation is noted over the knuckles, elbows, posterior neck, and palmar creases.
      2. The skin in pressure areas, belt line, also darkens.
   iii. Laboratory findings include:
      1. Eosinophilia
      2. Hyponatremia
      3. Hyperkalemia
      4. Hypoglycemia
   c. Diagnosis
   i. A low AM serum cortisol level with an elevated ACTH level is diagnostic.
   ii. Computed tomography (CT) scan of the adrenals may be needed to evaluate for tuberculosis of the adrenal glands.
   d. Treatment
   i. Hydrocortisone is the drug of choice.
   ii. If not resulting in adequate salt-retaining effect then fludrocortisone may be added.
V. Glucocorticoids
   a. General
   i. Anti-seizure medications enhance metabolism of glucocorticoids, making them less potent.
   ii. Glucocorticoid activity (see Table 7-5).
   b. Side effects
   i. Prolonged therapy or high doses may lead to a variety of side effects.
      1. Decrease risk of side effects when:

(a) Dose equal to or less than the normal daily production.
(b) Duration of therapy less than 3 weeks
(c) Single AM dose less suppressive.
   2. See Table 7-6 for common side effects.
VI. Primary hyperaldosteronism
   a. General
   i. Due to unilateral adrenocortical adenoma (Conn syndrome) or bilateral cortical hyperplasia.
   ii. More common in women.
   b. Clinical manifestations
   i. Symptoms include muscle weakness, paresthesias, headache, polyuria, and polydipsia.
   ii. On physical examination hypertension is noted.
   iii. Laboratory tests reveal hypokalemia.

Table 7-5 • Glucocorticoid Activity

	Systemic Activity	Topical Activity
Hydrocortisone	1	1
Prednisone	4–5	1–2
Triamcinolone	5	1
Dexamethasone	30	5–10
Methylprednisolone	5	5

Table 7-6 • Side Effects of Glucocorticoids

Insomnia	Personality change
Weight gain	Muscle weakness
Polyuria	Kidney stones
Diabetes	Sex hormone suppression
Infection	Amenorrhea
Osteoporosis	Aseptic necrosis of bone

c. Diagnosis
  i. Before testing all antihypertensive medications must be stopped and all patients must have a high sodium intake during testing.
  ii. Diagnosis is made with noting a low plasma renin activity and an elevated 24-hour urine aldosterone level.
  iii. CT scan of the adrenal should be completed to evaluate for adrenal tumors.
d. Treatment
  i. Conn syndrome is treated with adrenalectomy or lifelong spironolactone therapy.
  ii. Bilateral adrenal hyperplasia is treated with spironolactone.
  iii. Complications seen are those noted with chronic hypertension.

DISEASES OF THE PITUITARY GLAND

I. General
  a. See Table 7-7 for summary of pituitary hormones.
II. Acromegaly/Gigantism
  a. General
    i. Due to excessive growth hormone.
      1. Is called gigantism if occurs before closure of epiphyses.
      2. Is called acromegaly if occurs after closure of epiphyses.
    ii. Acromegaly is almost always caused by pituitary adenoma.
  b. Clinical manifestations
    i. Physical findings include large, doughy hands, feet grow wider, facial features become coarse, mandible becomes more prominent, and tooth spacing widens.
    ii. Hypertension and cardiomegaly are common.
    iii. Increased risk of developing diabetes mellitus.
    iv. Headaches are common and temporal hemianopia may develop secondary to impingement of optic chiasm.

QUESTION

All of the following are side effects of glucocorticoids EXCEPT?
  A. Diabetes
  B. Weight loss
  C. Osteoporosis
  D. Muscle weakness

c. Diagnosis
  i. Laboratory findings include elevated prolactin levels (co-secreted by many growth hormone-secreting tumors).
  ii. After administration of glucose an elevated growth hormone level is noted in acromegaly.
  iii. Magnetic resonance imaging (MRI) may reveal a pituitary tumor.
d. Treatment
  i. Pituitary adenomas are removed by transnasal, transsphenoidal surgery.
  ii. Dopamine agonists can be used to shrink tumors.
  iii. Somatostatin analogs (octreotide and lanreotide) can be used to treat patients with acromegaly despite surgery.
III. Dwarfism/Short stature
  a. Short stature
    i. General
      1. See Table 7-8 for etiologies.
    ii. Clinical manifestations
      1. Familial short stature
        (a) Establish growth curves at or below the 5th percentile by age 2.
        (b) Otherwise healthy with a normal physical examination.
        (c) Have normal bone age and puberty occurs at the expected time.
      2. Constitutional delay
        (a) Children grow or develop at or below the 5th percentile at normal growth velocity.
          (i) Growth curve parallel to the 5th percentile.

NOTES

ANSWER B EXPLANATION: *Side effects of glucocorticoids include, weight gain, diabetes mellitus, infection, osteoporosis, personality changes, and avascular necrosis of bone.*

correct ☐   incorrect ☐

   (b) Have delay in puberty and skeletal maturation.
   (c) Child will likely mature to expected height for his/her family.
  3. Growth hormone deficiency

   (a) Children grow at a diminished velocity, less than 5 cm/year.
   (b) May have a history of birth asphyxia, neonatal hypoglycemia, microphallus, or midline defects.
  4. Primary hypothyroidism
   (a) Diagnosis with an elevated TSH.
  5. Chronic diseases
   (a) Due to lack of caloric intake or absorption.
   (b) Seen in children with cystic fibrosis, diabetes mellitus, chronic renal failure, inflammatory bowel disease, and celiac sprue.

Table 7-7 • Pituitary Hormones

Hormone	Releasing/Inhibiting Agent	Function
Anterior Pituitary		
Thyroid-stimulating hormone (TSH)	Thyroid-stimulating hormone releasing hormone (TRH)	Causes thyroid to release thyroid hormone.
Prolactin	Prolactin inhibitory hormone (PIH)	Promotes development of the breasts and secretion of milk.
Follicle-stimulating hormone (FSH)	Gonadotropin-releasing hormone (GnRH)	Causes growth of follicles in the ovaries prior to ovulation, also promotes formation of sperm in the testes.
Luteinizing hormone (LH)	Gonadotropin-releasing hormone (GnRH)	Plays a role in causing ovulation and causes secretion of female sex hormones by the ovaries and testosterone by the testes.
Growth hormone	Growth hormone-releasing hormone (GHRH)	Causes growth of almost all cells and tissues.
Adrenocorticotropin hormone (ACTH)	Corticotropin-releasing hormone (CRH)	Causes adrenal cortex to secrete adrenocortical hormone.
Posterior Pituitary	**Stimulus**	**Function**
Antidiuretic hormone (ADH)	Increase in blood osmolality.	Causes the kidneys to retain water.
Oxytocin	Breast stimulation and contraction of uterus during parturition.	Causes contraction of the uterus during birthing process and stimulates expression of milk from breasts.

NOTES

6. Turner syndrome
    (a) Results from having only one X chromosome.
    (b) Clinical features include webbed neck, low hairline, short stature, multiple pigmented nevi, and a shield-shaped chest.
    (c) 100% of patients have gonadal dysgenesis.
    (d) Renal anomalies, such as duplication of collecting system and horseshoe kidney, are common.
7. Medications
    (a) Chronic use of medications, such as steroids, dextroamphetamine, and methylphenidate, may result in poor growth.
  b. Dwarfism
    i. General
      1. Prototype is achondroplasia.
      2. Majority of cases result from new gene mutations.
    ii. Clinical manifestations
      1. Physical examination reveals short limbs, long narrow trunk, large heads with midface hypoplasia, and prominent brows.

2. Patients have delayed developmental milestones and have normal intelligence.
    iii. Diagnosis
      1. Mutation in the FGFR3 gene is noted.
    iv. Treatment
      1. Complications include neurologic complications, bowing of legs, obesity, dental problems, and frequent ear infections.
      2. Surgery utilized to correct orthopedic problems.
      3. Use of growth hormone is controversial.
IV. Diabetes insipidus
  a. General
    i. Due to deficiency of or resistance to vasopressin.

Table 7-8 • Causes of Short Stature		
Normal Causes	**Pathologic Disproportionate**	**Pathologic Proportionate**
Familial (Genetic)	Rickets	Prenatal Intrauterine growth retardation Placental dysfunction Intrauterine infections Teratogens Chromosomal abnormalities (Turner syndrome or trisomy 21)
Constitutional	Achondroplasia	Postnatal Malnutrition Chronic disease Drugs Growth hormone deficiency Glucocorticoid excess

NOTES

ANSWER **C** EXPLANATION: *Acromegaly is due to excessive production of growth hormone.*

correct ☐   incorrect ☐

ii. Etiologies
1. Deficiency of vasopressin (central diabetes insipidus)
   (a) Primary
       (i) May be familial with no sign of organic lesion.
   (b) Secondary
       (i) Due to damage to the hypothalamus.
2. Nephrogenic diabetes insipidus
   (a) Due to defect in kidney tubules that interferes with water reabsorption.
   (b) Clinical manifestations
       (i) Symptoms include intense thirst (craving for ice water) and polyuria.
           (1) Volume of ingested fluid varies from 2–20 L and equally large volumes of urine.
       (ii) May present with hypernatremia and dehydration.
       (iii) There is no single laboratory test for diagnosis of diabetes insipidus.
           (1) Urine specific gravity typically less than 1.005.
   c. Diagnosis
      i. Diagnosis based on clinical picture with polyuria and dehydration.
      ii. A vasopressin challenge test can be used to diagnose central diabetes insipidus.
      iii. Vasopressin levels can be measured to diagnose nephrogenic diabetes insipidus.
   d. Treatment
      i. Desmopressin acetate is the treatment of choice for central diabetes insipidus.
         1. Given intranasally as needed for thirst and polyuria.
      ii. Central and nephrogenic diabetes insipidus may respond to hydrochlorothiazide.

iii. Avoid thioridazine and lithium since they may cause polyuria.
V. Hyperprolactinemia
   a. General
      i. Main role of prolactin is in lactation.
      ii. Prolactin, plus the effects of estrogen and progesterone allow breast development to take place.
      iii. The control of the secretion of prolactin is under inhibitory control.
         1. Prolactin inhibitory factor (PIF) is dopamine.
      iv. Etiologies are in three groups:
         1. Physiologic: exercise, pregnancy, puerperium, stress, and suckling.
         2. Pharmacologic: estrogens, cimetidine, ranitidine, methyldopa, metoclopramide, phenothiazine, protease inhibitors, risperidone, selective serotonin reuptake inhibitors (SSRIs), and tricyclic antidepressants.
         3. Pathologic: acromegaly, chronic chest wall stimulation, cirrhosis, hypothyroidism, prolactin-secreting tumors, renal failure, and systemic lupus erythematosus (SLE).
   b. Clinical manifestations
      i. More common in females and sporadic in nature.
      ii. Increased levels may result in hypogonadotropic hypogonadism.
         1. Men may have erectile dysfunction, gynecomastia, and decreased libido.
         2. Women may have oligomenorrhea or amenorrhea and galactorrhea.
      iii. Large tumors may cause headache and visual symptoms.
   c. Diagnosis
      i. Rule out conditions known to cause hyperprolactinemia.
         1. Liver function tests for cirrhosis.
         2. Beta-human chorionic gonadotropin (beta-hCG) for pregnancy.
         3. TSH for hypothyroidism.
         4. Blood urea nitrogen (BUN) and creatinine for renal failure.

NOTES

    ii. MRI of the pituitary to evaluate for tumor.

  d. Treatment

    i. Stop all medications known to increase prolactin levels if possible.

    ii. Dopamine agonists

      1. Initial treatment of choice for patients with large tumors or those desiring normal sexual function and fertility.

        (a) Cabergoline

        (b) Bromocriptine

        (c) Pergolide

      2. Side effects include fatigue, nausea, dizziness, and orthostatic hypotension.

    iii. Surgery

      1. Reserved for large tumors causing visual symptoms.

    iv. Radiation therapy

      1. Reserved for patients who have rapid growing tumors despite other treatment.

DIABETES MELLITUS

I. General

  a. Leading cause of blindness, end-stage renal disease, and nontraumatic limb amputation in the United States.

  b. Diabetes increases risk for cardiovascular, cerebral, and peripheral vascular disease.

  c. Diabetes is a major factor in neonatal morbidity and mortality.

  d. Long-term complications are noted in type 1 and type 2 diabetes.

    i. Microvascular disease more common in type 1.

    ii. Macrovascular disease more common in type 2.

    iii. See Table 7-9 for complications noted in diabetes mellitus.

II. Type 1

  a. General

    i. Formally known as insulin-dependent diabetes.

    ii. Patients have little or no insulin secretion capacity.

QUESTION

Which of the following clinical manifestations is noted in patients with hyperprolactinemia?

  A. Muscle weakness

  B. Headache

  C. Hirsutism

  D. Obesity

Table 7-9 • Complications of Diabetes Mellitus

Eyes
Diabetic retinopathy
Cataracts
Renal
Glomerulosclerosis
Renal tubular necrosis
Pyelonephritis
Neurologic
Peripheral neuropathy
Autonomic neuropathy (gastroparesis, erectile dysfunction, postural hypotension)
Cardiovascular
Heart disease (myocardial infarction, cardiomyopathy)
Skin
Lower extremity ulcers
Infectious
Malignant otitis externa

NOTES

ANSWER **B** EXPLANATION: *Hyperprolactinemia, due to a pituitary adenoma, may present with headache and visual changes.*

correct ❑   incorrect ❑

iii. An autoimmune disease associated with a specific HLA gene and presence of autoantibodies to islet cells of the pancreas.
b. Clinical manifestations
   i. At time of presentation patients appear very ill.
   ii. Symptoms appear abruptly and include polyuria, polydipsia, polyphagia, and weight loss.
     1. May also present with ketoacidosis.
   iii. Laboratory findings include:
     1. Glycosuria
     2. Elevated glycosylated hemoglobin
       (a) Reflects state of glycemia over the preceding 10–12 weeks.
     3. Ketonuria
       (a) May also be noted in starvation, high-fat diets, alcoholic ketoacidosis, and fever.
     4. Proteinuria
     5. Microalbuminuria
       (a) Presence of microalbumin is an early predictor of diabetic nephropathy.
c. Diagnosis
   i. Based on the following:
     1. Symptoms of diabetes (polyuria, polydipsia, unexplained weight loss) plus random plasma glucose greater than 200 mg/dL.
     2. Fasting plasma glucose greater than 126 mg/dL.
     3. Two-hour (post-standard 75-g glucose tolerance test) plasma glucose greater than 200 mg/dL.
   ii. Impaired fasting glucose
     1. Refers to a patient with fasting plasma glucose greater than 110 mg/dL but less than 126 mg/dL.
   iii. Impaired glucose tolerance
     1. Refers to a patient with 2-hour plasma glucose greater than 140 mg/dL but less than 200 mg/dL.

d. Treatment
   i. Prevention of long-term complications is vital.
   ii. Diet
     1. Balance caloric intake with energy expenditure.
     2. Must match carbohydrate intake with insulin dosing.
     3. Limit cholesterol to 300 mg/day.
     4. Daily protein intake 10%–20% of total calories.
     5. Restrict saturated fats to 10% of total calories.
     6. Restrict sodium to less than 2.4 g/day.
   iii. Insulin
     1. Insulin replacement along with lifestyle changes is required.
     2. Are many different insulin regimens and each should be tailored to the individual patient.
     3. Frequent monitoring of plasma glucose levels is required to assist patients with maintaining adequate control of blood glucose.
     4. See Table 7-10 for summary of insulin preparations.
   iv. Complications
     1. Diabetic ketoacidosis
       (a) Due to increased lipolysis, decreased glucose uptake, and increased proteolysis.
         (i) Results in hyperglycemia, ketonuria, and acidosis.

Table 7-10 • Summary of Insulin Preparations

Class	Type	Onset	Peak	Duration
Ultra short-acting	Lispro or Aspart	5–15 min	1–2 hr	3–4 hr
Short-acting	Regular	15–30 min	2–4 hr	5–8 hr
Intermediate-acting	NPH or Lente	2–4 hr	5–10 hr	18–24 hr
Long-acting	Ultralente	4–6 hr	8–16 hr	24–36 hr
	Glargine	2–4 hr	No peak	>30 hr

NOTES

(b) Precipitating factors include infections, inadequate insulin treatment, and myocardial ischemia/infarction.

(c) Clinical signings include abdominal pain, nausea/vomiting, tachycardia, dehydration, and fruity breath odor.

(d) Laboratory results reveal hyperglycemia (250–1000 mg/dL), presence of ketones in blood and urine, elevated anion gap metabolic acidosis (bicarbonate <18 mEq/L and pH <7.30), and electrolyte abnormalities.

(e) Treatment consists of IV fluids, regular insulin, correction of electrolyte abnormalities, and treatment of underlying cause.

III. Type 2
  a. General
    i. Accounts for 90% of all cases of clinical diabetes.
    ii. Patients retain some endogenous insulin secretion ability, but levels are low relative to glucose levels and level of insulin resistance.
    iii. High rate of genetic influence, not related to HLA genes, and also associated with high-fat diets, obesity, and decreased physical activity.
  b. Clinical manifestations
    i. Insidious onset of symptoms and may be mild or symptomatic.
    ii. Symptoms include polyuria, polydipsia, blurry vision, fatigue, weakness, and dizziness.
      1. May present with symptoms of chronic complications such as vascular or neurologic disease.
    iii. Laboratory findings include:
      1. Glycosuria
      2. Elevated glycosylated hemoglobin
        (a) Reflects state of glycemia over the preceding 10–12 weeks.
      3. Ketonuria
        (a) May also be noted in starvation, high-fat diets, alcoholic ketoacidosis, and fever.
      4. Proteinuria
      5. Microalbuminuria
        (a) Presence of microalbumin is an early predictor of diabetic nephropathy.

c. Diagnosis
  i. Based on the following:
    1. Symptoms of diabetes (polyuria, polydipsia, unexplained weight loss) plus random plasma glucose greater than 200 mg/dL.
    2. Fasting plasma glucose greater than 126 mg/dL.
    3. Two-hour (post-standard 75-g glucose tolerance test) plasma glucose greater than 200 mg/dL.
  ii. Impaired fasting glucose
    1. Refers to a patient with fasting plasma glucose greater than 110 mg/dL but less than 126 mg/dL.
  iii. Impaired glucose tolerance
    1. Refers to a patient with 2-hour plasma glucose greater than 140 mg/dL but less than 200 mg/dL.

d. Treatment
  i. Diet
    1. Even modest weight loss in the obese patient will improve glycemic control.
    2. Diet high in carbohydrates (>50%) may improve insulin action and glycemia control in mild fasting hyperglycemia.
      (a) In patients with severe fasting hyperglycemia or elevated triglycerides, a diet with reduced (<45%) carbohydrates is indicated.
    3. Limit cholesterol to 300 mg/day.
    4. Daily protein intake should be 10%–20% of total calories.
    5. Restrict saturated fats to 10% of total calories.
    6. Restrict sodium to less than 2.4 g/day.
  ii. Oral antidiabetic medications
    1. Indicated in patients who fail treatment with diet and exercise.
    2. See Table 7-11 for summary of antidiabetic medications.
  iv. Monitoring
    1. Regular self-monitoring allows patients to maintain tight control of blood sugar levels.
  v. Complications
    1. Hyperosmolar hyperglycemic state
      (a) Most commonly noted in the elderly with diabetes mellitus type 2.

NOTES

Table 7-11 • Oral Antidiabetic Medications

Drug	Classification	Mechanism of Action	Site of Metabolism	Duration of Action (Hours)	Side Effects
Chlorpropamide	1st Generation sulfonylurea	Increase pancreas insulin secretion	Kidney	>60	Hypoglycemia Weight gain
Glimepiride	2nd Generation sulfonylurea	Increase pancreas insulin secretion	Liver	24	Hypoglycemia Weight gain
Glipizide	2nd Generation sulfonylurea	Increase pancreas insulin secretion	Liver	12–24	Hypoglycemia Weight gain
Glyburide	2nd Generation sulfonylurea	Increase pancreas insulin secretion	Liver	Up to 24	Hypoglycemia Weight gain
Tolazamide	1st Generation sulfonylurea	Increase pancreas insulin secretion	Liver	12–24	Hypoglycemia Weight gain
Tolbutamide	1st Generation sulfonylurea	Increase pancreas insulin secretion	Liver	6–12	Hypoglycemia Weight gain
Repaglinide	Meglitinide analog	Increase pancreas insulin secretion	Liver	<4	Hypoglycemia Weight gain
Metformin	Biguanides	Decreases hepatic glucose production	Kidney	Up to 24	Abdominal pain Nausea Diarrhea Lactic acidosis
Pioglitazone	Thiazolidinediones	Decrease peripheral insulin resistance	Liver	24	Fluid retention Weight gain Congestive heart failure (CHF)
Rosiglitazone	Thiazolidinediones	Decrease peripheral insulin resistance	Liver	Up to 24	Fluid retention Weight gain CHF
Acarbose	Alpha-glucosidase inhibitors	Decrease postprandial digestion of glucose	Gut	Local effect	Abdominal pain Nausea Diarrhea
Miglitol	Alpha-glucosidase inhibitors	Decrease postprandial digestion of glucose	Kidney	Local effect	Abdominal pain Nausea Diarrhea

NOTES

(b) Etiology not fully understood, but patients have severe dehydration with hyperglycemia.

(c) Symptoms include severe dehydration and alterations in mental status.

(d) Laboratory results reveal severe hyperosmolarity (>320 mOsm/L), hyperglycemia (>600 mg/dL).
   [i] Severe acidosis and ketosis are rare.

(e) Treatment consists of IV fluids, regular insulin, correction of electrolyte abnormalities, and treatment of the underlying cause.

(f) See Table 7-12 for comparison of insulin shock, diabetic ketoacidosis (DKA), and hyperosmolar shock.

VII. Hypoglycemia
   a. General
      i. There are two types, fasting and postprandial.
      ii. Etiologies
         1. See Table 7-13.
   b. Clinical manifestations
      i. Symptoms begin when blood sugar level at 60 mg/dL.

QUESTION

Which of the following diabetic medications should be avoided in patients at risk for developing lactic acidosis?

   A. Glipizide (Glucotrol)
   B. Metformin (Glucophage)
   C. Acarbose (Precose)
   D. Pioglitazone (Actos)

---

   1. Impaired brain function when blood sugar at 50 mg/dL.
   ii. Symptoms include sweating, palpitations, hunger, tremor, weakness, headache, lightheadedness, confusion, seizures, and coma.
   iii. In a patient with insulinoma note the following:
      1. Symptoms develop in early morning or after missing a meal.
      2. Symptoms include blurry vision, headache, slurred speech, and weakness.

Table 7-12 • Comparison of Acute Complications of Diabetes Mellitus

Feature	Insulin Shock	Diabetic Ketoacidosis	Hyperosmolar Shock
Insulin	Excessive	Insufficient	Normal or increased
Onset	Rapid	Gradual (days)	Gradual (days)
Skin	Cold sweats, pale	Dry, flushed	Dry, flushed
Respirations	Normal or shallow	Slow and deep	Typically normal
Heart rate	Rapid	Rapid	Typically normal
Blood pressure	Normal	Low	Normal
Blood glucose	Very low	High	Very high
pH	Normal	Low	Normal
Acetone	Absent	Positive	Absent

NOTES

ANSWER B EXPLANATION: *Metformin should be avoided in patients with lactic acidosis or at risk of developing lactic acidosis. Other side effects include abdominal pain, nausea, and diarrhea.*

correct ☐   incorrect ☐

c. Diagnosis
   i. Prolonged fasting in the hospital until hypoglycemia is noted is the most dependable means of making the diagnosis.
   ii. Diagnosis of insulinoma is based on noting elevated insulin levels during a time of hypoglycemia.

Table 7-13 • Etiology of Hypoglycemia
Fasting hypoglycemia
Endocrine disorders
Addison's disease
Myxedema
Hypopituitarism
Liver failure
Renal failure
Pancreatic B-cell tumor
Administration of insulin or sulfonylureas
Postprandial hypoglycemia
Postgastrectomy
Functional
Alcohol-related hypoglycemia
Autoimmune
Antibodies to insulin or insulin receptors

d. Treatment
   i. Dextrose is used in the treatment of the patient with hypoglycemia due to administration of excess insulin.
   ii. Treatment of the patient with an insulinoma is surgical resection of the tumor, frequent feedings, and the use of diazoxide.

LIPID DISORDERS

I. Hypercholesterolemia
   a. General
      i. Linked to the development of atherosclerosis.
      ii. Due to elevations in low-density lipoprotein (LDL).
         1. Elevations of LDL are associated with increased risk of atherosclerotic heart disease.
         2. Elevations of high-density lipoproteins (HDL) are associated with a decreased risk of atherosclerotic heart disease.
      iii. Normal range (see Table 7-14)
      iv. Etiology
         1. Familial hypercholesterolemia
            (a) Autosomal dominant disorder due to defective or absence of LDL receptors.
            (b) See Table 7-15.
         2. Nephrotic syndrome
         3. Hypothyroidism
         4. Obstructive liver disease

Table 7-14 • Normal Range for Fasting Lipids			
Lipid	Acceptable (mg/dL)	Borderline (mg/dL)	Unacceptable (mg/dL)
Cholesterol	<200	200–239	>240
LDL	<130 (primary) <100 (secondary)		>160 >100
HDL	≥60		<40
Triglyceride	<150	150–500	>500

Table 7-15 • Types of Hyperlipidemia

Type	Lipids Elevated	Subtype Elevated	Coronary Artery Disease Risk
I	Triglycerides	Chylomicrons	Normal
IIA	Cholesterol	LDL	Very high
IIB	Cholesterol and triglycerides	VLDL and LDL	Very high
III	Cholesterol and triglycerides	Beta-VLDL and LDL	Very high
IV	Triglycerides	VLDL	Varies
V	Triglycerides	VLDL and chylomicrons	Moderate

b. Clinical manifestations
  i. Xanthomas noted on Achilles tendon, patellar tendon, and extensor tendons of the hand.
c. Diagnosis
  i. Laboratory tests reveal elevated LDL cholesterol.
  ii. Plasma cholesterol levels typically greater than 300 mg/dL.
d. Treatment
  i. Dietary
    1. Limit cholesterol intake to less than 300 mg/day.
    2. Limit total dietary fats to 30% and saturated fats to less than 10% of total calories.
  ii. Medications
    1. Bile-acid binding agents
      (a) Bind bile acids/cholesterol and promote loss in the stool.
      (b) Also increase LDL receptor expression and directly remove LDL particles.
      (c) Side effects include constipation and bloating.

      (d) Agents can interfere with absorption of numerous medications including glycosides, thiazides, warfarin, tetracycline, thyroxine, and iron salts.
    2. HMG-CoA reductase inhibitors (statins)
      (a) Directly inhibits cholesterol biosynthesis.
      (b) Side effects include myositis.
    3. Nicotinic acid (niacin)
      (a) Inhibit release of lipoproteins from the liver.
      (b) Side effects include flushing.
II. Hypertriglyceridemia
  a. General
    i. Linked to the development of pancreatitis.
    ii. Due to elevations in very low-density lipoprotein (VLDL) and chylomicrons.
    iii. Etiology
      1. Familial hypertriglyceridemia
        (a) Autosomal dominant disorder.
      2. Diabetes mellitus
      3. Uremia
      4. Sepsis
      5. Obesity
      6. SLE
      7. Alcohol
  b. Clinical manifestations
    i. Are typically asymptomatic and without signs of xanthomas.
    ii. May have signs and symptoms of pancreatitis.
    iii. Diagnosed with routine blood screening.
  c. Diagnosis
    i. Marked elevations in triglycerides, normal or low LDL levels, and decreased levels of HDL cholesterol.
  d. Treatment
    i. Treatment plan should begin with weight loss, increased physical activity, low-fat diet, and restriction of alcohol.
    ii. Medications
      1. Fibric acid derivations
        (a) Reduce hepatic triglyceride production and increased HDL synthesis.
        (b) Side effects include cholelithiasis and drug-induced hepatitis.

NOTES

Question 1

Which of the following presents with truncal fat distribution, moon facies, and hypertension?

- A. Hypoparathyroidism
- B. Cushing's disease
- C. Grave's disease
- D. Diabetes mellitus type II

Question 2

A 45-year-old presents with a history of weakness, orthostatic hypotension and hyperpigmentation. Which of the following laboratory tests would assist in making the correct diagnosis?

- A. 24 hour urine for catecholamines
- B. Thyroid simulating hormone
- C. Glucose tolerance test
- D. ACTH level

Question 3

A 35-year-old female presents for evaluation of headache, vision changes, and delayed menses. On physical examination bitemporal homonymous hemianopsia by confrontation is noted along with nipple discharge. Her pelvic examination is normal. Which of the following is the most likely diagnosis?

- A. Ovarian failure
- B. Hypothyroidism
- C. Addison's disease
- D. Pituitary adenoma

Question 4

A 55-year-old presents with severe palpitations and fever. Thyroid studies reveal an elevated free T4 and TSH level which is undetectable. Which of the following is the most appropriate management of this patient pending further evaluation?

- A. Aspirin
- B. Propranolol (Inderal)
- C. Cardiac pacing
- D. No treatment is indicated

Question 5

Glucophage (Metformin) is contraindicated in which of the following conditions?

- A. Lactic acidosis
- B. Stable angina
- C. Pregnancy
- D. Obesity

Question 6

In the diabetic patient the daily protein intake should be limited to what percent of total calories?

- A. 5–10
- B. 10–20
- C. 20–30
- D. 30–40

NOTES

Question 7

Which of the following inhibits ACTH secretion?

    A. Aldesterone
    B. Cortisol
    C. Glucose
    D. Calcium

Answer 1

ANSWER **B** EXPLANATION: *Cushing's disease or syndrome typically presents with centripetal weight gain, moon facies, striae, hypertension, and proximal muscle weakness.*

Topic: Cushing's syndrome

correct ☐   incorrect ☐

Answer 2

ANSWER **D** EXPLANATION: *Addison's disease (acute corticoadrenal insufficiency) presents with headache and abdominal pain. On physical examination orthostatic hypotension and hyperpigmentation are noted. Plasma ACTH levels are elevated in primary disease and diagnosis can be made by cosyntropin stimulation test.*

Topic: Acute corticoadrenal insufficiency

correct ☐   incorrect ☐

Answer 3

ANSWER **D** EXPLANATION: *Large pituitary adenomas present with headache and visual changes. Production of increased amounts of prolactin will lead to nipple discharge.*

Topic: Hyperprolactinemia

correct ☐   incorrect ☐

Answer 4

ANSWER **B** EXPLANATION: *Hyperthyroidism presents with palpitations, diarrhea, fever, and other signs of increased metabolism. Laboratory testing reveals an elevated T4 and decreased TSH. Early on treatment consists of symptomatic control, such as beta-blockers (propranolol) for control of palpitations. Aspirin is contraindicated due to causing increase release of thyroid hormone.*

Topic: Hyperthyroidism

correct ☐   incorrect ☐

Answer 5

ANSWER **A** EXPLANATION: *Glucophage (metformin), a biguanides, works by decreasing hepatic glucose production. Contraindications include renal failure and lactic acidosis.*

Topic: Diabetes mellitus Type 2

correct ☐   incorrect ☐

NOTES

Answer 6

ANSWER **B** EXPLANATION: *Dietary management is important in the management of the diabetic patient. Cholesterol should be limited to 300 mg per day, protein limited to 10-20% of total calories, restrict saturated fats to 10% of total calories and restrict sodium to less than 2.4 g per day.*

Topic: Diabetes mellitus

correct ☐   **incorrect** ☐

Answer 7

ANSWER **D** EXPLANATION: *ACTH is released by the anterior pituitary and leads to the release of cortisol and release is suppressed by negative feed back of cortisol.*

Topic: Adrenal gland

correct ☐   **incorrect** ☐

NOTES

Neurologic System

8

EXAM BLUEPRINT TOPICS

Alzheimer's Disease
Cerebral Palsy
Diseases of Peripheral Nerves
Bell's palsy
Diabetic peripheral neuropathy
Guillain-Barré syndrome
Myasthenia gravis
Headaches
Cluster headache
Migraine
Tension headache
Infectious Disorders
Encephalitis
Meningitis—bacterial
Movement Disorders
Amyotrophic lateral sclerosis (Lou Gehrig's disease)
Essential tremor
Huntington's disease
Parkinson's disease
Multiple Sclerosis
Seizure Disorders
Generalized convulsive disorder
Status epilepticus
Vascular Diseases
Cerebral aneurysm
Normal pressure hydrocephalus
Stroke
Subarachnoid hemorrhage

I. Alzheimer's disease
  a. General
    i. A progressive dementia with insidious onset and characterized by atrophy of the cerebral cortex.
    ii. A very common cause of dementia.
      1. Female-to-male ratio is 2:1.
    iii. Genetic mutations have been implicated.
      1. Increased risk if first-degree relative is affected with the disease.
    iv. A mean of 10 years passes from onset of disease to death.
    v. See Table 8-1 for various etiologies of degenerative dementias.
  b. Clinical manifestations
    i. Patient is typically older than 65 years and presents with the following:
      1. Early stage
        (a) Memory loss
          (i) Have difficulty learning new material and impaired recent memory.
        (b) Word-finding problems
          (i) Word finding pauses with diminished verbal fluency.
        (c) Visuospatial disturbances
          (i) Decline in drawing and driving.
      2. Intermediate stage
        (a) Develop aphasia, apraxia, and behavioral problems.
        (b) Sleep–wake cycle disturbances.
        (c) Decline in activities of daily living.
        (d) May wander, get lost, and have increased risk for falls.
      3. Terminal stage
        (a) Further cognitive decline, motor abnormalities, and both urinary and fecal incontinence.
        (b) Recent and remote memory totally lost.
        (c) May be unable to swallow and eat.
  c. Diagnosis
    i. Definitive diagnosis can be proven only at autopsy with the demonstration of neurofibrillary tangles and senile plaques.

NOTES

Table 8-1 • Degenerative Dementias		
Neurodegenerative	**Traumatic**	**Infectious**
Alzheimer's disease	Punch drunk	AIDS encephalopathy
Lewy body disease		Progressive multifocal leukoencephalopathy
Huntington's disease		Creutzfeldt-Jacob disease
Parkinson's disease		
Pick's disease		

ii. Evaluate each patient to exclude other possible causes of dementia.
1. This includes evaluating serum chemistries, vitamin B_{12}, thyroid-stimulating hormone (TSH), and cerebrospinal fluid (CSF) studies.
d. Treatment
i. There is no cure. Treatment is palliative only.
ii. Education and counseling, support groups, for family and caregivers is essential.
iii. Medications for specific behavioral problems.
1. Delusions
(a) Risperidone, olanzapine, or quetiapine can be used.
(b) Haloperidol should be avoided due to side effects.
2. Agitation
(a) Trazodone, divalproex, or carbamazepine can be used.
(b) Anticholinergic agents are contraindicated due to possible worsening of dementia.
iv. Medications for Alzheimer's disease
1. Acetylcholinesterase inhibitors will improve cognition, activities of daily living, and apathy.
(a) Donepezil
(b) Rivastigmine
(c) Galantamine

2. Side effects of the acetyl-cholinesterase inhibitors include nausea, vomiting, diarrhea, and muscle cramps.
II. Cerebral palsy
a. General
i. A nonprogressive disorder of movement and posture that results from a lesion of the immature brain.
ii. Most common movement disorder of children.
1. Will note delay in motor milestones.
iii. Risk factors include premature birth, birth asphyxia, intrauterine growth retardation, infection, or trauma.
b. Clinical manifestations
i. Presentation varies with infants being initially hypotonic and older patients divided into two groups.
1. Pyramidal (spastic)
(a) Tone remains constant despite activity, with primitive and pathologic reflexes present, and note significant hyperreflexia.
(b) Four types
(i) Diplegia: bilateral lower extremity spasticity
(ii) Quadriplegia: all limbs severely involved, lower extremities more than upper.
(iii) Hemiplegia: one side involved, upper extremity more than lower.
(iv) Bilateral hemiplegia: all limbs severely involved, upper extremities more than lower.
2. Extrapyramidal
(a) Tone is variable depending on level of arousal, primitive reflexes noted, and hyperreflexia may or may not be present.
(b) Three types
(i) Ataxic: have difficulty coordinating purposeful movements.
(ii) Choreoathetoid and dystonic have uncontrollable jerking, writhing, and posturing movements.

NOTES

    ii. Associated neurologic deficits are common.
       1. Seizures, mental retardation, hearing and vision problems are common.
  c. Diagnosis
    i. Based on clinical presentation.
  d. Treatment
    i. A multidisciplinary approach is needed to maximize function and minimize impairment.
    ii. No cure is available.
III. Diseases of the peripheral nerves
  a. Bell's palsy
    i. General
       1. Unilateral facial paralysis (cranial nerve 7) of unknown etiology.
         (a) May be a link to herpes simplex virus.
       2. Prognosis is excellent.
    ii. Clinical manifestations
       1. Typically note facial paralysis in the morning, and disease appears to come on over night.
       2. Patient will have trouble closing eye on affected side.
       3. Paralysis may be preceded by pain behind the ear.
       4. On physical examination, note seventh cranial nerve palsy, loss of taste on the anterior two thirds of the tongue, and hyperacusis.
    iii. Diagnosis
       1. One of exclusion.
       2. Rule out herpes zoster oticus (Ramsay Hunt syndrome).
         (a) May note herpetic lesions in the external auditory canal.
    iv. Treatment
       1. Most cases resolve without treatment.
       2. Protect the eye from drying.
       3. With link to herpes simplex infection acyclovir may be considered early in the treatment.
  b. Diabetic peripheral neuropathy
    i. General
       1. Symptomatic, possibly disabling neuropathy seen in nearly one half of diabetic patients.
       2. Can have peripheral and/or autonomic neuropathy.

QUESTION

Which of the following is an acetylcholinesterase inhibitor used in the treatment of Alzheimer's disease?

  A. Donepezil (Aricept)
  B. Risperidone (Risperdal)
  C. Haloperidol (Haldol)
  D. Trazodone (Desyrel)

    ii. Clinical manifestations
       1. Focal neuropathy
         (a) Begin suddenly and present with pain.
         (b) Self-limited, lasting 6 to 8 weeks.
         (c) Treatment aimed at pain control.
       2. Sensorimotor polyneuropathy
         (a) Most common neurologic syndrome seen in diabetes.
         (b) Effects distal sensorimotor nerves of the hands and feet.
         (c) Patients report numbness or tingling in a stocking-glove pattern.
         (d) Pain is common and may be described as burning or gnawing.
         (e) Physical examination findings include loss of vibratory sensation, light touch, two-point discrimination, and thermal sensitivity.
       3. Autonomic
         (a) May affect many different organ systems.
           (i) Cardiac symptoms include resting tachycardia, decreased heart rate variability, and prolonged QTc.
           (ii) Vascular symptoms include postural hypotension.
           (iii) Gastrointestinal symptoms include constipation and gastroparesis.
           (iv) Genitourinary symptoms include bladder hypotonia, incontinence, and erectile dysfunction.

NOTES

ANSWER A EXPLANATION: *Donepezil, an acetylcholinesterase inhibitor, is used in the treatment of Alzheimer's disease.*

correct ☐   incorrect ☐

iii. Diagnosis
  1. A complete history and physical examination are needed.
     (a) Neurologic examination must include a detailed sensory examination.
  2. Nerve conduction studies and electromyography may be needed.
iv. Treatment
  1. Tight glycemic control is the best early treatment.
     (a) Tight blood sugar control can slow the onset of disease by 60% to 70%.
  2. Treatment of autonomic symptoms
     (a) Gastroparesis treated with metoclopramide.
     (b) Genitourinary complaints treated with bethanechol or alpha-blockers.
     (c) Erectile dysfunction can be treated with sildenafil.
        (i) Sildenafil should be avoided in patients with heart disease.
  3. Neuropathic pain control
     (a) Tricyclic antidepressants such as amitriptyline and desipramine.
     (b) Anticonvulsants such as carbamazepine and gabapentin.
     (c) Topical therapy such as capsaicin.
     (d) Long-term opiate use and pain specialist management may be needed in refractory cases.
c. Guillain-Barré syndrome
  i. General
     1. An acute or subacute polyradiculoneuropathy most likely due to an immune-mediated mechanism.
     2. Due to lymphocytic infiltration and macrophage-mediated demyelination and axonal degeneration.
     3. Typically follows some type of infection such as *Campylobacter*, infectious mononucleosis, cytomegalovirus (CMV), herpes, and *Mycoplasma*.
  ii. Clinical manifestations
     1. Initial symptoms include ataxia and tingling or a pins-and-needles sensation in the feet.
     2. Weakness then develops, typically involving the legs.
     3. On physical examination, the deep tendon reflexes are lost early, and weakness is noted in an ascending pattern.
  iii. Diagnosis
     1. Diagnosis based on history and physical examination of progressive weakness and areflexia.
     2. Spinal fluid studies may reveal an elevated total protein and normal cell count.
     3. Electromyogram (EMG) results are consistent with demyelination and decreased nerve conduction studies.
  iv. Treatment
     1. Typically requires hospitalization because of the risk for respiratory muscle involvement and need for ventilatory support.
     2. Treatment options include plasmapheresis and high doses of human immunoglobulin.
d. Myasthenia gravis
  i. General
     1. An acquired autoimmune disorder that causes a decrease in acetylcholine receptors at the motor endplate.
     2. Fluctuating weakness of commonly used voluntary muscles that results in increased weakness with activity of affected muscles.
     3. Occurs at all ages, with women primarily affected in their 20s and males in their 50s or 60s.
  ii. Clinical manifestations
     1. In early stages, the disease affects the eye muscles, causing ptosis and diplopia.

NOTES

(a) Other facial muscles may be affected, resulting in loss of facial expression, jaw drop, and choking on food.
2. Limb muscle involvement leads to abnormal fatigability.
(a) Patients will have trouble combing hair, climbing stairs, or lifting objects repeatedly.
3. Deep tendon reflexes are normal.
iii. Diagnosis
1. Based on history and physical examination findings.
2. Anticholinesterase challenge test in which intravenous (IV) edrophonium or intramuscular (IM) neostigmine results in improved strength in seconds to minutes.
3. EMG reveals a decrease in action potentials amplitude over a number of muscle contractions.
4. Serology testing may reveal presence of antibodies to acetylcholine receptor binding sites.
iv. Treatment
1. Anticholinesterase drugs such as pyridostigmine bromide and neostigmine bromide are the cornerstone of treatment.
2. Other treatment options include alternate-day prednisone treatment, thymectomy, azathioprine, plasmapheresis, and IV immunoglobulin.
3. Aminoglycosides may exacerbate the disease and should be avoided.

IV. Headaches
a. Cluster headache
i. General
1. Recurrent episodes of frequent headaches separated by periods of being headache free.
2. Cause is unknown.
3. More common in males than females by a 6:1 ratio.
4. Headaches may cease during pregnancy.
ii. Clinical manifestations
1. History of recurrent episodes of unilateral, orbital, supraorbital, or temporal pain.

QUESTION

Which of the following cranial nerves is involved in Bells' palsy?
A. V
B. VI
C. VII
D. VIII

2. Accompanied by conjunctival injection, lacrimation, rhinorrhea, nasal congestion, or ptosis.
3. Attacks last 15 minutes to 3 hours and can occur every other day, up to 8 times per day.
iii. Diagnosis
1. Based on history.
2. Rule out other causes of headache.
iv. Treatment
1. High-flow oxygen can serve as effective treatment.
2. Classic treatment is ergotamine tartrate.
3. Other options include sumatriptan and lithium carbonate.
b. Migraine
i. General
1. Affects females more than males, primarily between ages 25 and 45 years.
2. Increased risk for migraine in patients with relatives with migraines.
3. May be brought on by certain triggers.
(a) See Table 8-2

Table 8-2 • Migraine Headache Triggers	
Stress	Lack of sleep/fatigue
Menses	Glare
Oral contraceptives	Weather changes
Alcohol	Physical exertion
Foods (cheeses and chocolate)	Head trauma

NOTES

ANSWER C EXPLANATION: *Bells' palsy involves cranial nerve VII, with symptoms including facial palsy and loss of taste sensation on the anterior two=thirds of the tongue.*

correct ☐   incorrect ☐

ii. Clinical manifestations
  1. May have prodrome symptoms 24 to 48 hours before headache attack.
    (a) Symptoms include hyperactivity, mild euphoria, lethargy, depression, and craving for certain foods.
  2. Migraine may or may not have an aura.
    (a) Aura includes homonymous visual disturbances (scotoma), unilateral numbness, unilateral weakness, or ataxia.
  3. Headache lasts 4 to 72 hours and described as unilateral throbbing pain that is moderate to severe in intensity.
  4. Associated symptoms include nausea and vomiting, photophobia, and phonophobia.
  5. Headache is intensified with physical activity.
iii. Diagnosis
  1. Diagnosis based on history and physical examination.
  2. Diagnostic testing used to rule out other causes of headache.
iv. Treatment
  1. Acute treatment
    (a) Nonpharmacologic therapy includes behavior modification, biofeedback, hypnosis, and meditation.
    (b) Abortive pharmacologic therapy includes the following:
      (i) Mild attacks
        (1) Acetaminophen
        (2) Nonsteroidal anti-inflammatory drugs (NSAIDs)
      (ii) Moderate attacks
        (1) Butalbital with caffeine and aspirin

        (2) Dihydroergotamine
        (3) 5-HT receptor agonists (sumatriptan)
        (4) Ergotamine
      (iii) Severe attacks
        (1) Dihydroergotamine
        (2) Meperidine
      (iv) Vasoconstrictive agents, such as 5-HT receptor agonists, should be avoided in patients with uncontrolled hypertension or coronary artery disease.
  2. Preventive treatment
    (a) Recommended if headache limits normal daily activities more than 3 or more days per month, headaches are severe or are associated with a complication.
    (b) Treatment options include:
      (i) β-Adrenergic blockers
      (ii) NSAIDs
      (iii) Tricyclic antidepressants
      (iv) Calcium channel antagonists
      (v) Anticonvulsants
c. Tension headache
  i. General
    1. Most common type of primary headache disorder.
    2. More common in females than males and typically begins in the second decade of life.
  ii. Clinical manifestations
    1. Patients have recurrent attacks of diffuse, tight, bandlike, bilateral, mild to moderate pain.
    2. Pain may last from minutes to days.
    3. Pain does not worsen with physical exertion, and there is no associated nausea, vomiting, or photophobia.
  iii. Diagnosis
    1. Based on history and physical examination and ruling out other causes.
  iv. Treatment
    1. Typically respond to acetaminophen and NSAIDs.
      (a) Frequent use of pain medications can lead to an increase in the number of headaches.

NOTES

2. Chronic tension headaches may require prophylactic treatment with tricyclic antidepressants.

V. Infectious disorders
  a. Encephalitis
    i. General
      1. Encephalitis is infection of the brain parenchyma.
      2. Etiology is typically viral and includes:
        (a) Enterovirus
        (b) Arboviruses
          (i) Transmitted by mosquitoes and ticks.
          (ii) Cause of:
            (1) California encephalitis
            (2) Eastern and Western equine encephalitis
            (3) St. Louis encephalitis
            (4) West Nile encephalitis
        (c) Herpes simplex virus
        (d) Cytomegalovirus
        (e) Rubella
        (f) Measles
      3. Incidence peaks in the late summer.
    ii. Clinical manifestations
      1. Patient presents with fever, malaise, myalgias, gastrointestinal and respiratory symptoms, and rash.
      2. Signs of meningeal irritation, such as headache, photophobia, and stiff neck, follow.
      3. May also develop seizures and decreased level of consciousness.
    iii. Diagnosis
      1. Computed tomography (CT) scan of the head should be performed first if suspect viral encephalitis.
      2. CSF testing is essential.
        (a) Gram stain is negative for bacteria.
        (b) Cell count reveals a WBC count typically greater than $50/mm^3$, with a majority of the cells being mononuclear leukocytes.
        (c) Glucose values are typically normal or slightly decreased.
        (d) Protein is typically greater than 100 mg/dL.
        (e) C-reactive protein is normal.

QUESTION

The physician assistant is concerned about a possible diagnosis of myasthenia gravis. Which of the following medications can be used to confirm the diagnosis?

A. Atropine
B. Edrophonium
C. Guanidine
D. Prednisone

    iv. Treatment
      1. Treatment is directed at symptomatic control.
        (a) Acetaminophen is the drug of choice for controlling fever and headache.
        (b) Anticonvulsants are not routinely indicated.
      2. Meningitis caused by herpes should be treated with antivirals, such as acyclovir.
      3. Full recovery typically occurs in 1 to 2 weeks for viral meningitis.
      4. Prognosis with encephalitis varies with the cause.
        (a) Eastern equine encephalitis has a high mortality rate, whereas California encephalitis has a low mortality rate.
  b. Meningitis—bacterial
    i. General
      1. Inflammation of the arachnoid, pia mater, and CSF.
      2. Bacterial meningitis is a medical emergency, requiring immediate diagnosis and antibiotic treatment.
      3. Etiology
        (a) See Table 8-3 for etiologies by age group.
      4. Clinical settings
        (a) Meningococcal meningitis noted in areas of crowded conditions such as classrooms, military, prison systems, or dormitories.

NOTES

ANSWER **B** EXPLANATION: *Anticholinesterase challenge test with IV edrophonium or IM neostigmine results in improved strength within seconds in patients with myasthenia gravis.*

correct ☐   incorrect ☐

(i) Meningococcal meningitis is the only type that occurs in outbreaks.
(b) Pneumococcal meningitis noted in patients with acute otitis media and pneumonia.
(c) *Staphylococcus aureus* meningitis noted as a complication of a neurosurgical procedure, trauma, or secondary to endocarditis.
ii. Clinical manifestations
1. Present with acute onset of fever, headache, vomiting, and stiff neck.
2. On physical examination, there is evidence of:
(a) Meningeal irritation noted by drowsiness, obtundation, stiff neck, Kernig's and Brudzinski's signs.
(i) With patient supine and hip and knee flexed to 90 degrees, further extension of the knee causes pain in the neck or hamstring. This is a positive Kernig's sign.

(ii) Flexing the neck of a supine patient resulting in flexion of the hip and knee is a positive Brudzinski's sign.
(b) Petechial or purpuric rash may be noted in meningococcal infection.
(c) Neurologic findings include:
(i) Cranial nerve abnormalities
(1) Typically cranial nerves 3, 4, 6, and 7.
(ii) Seizures
(iii) Brain swelling
(iv) Focal cerebral signs such as hemiparesis, dysphagia, and visual field defects.
(v) Papilledema is rare.
iii. Diagnosis
1. CSF should be obtained and examined.
(a) Gram stain should be evaluated for white blood cells and bacteria.
(b) Rapid antigen testing can be used to test for *Haemophilus influenzae, Streptococcus pneumoniae,* Group B *Streptococcus, Neisseria meningitidis,* and *Escherichia coli.*
(c) Cell count reveals a WBC count typically greater than $100/mm^3$, with a majority of the cells being polymorphonuclear leukocytes.
(d) Glucose values typically less than 40 mg/dL.
(e) Protein typically greater than 100 mg/dL.

Table 8-3 • Etiology of Meningitis Based on Age Group		
Neonates	**Children (Age < 15 yr)**	**Adults (Age > 15 yr)**
Streptococci group B	*Streptococcus pneumoniae*	*Streptococcus pneumoniae*
Gram-negative bacilli (*Escherichia coli*)	*Neisseria meningitidis*	*Listeria monocytogenes*
Listeria monocytogenes	*Haemophilus influenzae*	*Staphylococcus aureus* Gram-negative bacilli *Neisseria meningitidis*

NOTES

(f) Lactic acid levels are elevated.
(g) C-reactive protein is elevated.
2. Initial CT of the head is not indicated unless signs of mass effect of focal neurologic deficit on physical examination.
3. See Table 8-4 for laboratory results of the various etiologies of meningitis.
iv. Treatment
1. Bactericidal agents should be used whenever possible.

(a) Certain antibiotics should be avoided, such as first- and second-generation cephalosporins and clindamycin, because adequate levels cannot be achieved in the CSF.
(b) See Table 8-5 for antibiotic choice for selective bacteria causing meningitis.
2. Initial therapy for bacterial meningitis of unknown cause varies based on age group.
(a) See Table 8-6.

Table 8-4 • Laboratory Findings in Meningitis

Agent	Opening Pressure (mm H_2O)	WBC Count (mm^3)	Neutrophil (%)	Lymphocyte (%)	Protein	Glucose
Normal	<200	<5	None	100%	<50 mg/dL	>50 mg/dL
Bacterial	High	>100	>80	<20	>50 mg/dL	>50 mg/dL
Viral	High	>50	<50	>50	>50 mg/dL	<30 mg/dL
Fungal	High	>50	<50	>50	>50 mg/dL	<30 mg/dL

Table 8-5 • Antibiotic Choice for Selective Bacteria in Meningitis

Organism	First Choice	Second Choice	Duration of Therapy (Days)
Streptococcus pneumoniae	Penicillin G or ampicillin, or ceftriaxone	Vancomycin or chloramphenicol	10–14
Neisseria meningitidis	Penicillin G or ampicillin	Ceftriaxone	7
Haemophilus influenzae	Ampicillin or ceftriaxone	Third-generation cephalosporin or chloramphenicol	10
Listeria monocytogenes	Ampicillin or penicillin G	Trimethoprim-sulfamethoxazole	14–21
Staphylococcus aureus	Nafcillin	Vancomycin	14
Gram-negative bacilli	Cefotaxime or ceftazidime plus aminoglycoside	Meropenem plus aminoglycoside	21
Pseuadomonas aeruginosa	Cefepime plus tobramycin	Meropenem plus aminoglycoside	21

NOTES

Table 8-6 • Initial Therapy for Bacterial Meningitis of Unknown Cause

Age Group	First Choice	Second Choice
Neonate	Ampicillin plus cefotaxime	Ampicillin plus gentamycin
Children	Cefotaxime or ceftriaxone plus vancomycin	Ampicillin plus chloramphenicol or meropenem
Adults	Cefotaxime or ceftriaxone plus vancomycin	Meropenem
Elderly	Cefotaxime or ceftriaxone plus ampicillin plus vancomycin	Cefotaxime plus vancomycin plus trimethoprim-sulfamethoxazole

3. Chemoprophylaxis of close contacts of patients with meningococcal meningitis is needed.
   (a) Oral rifampin is the drug of choice.
      (i) Avoid in pregnant patients.
   (b) Oral ciprofloxacin, ofloxacin, or azithromycin can be used as alternatives.
4. Complications include hydrocephalus, deafness, seizures, and cranial nerve palsies.

VI. Movement disorders
  a. Amyotrophic lateral sclerosis (Lou Gehrig's disease)
    i. General
      1. Upper and lower motor neuron disorder of unknown cause that presents with progressive weakness.
      2. Most common motor neuron disease that typically affects patients older than 40 years and more males than females.
    ii. Clinical manifestations
      1. First sign is muscle weakness and atrophy in the hands.
      2. May also note fasciculations (including the tongue), spasticity, dysarthria, and dysphagia.
      3. Sensory systems, voluntary eye muscles, and urinary sphincter are spared from the disease.
      4. May note signs of both upper and lower motor neuron disease.
        (a) See Table 8-7.
    iii. Diagnosis
      1. Based on history and physical examination.

Table 8-7 • Signs of Upper and Lower Motor Neuron Disease

Upper Motor Neuron	Lower Motor Neuron
Spasticity	Flaccid paralysis
Hyperreflexia	Areflexia or hyporeflexia
Upward Babinski reflex	Fasciculations
Little or no muscle atrophy	Downward Babinski reflex
No fasciculations	Loss of muscle tone and atrophy

NOTES

2. EMG may show changes of chronic partial denervation with spontaneous abnormal activity in resting muscle in at least three limbs.

iv. Treatment
1. Riluzole may reduce progression of the disease for 3 to 6 months.
2. Supportive care with disease typically fatal in 3 to 5 years.

b. Essential tremor
   i. General
      1. Cause is unknown, but can be inherited in an autosomal dominant pattern.
   ii. Clinical manifestations
      1. May begin at any age and is enhanced by emotional stress.
      2. Typically involves the hands or head.
      3. Physical examination is normal except for the tremor.
      4. Patients lack the hypokinetic features and rigidity of Parkinson's disease.
   iii. Treatment
      1. Beta-blockers are the most effective in treating the tremor.
      2. Modest doses of alcohol may improve the tremor.

c. Huntington's disease
   i. General
      1. A genetic disorder characterized by choreiform movements, mental status decline, and personality changes.
      2. Onset of symptoms is typically age 30 to 50 years.
   ii. Clinical manifestations
      1. Presents with insidious onset of clumsiness and random, brief, fidgety movements
      2. Involuntary choreic movements
         (a) Worse with voluntary movements, increased by emotional stress, and disappear with sleep.
         (b) Gait is irregular, unsteady, and dancelike.
      3. Dementia
         (a) Includes memory loss and apathy.
      4. Personality changes
         (a) Include agitation, psychosis, irritability, and antisocial behavior.

QUESTION

A 19-year-old female presents with recurrent severe headaches for the past year. The headaches are unilateral, throbbing, and accompanied by nausea, vomiting, and light sensitivity. Physical exam is normal. Which of the following is the most likely diagnosis?

A. Chronic sinusitis
B. Cluster headache
C. Subarachnoid hemorrhage
D. Migraine

5. On physical examination, the reflexes are brisk, and the patient is not able maintain tongue protrusion.
6. Laboratory and CSF studies are normal.
7. CT or magnetic resonance imaging (MRI) of the brain reveals cerebral atrophy.

iii. Diagnosis
1. Based on history, especially family history, and physical examination.

iv. Treatment
1. There is no cure for the disease.
   (a) Genetic counseling, physical and occupational therapy, and nutritional counseling are important.
2. Initially movement disorder can be controlled with reserpine or haloperidol.
3. Death typically occurs about 15 years after onset of symptoms.

d. Parkinson's disease
   i. General
      1. A progressive, degenerative disease resulting from loss of dopaminergic neurons in the substantia nigra.
      2. Very common disorder, affecting males more than females.
      3. Mean age of onset is 55 years.
      4. Drug-induced parkinsonism can be noted with dopamine receptor antagonists, such as antiemetics, antipsychotics, and reserpine.

NOTES

ANSWER D E XPLANATION: *Migraine headaches are more common in females and present with severe, unilateral, throbbing pain accompanied by nausea and vomiting, light sensitivity, and preceded by an aura*

correct ☐ incorrect ☐

---

  ii. Clinical manifestations
    1. Classic triad of:
      (a) Tremor: a resting, pill-rolling tremor that decreases with movement.
      (b) Cogwheel rigidity
      (c) Bradykinesia
        (i) Account for the slowing of movements, lack of facial expression (masked facies), staring expression from decreased blinking, impaired swallowing, monotone speech, and micrographia.
    2. Also note postural instability.
    3. Gait is shuffling with short steps and decreased arm swing.
    4. Depression and dementia are common.
  iii. Diagnosis
    1. History and physical examination are typically diagnostic.
    2. CT scan of the brain is often done to rule out other pathology.
  iv. Treatment
    1. A progressive disorder without a cure.
    2. Treatment is life long and must include psychological support for patient and family.
    3. Medications
      (a) Levodopa plus carbidopa
        (i) Levodopa is metabolized to dopamine.
        (ii) Carbidopa inactivates enzymes that metabolize levodopa.
        (iii) Levodopa can suppress tremor, but more useful in controlling bradykinesia and rigidity.
        (iv) Over time, patients lose their response to levodopa.

        (v) Side effects include nausea and vomiting, hypotension, dyskinesias, and confusion.
      (b) Dopamine agonist
        (i) Bromocriptine and pergolide
          (1) Side effects include anorexia, nausea, vomiting, and postural hypotension.
          (2) Avoid in patients with mental illness or recent myocardial infarction.
        (ii) Pramipexole and ropinirole
          (1) Side effects include fatigue, nausea, edema, confusion, and postural hypotension.
          (2) May also note excessive sleepiness.
      (c) Anticholinergics
        (i) More helpful with tremor and rigidity.
        (ii) Drugs include benztropine mesylate, procyclidine, and trihexyphenidyl.
        (iii) Side effects include dry mouth, nausea, constipation, palpitations, urinary retention, agitation, confusion, and increased intraocular pressure.
        (iv) Contraindicated in patients with narrow-angle glaucoma and prostatic hypertrophy.
      (d) Amantadine
        (i) Mode of action is unknown but appears to improve all the features of Parkinson's disease.
        (ii) Side effects are rare at the normal dose.
      (e) Selegiline
        (i) A monoamine oxidase B inhibitor that inhibits the breakdown of dopamine.
        (ii) Is not neuroprotective, but may delay the need for levodopa.
    4. Surgery
      (a) Stereotactic thalamotomy is done in cases of disabling tremor.

NOTES

VII. Multiple sclerosis
  a. General
    i. Cause is unknown, but mediated by immune-initiated inflammatory demyelination and axonal injury.
    ii. More common in the temperate zones of the world and decreases in incidence as move toward the equator.
    iii. Females are affected more often than males, and symptoms typically begin between the ages of 20 and 50 years.
  b. Clinical manifestations
    i. Common presenting symptoms include weakness, numbness, tingling, and unsteadiness in a limb.
      1. Heat may worsen the symptoms.
    ii. Visual symptoms are common and include diplopia, monocular vision loss, and blurry vision (optic neuritis).
    iii. Spasticity is common and consists of increased muscle tone, hyperreflexia, limb spasms, weakness, and loss of dexterity.
      1. Typically affects upper more than the lower extremities.
    iv. Lhermitte's sign is positive, sensation of electricity down the back with passive flexion of the neck.
    v. Pattern of disease varies from relapsing-remitting, secondary and primary progressive, and progressive-relapsing.
  c. Diagnosis
    i. Based on clinical features and laboratory results.
    ii. Laboratory tests reveal the following.
      1. CSF
        (a) Increased CSF immunoglobulin levels
          (i) Discrete oligoclonal bands.
        (b) CSF protein is normal or mildly elevated.
        (c) CSF cell count is less than 50 mononuclear cells/mm^3.
        (d) Increased levels of myelin basic protein.
      2. Sensory evoked potentials
        (a) Loss of myelin slows conduction velocity and possible conduction blocks.

        (b) Visual evoked potentials are prolonged in multiple sclerosis.
      3. MRI scanning
        (a) Reveals multifocal, hyperintense lesions in the periventricular cerebral white matter, cerebellum, brain stem, and spinal cord.
  d. Treatment
    i. Treatment of common symptoms
      1. Spasticity treated with baclofen or diazepam.
        (a) Dystonic spasms, brief, painful posturing of the extremities, are treated with carbamazepine or phenytoin.
      2. Fatigue treated with amantadine.
      3. Depression treated with serotonin reuptake inhibitors.
    ii. Treatment of multiple sclerosis
      1. A brief course of IV corticosteroids can be helpful in an acute relapse.
      2. Immunomodulatory therapy, interferon β-1b (Betaseron), reduces the frequency and severity of relapses, slows the progression of the disease, and reduces number of brain lesions.
VIII. Seizure disorders
  a. General
    i. Seizure disorders exhibit sudden, excessive, and disorderly discharge of cerebral neurons that result in abnormal movements or perceptions that are of short duration but tend to recur.

NOTES

ii. Classification
1. Partial
   (a) Simple
       (i) Confined to single locus in the brain.
       (ii) Patients often have abnormal activity of a single limb and do not lose consciousness.
       (iii) May be followed by a transient neurologic deficit (Todd's paralysis).
       (iv) Can occur at any age.
   (b) Complex
       (i) Patients have complex sensory hallucinations, mental distortion, and loss of consciousness.
       (ii) Motor dysfunction includes chewing movements and lip smacking.
2. Generalized
   (a) Tonic–clonic
       (i) Have loss of consciousness, followed by tonic (stiffening) then clonic (rhythmic jerking) phases.
       (ii) Urinary incontinence is common.
       (iii) Followed by postictal period.
   (b) Absence
       (i) Have brief, abrupt, and self-limiting loss of consciousness.
       (ii) Patients typically stare, then exhibit rapid eye blinking that lasts 3 to 5 seconds.
       (iii) No postictal period.
   (c) Myoclonic
       (i) Have short periods of muscle contraction that may reoccur for several minutes.
       (ii) No loss of consciousness.

3. Febrile
   (a) Consist of generalized tonic–clonic seizures of short duration and accompanied by high fever.
   (b) Occur between 6 months and 4 years of age.
iii. Clinical manifestations
1. A detailed history is vital in making the diagnosis.
2. Physical examination is typically normal.
iv. Diagnosis
1. Electroencephalography (EEG) is the most important test in diagnosing seizures.
   (a) Note epileptiform abnormalities on the EEG.
2. MRI should be obtained on all adults with new-onset seizures to rule out other abnormalities.
v. Treatment
1. No treatment can cure epilepsy, but can control frequency of seizures.
2. Drug levels monitored to minimize side effects.
3. About 70% of patients will achieve a 5-year remission of seizures.
4. Driving precautions must be taken in patients with seizure disorders.
5. See Table 8-8 for treatment of seizure disorders.
6. See Table 8-9 for summary of antiepileptic medications.
b. Status epilepticus
   i. General
   1. A single seizure lasting 90 minutes or multiple seizures that occur without regaining consciousness between episodes.
   2. Most common cause is a patient with known seizure disorder who has subtherapeutic levels of antiseizure medications.
   ii. Clinical manifestations
   1. Present most commonly with tonic–clonic seizures, but other types are possible.

NOTES

Table 8-8 • Antiepileptic Agent Selection		
Type of Epilepsy	**Preferred Agent**	**Alternative Agent**
Partial		
Simple	Phenytoin Carbamazepine	Phenobarbital Primidone
Complex	Phenytoin Carbamazepine	Primidone
Generalized		
Tonic-clonic	Phenytoin Carbamazepine	Phenobarbital Primidone Valproic acid
Absence	Ethosuximide	Valproic acid Clonazepam
Myoclonic	Valproic acid Clonazepam	
Febrile	Phenobarbital	Primidone

   iii. Diagnosis
     1. Rule out other causes, such as alcohol withdrawal, metabolic abnormalities, febrile, tumor, anoxia, or trauma.
       (a) Drug screen, chemistry profile, lumbar puncture, and CT/MRI are typically ordered.
     2. EEG should be obtained to make the diagnosis.
   iv. Treatment
     1. Treatment should be started immediately.
     2. Prognosis varies with etiology.
       (a) Death occurs in up to 10% of adults.
     3. Treatment protocol
       (a) Thiamine and glucose
       (b) Lorazepam or diazepam, can repeat once.

       (c) Phenytoin or fosphenytoin should be started immediately.
       (d) If seizures continue, repeat fosphenytoin at lower dose.
       (e) If after 30 minutes seizures continue, patient should be intubated and then started on pentobarbital, midazolam, or propofol.

IX. Vascular diseases
  a. Cerebral aneurysm
    i. General
      1. Thin-walled outpouchings that protrude from the arteries.
      2. Different types
        (a) Saccular (berry)
          (i) Most common intracranial aneurysm.
          (ii) Typically located on circle of Willis or major branches.
        (b) Fusiform
          (i) Elongated dilations of large arteries.
          (ii) Associated with atherosclerosis.
          (iii) Typically develop in the basilar artery.
        (c) Mycotic
          (i) Due to infected emboli.
          (ii) Frequently multiple and found in the distal cerebral arteries.
    ii. Clinical manifestations
      1. Signs and symptoms vary depending on the location of the aneurysm and compression of surrounding structures.
    iii. Diagnosis
      1. CT scan, magnetic resonance arteriography, or angiography is commonly used to make diagnosis.
    iv. Treatment
      1. Saccular aneurysms treated by surgical clipping.
      2. Fusiform aneurysms are treated with total occlusion.
  b. Normal pressure hydrocephalus
    i. General
      1. Dilatation of the cerebral ventricles and secondary to prior CNS insult.

NOTES

Table 8-9 • Summary of Antiepileptic Medications

Drug	Mechanism of Action	Side Effects	Notes
Phenytoin	Stabilize neuronal cells by decreasing flux of sodium ions	Nystagmus Ataxia Nausea/vomiting Gingival hyperplasia	Teratogenic—cleft lip and palate, and congenital heart disease
Carbamazepine	Blocks sodium channels, reducing abnormal impulses	Stupor or coma Respiratory depression Drowsiness Vertigo/ataxia Nausea/vomiting Aplastic anemia	
Phenobarbital	Unknown	Sedation Vertigo/ataxia Nystagmus Nausea/vomiting Rash	
Primidone	Unknown	Sedation Vertigo/ataxia Nystagmus Nausea/vomiting Rash	
Valproic acid	Enhances GABA action at inhibitory synapses, reducing abnormal discharge in the brain	Nausea/vomiting Sedation Ataxia Tremor Hepatic toxicity	Monitor liver function tests May cause thrombocytopenia and bleeding
Ethosuximide	Reduces propagation of abnormal electrical activity	Nausea/vomiting Drowsiness Dizziness Agitation	Stevens-Johnson syndrome may occur Aplastic anemia
Gabapentin	Unknown	Fatigue Somnolence Dizziness Ataxia	
Lamotrigine	Blocks sodium channels and prevents repeat firing	Diplopia Drowsiness Ataxia Rash	

NOTES

(a) Insults include subarachnoid hemorrhage, trauma, infection, or tumors.
2. Typically seen in adults older than 60 years, and incidence higher in males than females.
ii. Clinical manifestations
1. Present with wide-based, shuffling gait (apraxia), dementia, and urinary incontinence.
2. Also note weakness, malaise, and lethargy.
iii. Diagnosis
1. Based on history and physical examination.
2. Lumbar puncture reveals an elevated opening pressure.
3. CT scan or MRI shows enlarged ventricles.
iv. Treatment
1. Removal of CSF provides temporary relief.
2. Ventriculoperitoneal shunt is the treatment of choice.
c. Stroke
i. General
1. Multiple types of strokes
(a) Ischemic
(i) Caused by insufficient blood flow to part or all the brain.
(ii) Neurologic deficit lasts longer than 24 hours.
(1) If less than 24 hours, symptoms termed a transient ischemic attack.
(iii) No extravasated blood into the brain.
(iv) Account for 60% to 65% of all strokes.
(v) Two types of ischemic strokes
(1) Thrombosis
[a] Occlusion forms locally at the site.
(2) Embolic
[a] Due to piece of clot breaking off from other location and traveling to the brain.

[b] Sources include mural thrombi, valvular heart disease, and arrhythmias (atrial fibrillation).
(b) Hemorrhagic
(i) Extravasation of blood into the brain.
(ii) Account for 15% of all strokes.
(c) Small vessel (lacunar)
(i) Caused by occlusion of small arterioles.
(ii) Account for 20% of all strokes.
(iii) Typically due to long-standing hypertension.
2. Risk factors for stroke include:
(a) Increasing age
(b) Atrial fibrillation
(c) Hypercoagulable states
(d) Hypertension
(e) Smoking
(f) Diabetes
(g) Elevated serum lipids
(h) Recent myocardial infarction
(i) Carotid stenosis
(j) Transient ischemic attack (TIA)
ii. Clinical manifestations
1. Signs and symptoms depend on location within the brain that has been deprived of blood flow.
2. See Table 8-10 for summary of clinical manifestations.
iii. Diagnosis
1. Neurologic examination will suggest location and size of stroke.

NOTES

ANSWER D EXPLANATION: *Status epilepticus, a seizure lasting 90 minutes or multiple seizures without regaining consciousness, are acutely treated with lorazepam or diazepam.*

correct ☐   incorrect ☐

Table 8-10 • Clinical Manifestations of Stroke	
Occluded Blood Vessel	**Clinical Manifestations**
Internal carotid artery	Ipsilateral blindness
Anterior cerebral artery (rare)	Upper motor neuron weakness Neglect of contralateral leg Urinary incontinence Transcortical motor aphasia
Middle cerebral artery (common)	Contralateral weakness Sensory loss face and arm Expressive aphasia (if dominant side) Anosognosia and spatial disorientation (if non-dominant side)
Posterior cerebral artery	Highly variable Difficulty reading and performing calculations Memory impairment
Vertebral artery	Vertigo Nausea/vomiting Nystagmus Ipsilateral cerebellar ataxia
Basilar artery	Bilateral sensory Cerebellar dysfunction Cranial nerve abnormalities Paralysis/weakness of all extremities Impaired vision

2. Electrocardiogram (EKG) indicated to rule out arrhythmia.
3. Carotid Doppler and echocardiogram indicated to rule possible embolic source.
4. CT scan, noncontrast, is the standard initial study.
    (a) Evaluate for possible hemorrhage.
5. MRI is more sensitive for detecting early ischemia.
6. MRI angiography taking the place of cerebral angiography.
iv. Treatment
   1. Modify risk factors
       (a) Carotid endarterectomy for carotid stenosis.
       (b) Aspirin or anticoagulation for patients with atrial fibrillation or hypercoagulable states.
       (c) Control hypertension.
   2. Thrombolytic therapy is the only effective method for the acute treatment of ischemic stroke.
       (a) Must be started within 3 hours after onset of stroke.
       (b) CT must be obtained to rule out hemorrhage.
       (c) Blood pressure must be less than 180 mm Hg systolic or 110 mm Hg diastolic.
           (i) If elevated must lower before starting thrombolytic therapy.
       (d) Contraindications include:
           (i) Major surgery or trauma in last 2 weeks.
           (ii) Evidence of gastrointestinal bleeding.
   3. Hemorrhagic stroke treated with mannitol, hyperventilation, and head elevation to decrease increased intracranial pressure.
   4. Prophylactic heparin indicated, unless other contraindications, to decrease risk for pulmonary embolism or deep venous thrombosis.

NOTES

d. Subarachnoid hemorrhage
   i. General
      1. Rupture of vessels on or near the surface of the brain or ventricles.
      2. Mainly affects young adults; males and females are affected equally.
      3. Trauma is the most common cause of subarachnoid hemorrhage.
         (a) Rupture of an aneurysm is most common nontraumatic cause.
         (b) Arteriovenous malformations are another cause.
      4. Risk factors include:
         (a) Smoking
         (b) Binge drinking
         (c) Phenylpropanolamine or other sympathomimetics.
   ii. Clinical manifestations
      1. Patients describe pain as the worst headache of their life.
      2. Rapidly developing pain and stiff neck.
      3. Blood pressure may be elevated, and there may be mental status changes.
      4. On physical examination, focal neurologic deficit is not noted unless compression of surrounding brain structures.
      5. Funduscopic examination reveals well-circumscribed, bright red, preretinal hemorrhages.
   iii. Diagnosis
      1. Diagnosed by CT scan, which reveals an area of high attenuation consistent with bleeding.
      2. If CT negative, and suspicion high, lumbar puncture is indicated.
         (a) Will note a constant number of red blood cells in each tube.
         (b) In a traumatic tap, the number of red blood cells will decrease with each following tube.
         (c) Opening pressure is also elevated.
      3. Cerebral angiography is the definitive study to identify the source of the bleed.
   iv. Treatment
      1. Maintain airway, breathing, and circulation.
      2. Control blood pressure.
      3. Surgery may be needed depending on the cause.
      4. Overall mortality is 45%, with 10% dying before reaching the hospital.
      5. Medical complications include rebleeding, vasospasm, hydrocephalus, seizures, and hyponatremia.

Table 8-11 • Comparison of Epidural, Subdural, and Subarachnoid Hematomas

Hematoma	Vessel	Mechanism	Presentation
Epidural	Artery	Skull fracture	Spinal fluid rhinorrhea Unconsciousness followed by resolution and then later unconsciousness
Subdural	Venous	Head injury	Symptoms develop later after injury with headache, confusion, coma, and hemiparesis
Subarachnoid	Artery	Aneurysm	Worst headache of life Stiff neck and delirium

NOTES

Question 1

Which of the following physical examination finding is typically noted in Parkinson's disease?

   A. Bilateral visual field defects.
   B. Intermittent blank staring episodes.
   C. Cog wheeling of an upper extremity.
   D. Sensory loss over chest dermatomes.

Question 2

A 65-year-old patient with a history of hypertension and COPD presents with left facial drooping and weakness on the right side of the body. Which of the following is first best step in the evaluation of this patient?

   A. Cerebral CT scan
   B. Chest x-ray
   C. Carotid ultrasound
   D. Neurology consult

Question 3

A 50-year-old female is brought into the emergency room after suffering a seizure while eating supper. The patient developed convulsive jerking in the left arm and leg that last approximately 5 minutes. The patient also lost consciousness for 2-3 minutes. The patient has no prior history of seizures. Which of the following is the most likely diagnosis?

   A. Complex partial seizure
   B. Absence seizure
   C. Tonic-clonic seizure
   D. Myoclonic seizure

Question 4

A 15-year-old male presents to the emergency department with a history of being hit on the side of the head with a baseball bat. He is a little slow to respond, but is not lethargic. He is otherwise in good health. Physical exam is completely normal with the exception of a small collection of blood posterior to the left ear, near the site of the impact. Which of the following is the next best step in the evaluation of this patient?

   A. Cerebral angiography
   B. CT scan of the skull
   C. MRI of the brain
   D. Lumbar puncture

Question 5

A 70-year-old presents with neck stiffness and headache. Lumbar puncture laboratory testing reveals 500 WBCs with 100% neutrophils, total protein 230 mg/dl, and glucose 40 mg/dl. Which of the following is the best treatment option for this patient?

   A. Ceftriaxone (Rocephin)
   B. Ceftriaxone and ampicillin
   C. Acyclovir (Zovirax)
   D. Acyclovir and amphotericin B

Question 6

A patient presents with a history of debilitating migraine headaches 4 to 5 days per month. Which of the following medications can be used as prophylactic treatment for migraine headaches?

   A. Sumatriptan (Imitrex)
   B. Ergotamine tartrate (Cafergot)
   C. Desipramine (Norpramin)
   D. Acetaminophen (Tylenol)

NOTES

Question 7

Which of the following cranial nerves is affected in Bell's palsy?

- A. Abducens
- B. Trigeminal
- C. Oculomotor
- D. Facial

Answer 1

ANSWER C *Explanation: Parkinson's disease classically presents with the triad of tremor, bradykinesia, and cogwheel rigidity.*

Topic: Parkinson's disease

correct ☐   incorrect ☐

Answer 2

ANSWER A *Explanation: Evaluation of the possible stroke patient begins with a CT scan to evaluate for possible hemorrhage. Carotid ultrasound may be needed later to evaluate for possible embolic source.*

Topic: Stroke

correct ☐   incorrect ☐

Answer 3

ANSWER C *Explanation: Tonic-clonic seizures present with tonic (stiffening) and then clonic (rhythmic jerking) phases. Urinary incontinence and loss of consciousness are common.*

Topic: Seizure disorders

correct ☐   incorrect ☐

Answer 4

ANSWER B *Explanation: Any patient with trauma to head must have subarachnoid, epidural, or subdural hemorrhage ruled out. CT scan of the skull and brain are the test of choice in the evaluation of patients with head trauma.*

Topic: Subarachnoid hemorrhage

correct ☐   incorrect ☐

Answer 5

ANSWER B *Explanation: Bacterial meningitis in the elderly may be caused by Streptococcus pneumoniae, Neisseria meningitidis, and Listeria monocytogenes. Treatment in the elderly must include ceftriaxone and ampicillin to cover the most common organisms.*

Topic: Meni

correct ☐   incorrect ☐

NOTES

Answer 6

ANSWER C *Explanation: Preventive treatment is indicated if headache limits normal daily activities three or more days per month, headaches are severe, or associated with complications. Treatment options include beta-blockers, NSAIDS, and tricyclic antidepressants. Sumatriptan, ergotamine, and acetaminophen are used for acute treatment.*

Topic: Headache

correct ❑   **incorrect** ❑

Answer 7

ANSWER D *Explanation: Bell's palsy is due to unilateral paralysis of cranial nerve seven, the etiology is unknown.*

Topic: Bell's palsy

correct ❑   **incorrect** ❑

NOTES

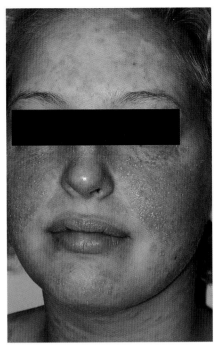

Plate 1. Facial Rash in SLE.
With permission from Bolognia, J.L.,
Lorizzo, J.L., & Rapini, R.P. (2003).
Dermatology. Edinburgh: Mosby. pg. 603.
fig 43.4.

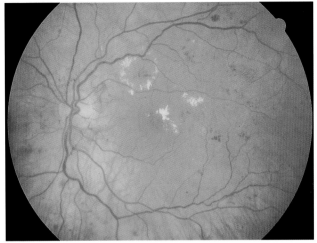

Plate 2. Diabetic Retinopathy
With permission from Goldman, (2004) Cecil's Textbook of
Medicine. 22nd ed. pg. 2418. Fig 465-15.

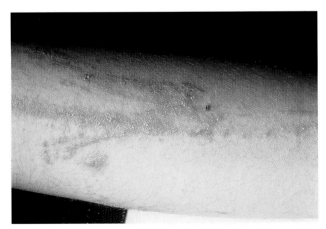

Plate 3. Contact dermatitis (Poison ivy)
With permission from Bolognia, J.L., Lorizzo, J.L., &
Rapini, R.P. (2003). *Dermatology.* Edinburgh: Mosby. pg. 227,
fig. 15.1.

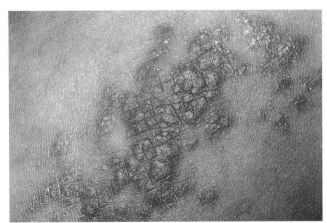

Plate 4. Lichen planus.
With permission from White, G.M. & Cox, N.H. (2002).
Diseases of the Skin: A Color Atlas and Text. Edinburgh: Mosby.
pg. 68, fig. 5.2c.

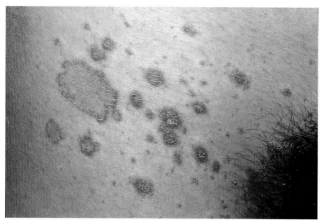

Plate 5. Pityriasis rosea
With permission from White, G.M. & Cox, N.H. (2002). *Diseases of the Skin: A Color Atlas and Text.* Edinburgh: Mosby. pg. 66, fig. 4.44a

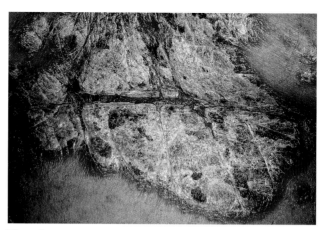

Plate 6. Psoriasis
With permission from Bolognia, J.L., Lorizzo, J.L., & Rapini, R.P. (2003). Dermatology. Edinburgh: Mosby. pg. 129, fig. 9.1.

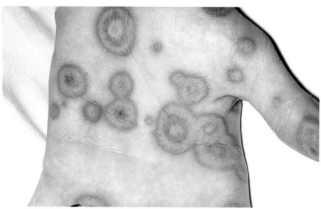

Plate 7. Erythema multiforme
With permission from White, G.M. & Cox, N.H. (2002). *Diseases of the Skin: A Color Atlas and Text.* Edinburgh: Mosby. pg. 116, fig. 8.28.

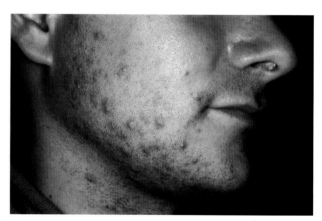

Plate 8. Acne
With permission from Bolognia, J.L., Lorizzo, J.L., & Rapini, R.P. (2003). *Dermatology.* Edinburgh: Mosby. pg. 533, fig. 38.6.

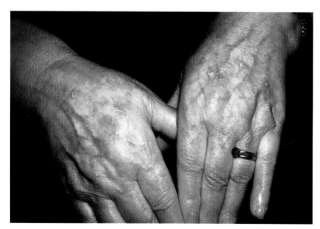

Plate 9. Actinic keratosis
With permission from Bolognia, J.L., Lorizzo, J.L., & Rapini, R.P. (2003). Dermatology. Edinburgh: Mosby. pg. 1681, fig. 109.2.

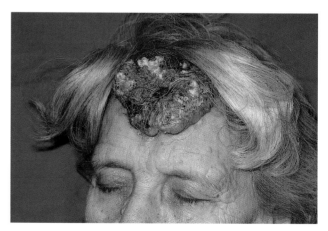

Plate 10. Basal cell carcinoma
With permission from White, G.M. & Cox, N.H. (2002). *Diseases of the Skin: A Color Atlas and Text.* Edinburgh: Mosby. pg. 469, fig. 29.34.

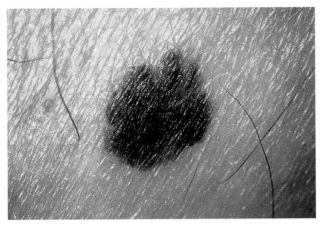

Plate 11. Melanoma
With permission from Bolognia, J.L., Lorizzo, J.L., & Rapini, R.P. (2003). Dermatology. Edinburgh: Mosby. pg. 1793, fig. 114.6.

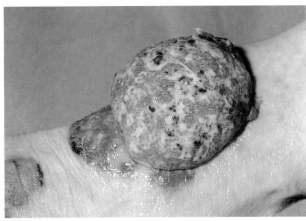

Plate 12. Squamous cell carcinoma
With permission from White, G.M. & Cox, N.H. (2002). *Diseases of the Skin: A Color Atlas and Text.* Edinburgh: Mosby. pg. 474, fig. 29.55.

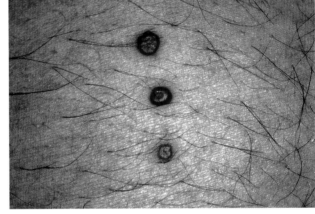

Plate 14. Molluscum contagiosum
With permission from Bolognia, J.L., Lorizzo, J.L., & Rapini, R.P. (2003). Dermatology. Edinburgh: Mosby. pg. 1267, fig. 81.12A.

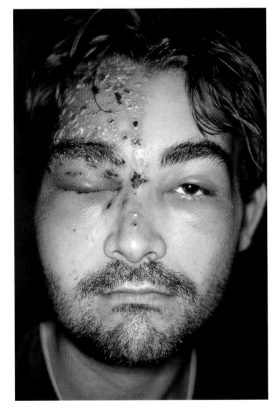

Plate 13. Herpes Zoster
With permission from Bolognia, J.L., Lorizzo, J.L., & Rapini, R.P. (2003). Dermatology. Edinburgh: Mosby. pg. 1243, fig. 80.12A.

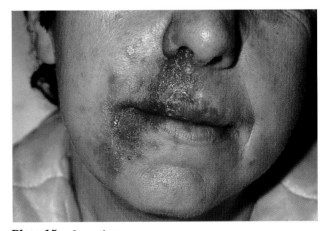

Plate 15. Impetigo
With permission from White, G.M. & Cox, N.H. (2002). *Diseases of the Skin: A Color Atlas and Text.* Edinburgh: Mosby. pg. 323, fig. 20.2.

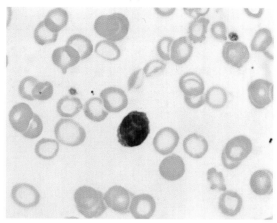

Plate 16.   Microcytic cells
With permission from Hoffman, R., Benz, E.J., Jr.,
Shattil, S.J., Furie, B., Cohen, H.J., Silberstein, L.E., &
McGlave, P. (2000). *Hematology: Principles and Practice.*
(3rd ed.). New York: Churchill Livingstone. color plate
155.14.

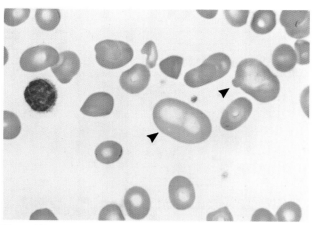

Plate 17.   Macrocytic cells
With permission from Hoffman, R., Benz, E.J., Jr., Shattil,
S.J., Furie, B., Cohen, H.J., Silberstein, L.E., & McGlave, P.
(2000). *Hematology: Principles and Practice.* (3rd ed.). New
York: Churchill Livingstone. Color plate 155.15.

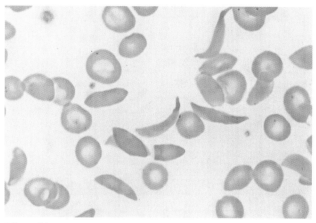

Plate 18.   Sickle cells
With permission from Hoffman, R., Benz, E.J., Jr., Shattil,
S.J., Furie, B., Cohen, H.J., Silberstein, L.E., & McGlave, P.
(2000). *Hematology: Principles and Practice.* (3rd ed.). New
York: Churchill Livingstone. Color plate 155.23

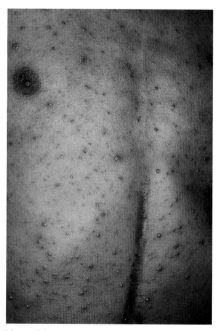

Plate 20.   Chicken pox
With permission from Bolognia, J.L.,
Lorizzo, J.L., & Rapini, R.P. (2003).
Dermatology. Edinburgh: Mosby. pg. 1242,
fig. 80.11A

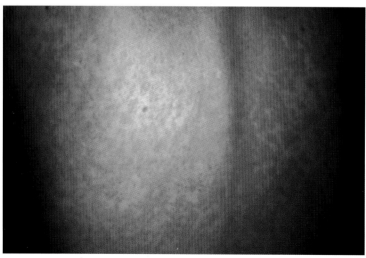

Plate 19.   Rubeola
With permission from Bolognia, J.L., Lorizzo, J.L., & Rapini, R.P.
(2003). *Dermatology.* Edinburgh: Mosby. pg. 1259, fig. 81.6

9

Psychiatry/Behavioral Science

EXAM BLUEPRINT OUTLINE

Anxiety Disorders
Panic disorder
Generalized anxiety disorder
Post-traumatic stress disorder
Phobias
Attention-Deficit Disorder
Autistic Disorder
Eating Disorders
Anorexia nervosa
Bulimia nervosa
Obesity
Mood Disorders
Adjustment
Depressive
Dysthymic
Bipolar
Personality Disorders
Antisocial
Avoidant
Borderline
Dependent
Histrionic
Narcissistic
Obsessive-compulsive
Paranoid
Schizoid
Schizotypal
Psychoses
Delusional disorder
Schizophrenia
Schizoaffective disorder
Somatoform Disorders
Substance Use Disorders
Alcohol abuse/dependence
Drug abuse/dependence
Tobacco use/dependence

Other Behavior/Emotional Disorders
Child abuse
Elder abuse
Domestic violence
Uncomplicated bereavement

I. Anxiety disorders
  a. Panic disorders
    i. General
      1. Characterized by recurrent unexpected panic attacks that occur with or without agoraphobia.
        (a) Agoraphobia is a condition in which patients fear places in which escape may be difficult.
      2. These can be disabling conditions.
      3. Occur more commonly in females with typical onset before 30 years of age.
      4. Etiology is unknown.
    ii. Clinical manifestations
      1. Onset is sudden, and disorders peak within minutes.
      2. May last 5 to 30 minutes.
      3. Must experience at least 4 of 13 typically symptoms of panic.
        (a) See Table 9-1.
      4. To make the diagnosis one of the following must occur for at least 1 month.
        (a) Persistent concern about future attacks
        (b) Worry about implications of the attacks
        (c) Significant change in behavior related to the attacks
    iii. Treatment
      1. Treatment includes cognitive-behavioral therapy and pharmacotherapy.

NOTES

Table 9-1 • *DSM-IV-TR* Criteria for Panic Attacks
Palpitations
Sweating
Tremulous or shaking
Shortness of breath
Chest pain
Nausea or abdominal discomfort
Dizziness, lightheadedness, faintness
Feeling of unreality or detached from oneself
Fear of dying
Fear of losing control
Sensation of choking

DSM-IV-TR, Diagnostic and Statistical Manual of Mental Disorders, 4th ed., Text revision. American Psychiatric Association, 2000.

      (a) Cognitive-behavioral therapy consists of relaxation exercises and desensitization.
      (b) Exposure therapy can be used in agoraphobia.
    2. Pharmacotherapy consists of the following medications.
      (a) Tricyclic antidepressants
        (i) Such as nortriptyline, imipramine, or desipramine.
      (b) Monoamine oxidase inhibitors
        (i) Such as tranylcypromine and phenelzine.
      (c) Selective serotonin reuptake inhibitors
        (i) Such as fluoxetine, sertraline, and paroxetine.
      (d) High-potency benzodiazepines
        (i) Such as alprazolam and clonazepam.
  b. Generalized anxiety disorder
    i. General

1. Characterized by intensive worry over almost every aspect of life associated with physical manifestations of anxiety.
2. Typical onset in early 20s.
3. Both genetic and environmental etiologies.
  ii. Clinical manifestations
    1. Patients have pervasive anxiety and worry excessively about every aspects of their life (job, school, health, marriage, and social) most days for at least 6 months.
    2. Must also have difficulty controlling the worry and must be associated with at least three of the following:
      (a) Difficulty concentrating
      (b) Easily fatigued
      (c) Irritability
      (d) Muscle tension
      (e) Restlessness
      (f) Sleep disturbances
    3. Do not have panic attacks, phobias, obsession, or compulsions.
  iii. Treatment
    1. Treat with benzodiazepine, buspirone, or beta-blockers.
    2. Relaxation techniques have also been used with some success.
c. Post-traumatic stress disorder
  i. General
    1. May occur at any age and begin hours to years after the initial trauma.
  ii. Clinical manifestations
    1. Patients have endured a traumatic event that they re-experience through repetitive images or dreams or through recurrent illusions or flashbacks.
    2. Patients will make effort to avoid recollections of the event through disassociation or numbing, or by actual avoidance of things that may evoke recall of the event.
    3. Also experience feelings of detachment from others and have difficulty sleeping or have an exaggerated startle response.
  iii. Treatment
    1. Treatment is with psychotherapy and symptom-directed medications.

NOTES

2. Medications include tricyclic antidepressants and monoamine oxidase inhibitors.
   d. Phobias
   i. General
   1. An anxiety disorder characterized by intense fear of a particular situation, for example, heights, or objects, such as snakes.
   2. The most common psychiatric disorder with onset typically in childhood.
   3. Phobias tend to run in families.
   4. Social phobia is a disorder in which patients have intense fear of being scrutinized in a social or public setting.
   ii. Clinical manifestations
   1. An irrational fear of a specific object, place, or situation that is out of proportion to any actual danger.
   2. To make the diagnosis:
   (a) This marked, persistent fear must be noted by the patient to be excessive and unreasonable and brought on by the presence or possible presence of the object or situation.
   (b) Exposure must invariably provoke the anxiety reaction.
   (c) Everyday activities must be impaired by the avoidance or distress over the feared object or situation.
   iii. Treatment
   1. Certain childhood phobias disappear spontaneously with age.
   2. Exposure therapy is the treatment of choice.
   3. Social phobia can be treated with cognitive-behavioral therapy.
   (a) Medications such as monoamine oxidase inhibitors, beta-blockers, selective serotonin reuptake inhibitors, and alprazolam can be helpful.
II. Attention-deficit disorder
   a. General
   i. Disorder runs in families.
   ii. Concurrent psychiatric disorders are common.
   iii. More common in boys than girls.
   iv. Etiology is unknown.

b. Clinical manifestations
   i. Frequently noted when child enters school.
   1. Present with discipline difficulties, incomplete chores and projects, forgetting assignments, and poor impulse control.
   ii. Symptoms must be present before 7 years of age.
   iii. Criteria for diagnosis include:
   1. Either inattention or hyperactivity-impulsivity.
   2. See Table 9-2.
   3. Some impairment occurs in at least two or more settings.
   4. Must be evidence of clinically significant impairment in social, academic, or occupational functioning.
   5. Symptoms do not occur due to some other psychiatric disorder.
   c. Treatment
   i. Treatment includes behavioral management, such as positive reinforcement, firm limit setting, and reduction in stimulation.
   ii. Medications include psychostimulants, such as methylphenidate or dextro-amphetamine.
   1. Side effects with long-term use of these medications may include weight loss and diminished body growth.
III. Autistic disorder
   a. General
   i. A very rare familial disorder with a male-to-female ratio of 3:1.
   ii. A number of patients with autistic disorder have fragile X chromosome and tuberous sclerosis.
   iii. One fourth of patients with autistic disorder have seizures, and three fourths have some form of mental retardation.
   b. Clinical manifestations
   i. Typically note abnormal development shortly after birth.
   ii. Characterized by the following:
   1. Impaired social interactions
   (a) Failure to develop a social smile, facial expressions, or eye contact.
   (b) As patient gets older, failure to develop nonverbal forms of

NOTES

Table 9-2 • Symptoms of Inattention and Hyperactivity-Impulsivity		
Inattention	**Hyperactivity**	**Impulsivity**
Fails to give close attention to work	Often fidgets or squirms	Often blurts out answers
Has difficulty sustaining attention to tasks	Often leaves seat when sitting is expected	Has difficulty waiting turn
Often does not seem to listen when spoken to	Often runs or climbs when inappropriate	Often interrupts or intrudes on others
Does not follow through on instructions	Often has difficulty playing quietly	
Has difficulty organizing tasks	Is often on the go	
Avoids or dislikes to engage in tasks that require sustained mental effort	Often talks excessively	
Often loses items		
Is distracted		
Is often forgetful in daily activities		

communication and lack of desire or skills to develop friendships.
2. Impaired ability to communicate
   (a) May be a delay or total lack of language development.
   (b) Those with language development show impaired ability to start or sustain conversation.
   (c) Language may also be abnormal in pitch, tone, and rhythm.
3. Restricted variety of activities and interests
   (a) Patient may be preoccupied with one or more restricted pattern of interest.
   (b) May also develop an inflexible adherence to specific nonfunctional routines, repetitive motor movements, and persistent preoccupation with parts of objects.

c. Treatment
   i. A chronic lifelong disorder with few of these individuals living independently.
   ii. Behavioral management techniques are used to reduce the rigid behaviors and improve social functioning.
   iii. Antiseizure medications are used in patients with seizure disorder.
   iv. Neuroleptics, such as haloperidol, are used to help decrease aggressive behaviors.
IV. Eating disorders
   a. Anorexia nervosa
      i. General
         1. Severe eating disorder characterized by low body weight.
         2. Diagnosed when body weight falls below 85% of ideal weight.
            (a) Weight loss must be due to behavior directed at maintaining a low weight or body image.

NOTES

3. Average age of onset is 17 and more common in females.
ii. Clinical manifestations
1. Patients generally have a high fear of losing control and trouble with self-esteem; past physical or sexual abuse may be a risk factor.
2. Diagnosis includes:
   (a) Refusal to maintain body weight at greater than 85% of ideal.
   (b) Intense fear of weight gain
   (c) Preoccupation with body image
   (d) Denial of medical risks of low weight
   (e) Generally do not have loss of appetite
   (f) Amenorrhea
3. Methods of weight loss include:
   (a) Intensive exercise
   (b) Restrict food intake
   (c) Binging and purging
iii. Treatment
1. Treatment of medical complications is vital.
2. Medications, such as antidepressants and selective serotonin reuptake inhibitors, are used to treat comorbid psychiatric illness and have little effect on anorexia.
3. Psychotherapy, supervised meals, weight monitoring, and disease education are very helpful
b. Bulimia nervosa
i. General
1. Eating disorder characterized by binge eating with the maintenance of body weight.
2. More common in females than males, with a 10:1 ratio.
ii. Clinical manifestations
1. Patients engage in binge eating and behaviors designed to avoid weight gain, but maintain their body weight.
2. Binges may be brought on by stress or altered mood states.
   (a) Will often eat to the point of physical discomfort.
3. Purging may follow and be done by vomiting, laxatives, diuretics, and enemas.

A 4-year-old patient is brought in by his mother who states, "He just doesn't get involved with people." While talking with the patient, the physician assistant notes the child has problem-maintaining eye contact and suffers from echolalia. Which of the following is the most likely diagnosis?

A. Attention deficit disorder
B. Anxiety disorder
C. Schizophrenia
D. Autism

4. Patients are overly concerned with body image and preoccupied with becoming fat.
iii. Treatment
1. Similar to treatment for anorexia nervosa.
2. Focus first on achieving control of eating behaviors.
3. Selective serotonin reuptake inhibitors are effective in the treatment of bulimia nervosa.
4. Complications
   (a) See Table 9-3.
c. Obesity
i. General
1. Obesity is the second leading cause of preventable death in the United States.
   (a) Obesity increases risk for type II diabetes, gallstones, coronary artery disease, breast cancer, and colon cancer.
2. About half of obese individuals engage in binge eating.
   (a) Obese binge eaters are more likely to suffer from anxiety disorders, social phobias, and alcohol or drug problems than nonbingers.
3. Obesity is more common in women and among minorities and low-income populations.
ii. Clinical manifestations
1. Based on body mass index (BMI).
   (a) See Table 9-4.

NOTES

ANSWER D EXPLANATION: *Autism presents with impaired social interactions, impaired ability to communicate, and restricted variety of activities and interests.*

correct ☐   incorrect ☐

Table 9-3 • Medical Complication of Eating Disorder

Behavior	Complication
Binge eating	Gastric distention
Diuretic use	Dehydration Electrolyte abnormalities
Laxative use	Constipation Dehydration Metabolic acidosis
Starvation	Anemia Bradycardia Edema Hypotension Hypothermia
Vomiting	Esophageal rupture Hypokalemia Metabolic alkalosis

Table 9-4 • Body Mass Index (BMI) and Weight-Associated Health Risk

BMI	Weight	Weight-Associated Health Risk
<25	Normal	Normal
25–30	Overweight	Low to moderate
31–35	Obese	High
35–40	Obese	Very high
>40	Morbidly obese	Extremely high

2. Must rule out medical conditions, such as hypothyroidism, as cause of obesity.
iii. Treatment
1. Evaluate and treat any medical complications of obesity.
2. Evaluate diet and exercise habits.
3. Diagnose and treat any comorbid psychiatric disorders.
4. Identify any psychological cause of obesity.
5. Consider antiobesity medications.
6. Consider surgical options.
V. Mood disorders
a. Adjustment
i. General
1. Changes in emotional state or behaviors that are response to an identified psychosocial stressor.
(a) This does not include responses to severe psychosocial stressors, such as major depression, or in response to bereavement.
ii. Clinical manifestations
1. Typically occur within 3 months of the stressor and resolve within 6 months.
iii. Treatment
1. Psychotherapy is the most common psychosocial treatment.
(a) Individual and family therapy are helpful as are self-help groups.
2. Patients often self-medicate themselves with alcohol, caffeine, and over-the-counter medications.
3. Treatment of depression or anxiety symptoms with medications is common.
b. Depressive
i. General
1. A unipolar disorder.
2. Female-to-male ratio is 2:1.
3. Incidence is greatest between the ages of 20 and 40 years.
4. Risk factors for major depression include interpersonal losses, actual or perceived.
ii. Clinical manifestations
1. Diagnosed after a single episode of major depression.
(a) Must have five or more of the following for at least 2 weeks:

NOTES

(i) Must have depressed mood or loss of interest or pleasure to make diagnosis.

(ii) See Table 9-5.

(b) Must not be due to a medical condition, bereavement, or substance induced.

2. Characterized by emotional changes, depressed mood, and vegetative changes, alterations in sleep, appetite, and energy.

(a) Must not meet the criteria for bipolar or etiologic mood disorder.

3. Is frequently recurrent.

iii. Treatment

1. Responds to psychotherapy and medications.

2. Antidepressants are very helpful.

3. Electroconvulsive therapy can be used in psychotic, severe, or disease refractory to treatment.

c. Dysthymic

i. General

1. A unipolar mood disorder.

Table 9-5 • Criteria for Major Depression

Criteria	Description
Appetite	Increased or decreased with weight loss or gain
Concentration	Decreased or increased indecisiveness
Energy	Fatigue almost all day
Guilt	Feelings of worthlessness or inappropriate guilt
Interest	Decrease in interest and pleasure in most activities
Mood	Depressed mood almost all day, every day
Psychomotor	Agitation
Sleep	Insomnia or hypersomnia
Suicide risk	Recurrent thoughts of suicide

QUESTION

Which of the following characterizes anorexia nervosa?

A. Loss of pubic hair

B. Amenorrhea

C. Bradycardia

D. Edema

2. Have a loss of interest or pleasure in most activities but do not have symptoms severe enough to meet the diagnosis of major depressive episode.

3. Somewhat more common in females.

ii. Clinical manifestations

1. Patients often complain of having felt depressed throughout their life.

2. Have a tendency to over-react to normal stressors with a depressive mood.

3. Patients have low self-confidence and lead limited social lives, have unstable relationships, and abuse drugs and alcohol.

4. At times, the patient may have a superimposed major depressive episode.

5. Essential feature is the chronic nature (greater than 2 years) of the depressed mood with interference of personal and social functioning.

iii. Treatment

1. Psychotherapy is the principal treatment for these patients.

2. Many may receive some relief with a trial of antidepressants.

d. Bipolar

i. General

1. Are three types of bipolar disorders, bipolar I, bipolar II, and cyclothymia.

(a) Bipolar I is the most serious of the three.

2. Bipolar I and cyclothymia have an equal male-to-female ratio, whereas bipolar II is more common in females.

ANSWER **B** EXPLANATION: *Anorexia nervosa is characterized by poor self-esteem, low body weight, fear of gaining weight, and amenorrhea.*

correct ☐   incorrect ☐

ii. Clinical manifestations
1. Bipolar I is diagnosed after one manic episode, and episodes are intermixed with depressive episodes.
   (a) First episode typically occurs in the early 20s.
   (b) The transition between mania and depression typically occurs without a period of euthymia.
   (c) If patient has mania induced by antidepressant medications, psychostimulants, electroconvulsive therapy (ECT), or phototherapy, the patient is diagnosed with substance-induced mood disorder, not bipolar disorder.
   (d) Criteria for mania.
      (i) Must have a clear period of persistently elevated mood lasting 1 week or severe enough to require hospitalization.
      (ii) Symptoms cannot be due to a medical condition.
      (iii) Symptoms must cause distress or impairment.
         (1) See Table 9-6.
2. Bipolar II is similar to bipolar I except that mania is absent and hypomania is present.
   (a) Hypomania is a milder form of elevated mood than mania.
   (b) Have same symptoms as mania but less severe, cause less impairment, and typically do not require hospitalization.
3. Cyclothymic is a recurrent, chronic, mild form of bipolar.
   (a) The mood typically moves between hypomania and dysthymia.
   (b) Cannot have a history of mania or major depression.

Table 9-6 • Criteria for Manic Episode

Criteria	Description
Activity	Increased goal-oriented activities
Attention	Easily distracted
Hedonism	Excessive involvement in pleasurable activities
Self-esteem	Highly inflated
Sleep	Decreased need for sleep
Speech	Pressured
Thoughts	Racing, flight of ideas

iii. Treatment
1. Treatment of acute mania is antipsychotics with benzodiazepines and mood stabilizers.
   (a) Mood stabilizers, such as lithium, are essential in prevention of recurrence of mania and depression.
2. In bipolar II, caution should be taken in treatment with antidepressants because they may promote severe or frequent hypomania episodes.
VI. Personality disorders
   a. General
      i. Three personality disorder clusters.
         1. See Table 9-7.

Table 9-7 • Classification of Personality Disorders

Odd and Eccentric	Dramatic and Emotional	Anxious and Fearful
Paranoid	Antisocial	Avoidant
Schizoid	Borderline	Dependent
Schizotypal	Histrionic Narcissistic	Obsessive-compulsive

ii. Pattern of symptoms of personality disorders typically established by adolescence or early adulthood.

iii. Patients usually remain in touch with reality.

iv. Criteria for personality disorders
   1. Patients show evidence of an enduring pattern of inner experiences and behavior that:
      • Deviates greatly from cultural expectations
      • Is inflexible and personally and socially pervasive
      • Causes distress or social or work impairments
      • Demonstrates stable pattern of experiences and behavior of long duration
      • Cannot be explained by other mental illness
      • Is not caused by substance use or medical condition

b. Types
   i. Antisocial
      1. General
         (a) Have a disregard for rules and laws and rarely experience remorse for their actions.
         (b) They are exploitative, lie frequently, endanger others, and are impulsive and aggressive.
         (c) Alcohol use is frequent in these patients.
   ii. Avoidant
      1. General
         (a) Patients desire relationships but avoid them because of anxiety produced by their sense of inadequacy.
         (b) Very sensitive to criticism; fear rejection and humiliation.
         (c) Avoid spending time with others; must have a strong guarantee of acceptance to engage in a relationship.
   iii. Borderline
      1. General
         (a) Patients suffer from instability in relationships, self-image, affect, and impulse control.

(i) Relationships are complicated with anger, fear of abandonment, and shifting idealization and devaluation.
(ii) Self-image is unstable with unpredictable changes in relationships, goals, and values.
(iii) Affect is unstable and reactive with anger, depression, and panic being common.
(iv) Impulse control is weak and results in unsafe behaviors.

iv. Dependent
   1. General
      (a) Patients are very needy and rely on others for emotional support and decision making.
      (b) Live in continual fear of separation from someone they depend on.
      (c) Very submissive and clinging.
v. Histrionic
   1. General
      (a) Characterized by excessive and superficial emotionality and a need to be the center of attention.
      (b) Wear dramatic clothing, emotional responses to what are insignificant events are exaggerated, and inappropriate flirtatious and seductive behaviors are common.
      (c) Often have a problem with intimacy, believe their relationships are more intimate than they actually are.

QUESTION

Which of the following is the most appropriate treatment for a 10-year-old boy with attention-deficit disorder?
   A. Amitriptyline (Elavil)
   B. Fluoxetine (Prozac)
   C. Imipramine (Tofranil)
   D. Methylphenidate (Ritalin)

NOTES

ANSWER **D** EXPLANATION: *Attention-deficit disorder is treated with psychostimulates, such as methylphenidate and dextroamphetamine.*

correct ☐   incorrect ☐

vi. Narcissistic
  1. General
    (a) Characterized by self-centeredness and entitlement with low self-esteem.
    (b) Patients demand attention and admiration and are extravagant.
    (c) Concern or empathy for others is lacking.
    (d) Have an intense envy for others they regard as more desirable, worthy, or able.

vii. Obsessive-compulsive
  1. General
    (a) Patients are perfectionists and require a great deal of control and order in every aspect of their lives.
    (b) Attention to small details impairs their ability to finish what they start.
    (c) Are cold and rigid in relationships and make frequent moral judgments.
    (d) Are devoted to work and avoid intimacy.

viii. Paranoid
  1. General
    (a) Are distrustful and suspicious.
    (b) Anticipate harm, betrayal, and deception.
    (c) Require emotional distance.
    (d) Must separate from paranoia associated with psychotic disorders.

ix. Schizoid
  1. General
    (a) These patients are loners, emotionally detached, and prefer to be left alone.
    (b) Have a profound difficulty in experiencing or expressing emotions.
    (c) Do seek out relationships.
      (i) May have a strong bond with a family member.

x. Schizotypal
  1. General
    (a) Similar to schizophrenia but less severe, and without sustained psychotic symptoms.
    (b) Have few relationships and demonstrate peculiar thought, affect, perception, and beliefs.
    (c) May be highly distrustful and often paranoid.

c. Treatment
  i. Personality disorders are typically resistant to treatment.
  ii. Psychodynamic-based therapy is used along with cognitive, behavioral, and family therapy.
    1. Dialectical behavioral therapy is helpful in the treatment of borderline personality disorders.
  iii. Medications are used to treat specific symptoms.
    1. Mood stabilizers for mood instability and impulsiveness.
    2. Benzodiazepines are used for anxiety.
    3. Selective serotonin reuptake inhibitors are used for depression, obsessive-compulsive symptoms, and eating disturbances.
    4. Antipsychotics, in low doses, are used for psychotic or paranoid symptoms.

VII. Psychoses
  a. Delusional disorder
    i. General
      1. Characterized by nonbizarre delusions without other psychotic symptoms.
      2. Disorder is rare and occurs typically in middle to late life.
      3. More common in females.
      4. The disease is chronic and unremitting.
    ii. Clinical manifestations
      1. Characterized by nonbizarre delusions about things that could happen in real life.
      2. Delusions must be present for at least 1 month, and other than the delusions, the patient's social adjustment is normal.

NOTES

3. Patients must not meet the criteria for schizophrenia.
4. Seven subtypes of delusional disorder.
   (a) See Table 9-8.

iii. Treatment
1. Antipsychotics are appropriate but may be ineffective.
2. Psychotherapy is the primary treatment.

a. Must maintain an alliance with the patient and not support or refute the delusion.

b. Schizophrenia
   i. General
      1. Patients have psychotic symptoms and social and/or occupational dysfunction.
      2. Must persist for at least 6 months.
      3. Typical onset in the early 20s for men and late 20s for women.
      4. Etiology is unknown.
         (a) May be due to hyperactivity in brain dopaminergic pathways.
      5. Are at a high risk for suicide.
         (a) Risk factors for suicide include:
             (i) Male gender
             (ii) Age less than 30 years
             (iii) Chronic course

Table 9-8 • Subtypes of Delusional Disorders

Subtype	Description
Erotomanic	Convinced that another person is in love with them
Grandiose	Convinced that they have special abilities or more important than reality indicates
Jealous	Convinced that their lover is unfaithful
Persecutory	Convinced that others are out to harm them or they are being conspired against
Somatic	Convinced that they have a body function disorder
Mixed	No single delusion is predominate
Unspecific	Cannot be determined or match a subtype

Q4

A patient presents with concerns over acquiring infections from coming in contact with people. This has lead to washing his hands approximately 100 times a day. Which of the following is the most likely diagnosis?

a) Phobia
b) Schizophrenia
c) Schizotypal personality
d) Obsessive-compulsive disorder

(iv) Prior depression
(v) Recent hospital discharge
6. Schizophreniform disorder is schizophrenia that fails to last 6 months and does not involve social withdrawal.

ii. Clinical manifestations
1. Patients generally have a history of abnormal premorbid functioning, which may include poor social skills, social withdrawal, and unusual thinking.
2. Characterized by:
   (a) Positive and negative symptoms
       (i) Positive symptoms are the presence of:
           (1) Hallucinations
           (2) Delusions
           (3) Bizarre behavior
       (ii) Negative symptoms are the presence of:
           (1) Decreased expression of emotion
           (2) Poverty of speech
           (3) Few friends, activities, or interests.
   (b) To make the diagnosis two or more of the following must be present:
       (i) Hallucinations
       (ii) Delusions
       (iii) Disorganized speech
       (iv) Grossly disorganized or catatonic behavior
       (v) Negative symptoms

NOTES

ANSWER D EXPLANATION: *Obsessive-compulsive disorder presents with a need for a great amount of control and suffer such attention to detail that is interferes with ability to finish what they start.*

correct ☐   incorrect ☐

      (vi) Plus
          (1) Social and occupational deterioration
          (2) Disease for at least 6 months
  iii. Treatment
     1. Antipsychotic agents (neuroleptics) are the primary treatment.
     2. Psychosocial treatments are critical to long-term management of patients.
       (a) Includes:
          (i) Stable reality-oriented psychotherapy
          (ii) Family support
          (iii) Psychoeducation
          (iv) Social and vocational skills training
          (v) Attention to details of living situation
  c. Schizoaffective disorder
    i. General
     1. Patients have psychotic episodes that resemble schizophrenia but with prominent mood disturbances.
       (a) Psychotic symptoms must persist for some time in absence of any mood syndrome.
     2. Age of onset is late teens to early 20s.
    ii. Clinical manifestations
     1. Have symptoms of schizophrenia and a major mood disturbance, such as a manic or depressive episode.
     2. Must have periods of time in which they have psychotic symptoms without a major mood disturbance.
       (a) Mood disturbances need to be present for a substantial part of the illness.

    iii. Treatment
     1. Treated with a combination of mood stabilizers and antipsychotic medications.
VIII. Somatoform disorders
  a. General
    i. Characterized by presence of physical signs or symptoms without medical cause.
    ii. More common in females.
    iii. Patients have a complex medical history and often have gone through multiple medical and surgical procedures.
  b. Clinical manifestations
    i. Diagnosed when a patient has multiple medical complaints that are not the result of medical illness.
    ii. Diagnostic criteria require the following:
     1. Pain in four different body sites or body functions
     2. Two gastrointestinal symptoms, other than pain
     3. One sexual symptom, other than pain
     4. One pseudoneurologic symptom, other than pain
     5. See Table 9-9.
    iii. Symptoms must have begun before age 30 years and have persisted for several years.
IX. Substance use disorders
  a. General
    i. Substance abuse defined as maladaptive pattern of substance use leading to significant clinical impairment and disease. Manifested by:
     1. Failures to fulfill major obligations at home, work, or school.
     2. Recurrent use of substances in situations in which it is physically dangerous.
     3. Recurrent legal problems related to substance use.
     4. Recurrent substance use despite recurrent social and personal problems caused by or related to the substance use.
    ii. Substance dependence defined as a maladaptive pattern of substance use leading to significant impairment or distress. Manifested by:
    1. Tolerance
    2. Withdrawal

NOTES

3. Repeated, unintended, excessive use
4. Persistent failed efforts to decrease use
5. Excessive time spent trying to obtain substances
6. Reduction in important activities
7. Continued use despite patient awareness that substance is the cause of many problems.

iii. CAGE screening for alcohol and drug use.
1. **C**ut down: "Do you think you should cut down your drinking or drug use?"
2. **A**nnoyed: "Have people annoyed you by criticizing your drinking or drug use?"
3. **G**uilty: "Have you felt bad about your drinking or drug use?"
4. **E**ye opener: "Have you had a drink or used drugs to steady your nerves in the morning?"

b. Alcohol abuse/dependence
i. Alcohol intoxication
1. General
(a) Defined by presence of the following during or shortly after alcohol ingestion.
(i) Slurred speech

QUESTION

Which of the following is noted in patients with personality disorders?

A. Anxiety
B. Delusions
C. Manic episodes
D. Maladaptive pattern of behavior

(ii) Unsteady/incoordination
(iii) Nystagmus
(iv) Impaired attention or memory
(v) Stupor or coma
(vi) Maladaptive behavior or psychological changes, such as impaired judgment or inappropriate behavior.

2. Diagnosis
(a) Must also consider other possible medical causes, such hypoglycemia or toxicity of other substances.

Table 9-9 • Somatoform Disorders	
Disorder	**Description**
Somatization disorder	Chronic multiple medical complaints that are not due to medical problems.
Undifferentiated somatization disorder	Less severe form of somatization disorder.
Conversion disorder	Complaints include sensory and voluntary motor function that are not due to a medical condition.
Pain disorder	Pain is major complaint. Medical cause may be present, but psychological factors play a role in expression and impact of pain.
Hypochondriasis	Preoccupation with having a serious disease, based on misunderstanding of body function.
Body dysmorphic disorder	Excessive concern with perceived defect in body appearance.

NOTES

ANSWER **D** EXPLANATION: *Patients with personality disorders usually remain in touch with reality and present with pattern of experiences or behaviors that deviate from cultural norm, inflexible, and cause distress or social impairment.*

correct ☐   incorrect ☐

  (b) Diagnosis confirmed with blood alcohol level.
 3. Treatment
   (a) Supportive care.
 ii. Alcohol dependence
  1. General
   (a) About 10% of Americans are heavy drinkers, drinking almost every day and becoming intoxicated multiple times per month.
   (b) Male-to-female ratio for alcohol dependence is 4:1.
   (c) Alcohol abuse becomes dependence when tolerance and withdrawal symptoms develop.
   (d) The alcohol-dependent patient:
    (i) Drinks larger amounts over longer time periods than intended.
    (ii) Spends much time obtaining alcohol.
    (iii) Reduces or stops participation in other activities.
    (iv) Have a persistent desire or unsuccessful efforts to decrease or control alcohol use.
  2. Clinical manifestations
   (a) Early diagnosis difficult due to patient denying or minimizing drinking.
   (b) May present with accidents, falls, blackouts, or difficulties with law enforcement.
   (c) Information from family is required to make the diagnosis.
   (d) Physical examination
    (i) Early findings include acne rosacea, palmar erythema, and hepatomegaly (painless).
    (ii) Late findings include cirrhosis, jaundice, ascites, testicular atrophy, and gynecomastia.
   (e) Neuropsychiatric complications of alcoholism includes Wernicke-Korsakoff syndrome.
    (i) Due to thiamine deficiency.
    (ii) Wernicke stage consists of nystagmus, ataxia, and mental confusion.
     (1) Resolve with thiamine treatment.
    (iii) Korsakoff stage is anterograde amnesia and confabulation.
     (1) May be irreversible in many patients.
   (f) Other manifestations include alcoholic hallucinations, dementia, peripheral neuropathy, depression, and suicide.
   (g) In the later stages, social and occupational impairment occur, leading to job loss and family estrangement.
  3. Diagnosis
   (a) Blood alcohol levels will confirm presence of alcohol in the blood.
   (b) Other lab changes include elevated mean corpuscular volume (MCV), elevated serum gamma-glutamyltransferase (GGT), and elevated high-density lipoprotein (HDL).
  4. Treatment
   (a) Alcohol intoxication
    (i) Supportive measures, all known alcohol-dependent patients should receive folate and thiamine.
   (b) Minor alcohol withdrawal
    (i) Begins within 12 to 18 hours after stopping alcohol intake and peaks at 24 to 48 hours.
     (1) Untreated, uncomplicated withdrawal lasts 5 to 7 days.
    (ii) Present with tremors, nausea, vomiting, tachycardia, and hypertension.

NOTES

(iii) Treatment goal is patient comfort and to prevent serious complications.
    (1) Treat with chlordiazepoxide or oxazepam.
(c) Major alcohol withdrawal
  (i) Alcohol-induced seizures
    (1) Begin within 8 to 36 hours and peaks 24 to 48 after stopping alcohol intake.
    (2) Treated with intravenous (IV) benzodiazepines and phenytoin.
  (ii) Alcohol hallucinations
    (1) Begin 48 hours after stopping alcohol intake and may last more than 1 week.
    (2) Characterized by vivid, unpleasant auditory hallucinations in the presence of a clear sensorium.
    (3) Treat with a neuroleptic.
  (iii) Alcohol withdrawal delirium (delirium tremens)
    (1) Life-threatening condition manifested by delirium, autonomic hyperarousal, and mild fever.
    (2) Begins 2 to 3 days after the abrupt stopping of alcohol.
    (3) Treated with IV benzodiazepines and supportive care.
(d) Alcohol rehabilitation
  (i) Goals are sobriety and treatment of psychopathology.
  (ii) Options include:
    (1) Alcoholics Anonymous
    (2) Inpatient and residential rehabilitation programs
      [a] Half of patients will relapse in first 6 months.
    (3) Medications
      [a] Treatment of depression and anxiety
      [b] Disulfiram (Antabuse)
      [c] Naltrexone

QUESTION

Which of the following subtypes of delusional disorders is described by the patient being convinced that another person is in love with them?

A. Persecutory
B. Grandiose
C. Erotomanic
D. Jealous

c. Drug abuse/dependence
  i. Sedative/hypnotic/anxiolytic use disorders
    1. General
      (a) Are cross-tolerant with alcohol.
    2. Clinical manifestations
      (a) Similar to alcohol manifestations.
      (b) Withdrawal delirium will start 3 to 4 days after stopping drug.
      (c) Overdose can cause respiratory compromise.
      (d) Diagnosed with drug blood levels.
      (e) Dependence presence of three or more of the symptoms listed in Table 9-10.
    3. Treatment
      (a) Detoxification begins with the slow tapering of medication doses.
      (b) After detoxification, rehabilitation is required.
  ii. Opioid use disorders
    1. General

Table 9-10 • **Signs and Symptoms of Withdrawal**	
Minor Withdrawal	**Major Withdrawal**
Anxiety	Coarse tremors
Apprehension	Hyperreflexia
Restlessness	Nausea and vomiting Orthostatic hypotension Seizures Sweating Weakness

NOTES

ANSWER C EXPLANATION: *Erotomanic delusional disorder is described by a patient being convinced that another person is in love with them.*

correct ☐   incorrect ☐

(a) Use produces a flush and intense pleasurable sensation that resembles orgasm.
(b) Addicts often have comorbid substance abuse disorders, antisocial or borderline personality disorders, and mood disorders.
(c) Withdrawal symptoms typically begin 10 hours after last dose.
2. Clinical manifestations
(a) Signs of intoxication occur immediately after use.
(i) Include pupillary constriction, respiratory depression, slurred speech, hypotension, bradycardia, and hypothermia.
(b) Symptoms of opiate withdrawal.
(i) See Table 9-11.
(c) Diagnosis confirmed by urine or serum toxicology testing.
3. Treatment
(a) Addicted patients should be gradually withdrawn using methadone.
(i) Withdrawal with short-acting drugs is 7 to 10 days and long-acting 2 to 3 weeks.
(b) Clonidine, a centrally acting alpha-2-agonist, is used to treat the autonomic symptoms of withdrawal.
(c) Rehabilitation is needed.
(d) Methadone maintenance is used in patients who demonstrate physiologic dependence.
iii. Central nervous system (CNS) stimulant disorders
1. General
(a) Includes cocaine and amphetamines.

(b) Cocaine has a rapid onset of action and short half-life, thus requires frequent dosing, whereas amphetamines have a longer onset of action and half-life.
(c) Withdrawal symptoms peak in 2 to 4 days.
2. Clinical manifestations
(a) Intoxication characterized by:
(i) Euphoria or hypervigilance
(ii) Tachycardia or bradycardia
(iii) Pupillary dilatation
(iv) Hypertension or hypotension
(v) Perspiration or chills
(vi) Nausea and vomiting
(vii) Weight loss
(viii) Psychomotor agitation or retardation
(ix) Confusion, seizures, or coma
(x) Respiratory depression and chest pain

Table 9-11 • Symptoms of Opiate Withdrawal	
Mild Withdrawal	**Severe Withdrawal**
Diarrhea	Abdominal pain/cramps
Dysphoric mood	Anxiety
Fever	Hot and cold flashes
Hypertension	Muscle aches
Insomnia	Nausea and vomiting
Pupillary dilatation	Seizures (with meperidine withdrawal)
Restlessness	
Rhinorrhea	
Sweating	
Tachycardia	
Yawning	

NOTES

(b) Cocaine intoxication can cause tactile hallucinations, agitation, impaired judgment, and transient psychosis.

(c) Amphetamine can cause agitation, impaired judgment, and transient psychosis.

(d) Withdrawal leads to fatigue, depression, nightmares, headache, sweating, muscle cramps, and hunger.

3. Treatment
   (a) Treatment consists of supportive care with rehabilitation being the goal.

d. Tobacco use/dependence
   i. General
      1. Approximately 25% of Americans smoke.
      2. Most tobacco use begins in adolescence, and risk factors include peer and parental influences, behavioral problems, personality characteristics, and genetics.
      3. Tobacco use is the major cause of death from cancer, cardiovascular disease, and pulmonary disease.
      4. Tobacco smoke may produce illness through systemic absorption of toxins and/or local pulmonary injury by oxidant gases.
   ii. Clinical manifestations
      1. Withdrawal symptoms include anxiety, irritability, difficulty concentrating, restlessness, hunger, craving tobacco, disrupted sleep, and depression.
   iii. Treatment
      1. Counseling and support systems.
      2. Medications
         (a) Nicotine
            (i) Replacement products include gum, nasal sprays, inhalers, and transdermal patch.
         (b) Bupropion
            (i) An antidepressant drug; excessive doses can cause seizures, and the drug should

not be used in patients with seizures or eating disorders.
(ii) Combination therapy, nicotine replacement plus bupropion, increases likelihood of cessation.

X. Other behavioral/emotional disorders
   a. Child abuse
      i. General
         1. Occurs at all levels of society.
            (a) Increased incidence in families in which alcohol is abused.
         2. Child abuse is defined as a nonaccidental serious physical injury, sexual exploitation or misuse, neglect, or serious mental injury in a child younger than 18 years old, as a result of commission or omission by a parent, guardian, or caregiver.
         3. There are four categories.
            (a) Physical abuse: refers to serious bodily injury.
            (b) Sexual abuse: includes exposure or involvement of children to sexual material or acts.
            (c) Neglect: result of failure to provide for the basic needs of a child.
            (d) Emotional abuse: is a coercive, demeaning behavior toward a child that interferes with normal development.
      ii. Clinical manifestations
         1. Diagnosis of abuse relies on physical evidence of abuse.
            (a) Includes multiple skin lesions in various stages of healing, subdural and subarachnoid bleeding, retinal hemorrhages, long bone and rib fractures, and spinal injuries.
               (i) Commonly noted in shaken baby syndrome.
         2. Munchausen syndrome by proxy
            (a) In this syndrome, the parent fabricates illness in the child, seeks medical treatment, and denies any knowledge of the cause of the disorder.

NOTES

(b) The child has many office visits, and the parent is very cooperative.

(c) Diagnosis is made when child is removed from parent and signs and symptoms resolve.

iii. Treatment
1. All possible cases of abuse must be investigated.
2. Strategies to improve the environment and reduce caregiver stress should be incorporated.
3. Family counseling and family support to resolve family dysfunction is beneficial.

b. Elder abuse
i. General
1. Approximately 10% of those older than 65 years are abused.
2. Defined as an act or omission that results in harm or threatened to the health or welfare of the elderly.
   (a) Mistreatment includes abuse or neglect.
      (i) This includes physical, psychological, financial, and material. Sexual abuse does not occur.
      (ii) Acts of omission include withholding food, medicine, clothing, and other necessities.
3. Family conflicts often underlie elder abuse.

ii. Clinical manifestations
1. Victims tend to be very old and fragile and often live with their assailant.
2. Signs of abuse include bruising, old and new fractures, and signs of malnutrition.

iii. Treatment
1. Patient safety is paramount.
2. Interventions include legal services, housing, medical, psychiatric, and social services.

c. Domestic violence
i. General
1. Occurs across all socioeconomic, racial, and cultural lines.
   (a) Increased risk in families with problems of substance abuse.
2. Occurs most commonly as part of a chronic maladaptive relationship within the couple.

ii. Clinical manifestations
1. Abused women frequently present with vague complaints of anxiety, depression, or somatic symptoms.
2. Trauma often directed at areas of the body not on public view.
3. Trauma typically occurs at home and rarely in front of individuals outside the household.
4. Most abusers (male) are possessive, jealous, and very dependent on their wives.
5. Victims often blame themselves for the abuse.

iii. Treatment
1. Patient safety is paramount.
2. Emergency shelter should be offered.

d. Uncomplicated bereavement
i. General
1. Develops immediately or within a few months of the loss and not considered a mental disorder.
2. Normal bereavement may lead to a major depressive disorder.

ii. Clinical manifestations
1. Feelings of sadness, preoccupation with thoughts of the deceased, tearfulness, irritability, insomnia, and difficulty concentrating are present.
2. Normal bereavement is limited to no longer than 6 months.

iii. Treatment
1. Antidepressants are not indicated.
2. Benzodiazepines are indicated for sleep.

NOTES

Psychiatric Drugs

Drug Name	Mechanism of Action	Therapeutic Use	Side Effects
ANTIPSYCHOTICS			
Thioridazine (Mellaril)	Block dopamine receptors	Antipsychotic	Sedation Hypotension Anticholinergic Pigmentary retinopathy
Chlorpromazine (Thorazine)	Block dopamine receptors	Antipsychotic	Sedation Hypotension
Perphenazine (Trilafon)	Block dopamine receptors	Antipsychotic	Extrapyramidal SE
Trifluoperazine (Stelazine)	Block dopamine receptors	Antipsychotic	Extrapyramidal SE
Haloperidol (Haldol)	Block dopamine receptors	Antipsychotic	Extrapyramidal SE
Fluphenazine (Prolixin)	Block dopamine receptors	Antipsychotic	Extrapyramidal SE
Clozapine (Clozaril)	Block dopamine and serotonin receptors	Antipsychotic	Sedation Hypotension Anticholinergic Agranulocytosis
Quetiapine (Seroquel)	Block dopamine and serotonin receptors	Antipsychotic	Sedation Cataracts
Olanzapine (Zyprexa)	Block dopamine and serotonin receptors	Antipsychotic	Sedation
Risperidone (Risperdal)	Block dopamine and serotonin receptors	Antipsychotic	Hypotensive QT prolongation
ANTIDEPRESSANTS			
Fluoxetine (Prozac)	Inhibit reuptake of serotonin	Mood disorders Panic disorder OCD Bulimia	Nausea Headache Insomnia/sedation Sexual dysfunction
Sertraline (Zoloft)	Inhibit reuptake of serotonin	Mood disorders Panic disorder Bulimia	Nausea Headache Insomnia/sedation Sexual dysfunction

(*continued*)

NOTES

Psychiatric Drugs—cont'd

Drug Name	Mechanism of Action	Therapeutic Use	Side Effects
Paroxetine (Paxil)	Inhibit reuptake of serotonin	Mood disorders Panic disorder Bulimia	Nausea Headache Insomnia/sedation Sexual dysfunction
Fluvoxamine (Luvox)	Inhibit reuptake of serotonin	Mood disorders Panic disorder Bulimia	Nausea Headache Insomnia/sedation Sexual dysfunction
Citalopram (Celexa)	Inhibit reuptake of serotonin	Mood disorders Panic disorder Bulimia	Nausea Headache Insomnia/sedation Sexual dysfunction
Nortriptyline (Pamelor)	Block presynaptic uptake of norepinephrine and serotonin	Mood disorders Panic disorder	Orthostatic hypotension Anticholinergic Cardiac toxicity Sexual dysfunction
Imipramine (Tofranil)	Block presynaptic uptake of norepinephrine and serotonin	Mood disorders Panic disorder	Orthostatic hypotension Anticholinergic Cardiac toxicity Sexual dysfunction
Desipramine (Norpramin)	Block presynaptic uptake of norepinephrine and serotonin	Mood disorders Panic disorder	Orthostatic hypotension Anticholinergic Cardiac toxicity Sexual dysfunction
Tranylcypromine (Parnate)	Inhibits presynaptic monoamine oxidase	Mood disorders Panic disorder	Orthostatic hypotension Insomnia/agitation Hypertensive crisis
Phenelzine (Nardil)	Inhibits presynaptic monoamine oxidase	Mood disorders Panic disorder	Orthostatic hypotension Daytime somnolence Hypertensive crisis

NOTES

Psychiatric Drugs—cont'd

Drug Name	Mechanism of Action	Therapeutic Use	Side Effects
Bupropion (Wellbutrin)	Inhibits uptake of dopamine and norepinephrine	Mood disorders Smoking cessation	Risk of seizures
Nefazodone (Serzone)	Serotonin-modulating	Depression	Postural hypotension Seizures Priapism
Venlafaxine (Effexor)	Inhibitors of serotonin and norepinephrine reuptake	Depression	Anxiety Insomnia Seizures
Mirtazapine (Remeron)	Modulator of norepinephrine	Mood disorders	Sedation
Trazodone (Desyrel)	Serotonin-modulating	Depression Insomnia	Sedation Priapism
MOOD STABILIZERS			
Lithium (Eskalith)	Alter intracellular messengers	Acute mania Bipolar disorder Depression	Ataxia Coarse tremor Confusion Sinus arrest Acne exacerbation Weight gain
Valproate (Depakene)	Augments GABA synthesis	Acute mania Bipolar disorder Seizures	Sedation Mild tremor and ataxia GI distress
Carbamazepine (Tegretol)	Alters sodium channels	Acute mania Bipolar disorder Seizures	Ataxia Sedation Dizziness Somnolence Agranulocytosis Nausea and vomiting
Lamotrigine (Lamictal)	Inhibits sodium channels	Bipolar disorder Seizures	Ataxia Blurred vision Dizziness Nausea and vomiting Stevens-Johnson syndrome

(continued)

NOTES

Psychiatric Drugs—cont'd

Drug Name	Mechanism of Action	Therapeutic Use	Side Effects
ANXIOLYTICS			
Alprazolam (Xanax)	Agonist at the CNS GABA receptor-augment GABA function	Anxiety disorders Akathisia Agitation Panic disorders	Sleepiness Depress respiratory system
Chlordiazepoxide (Librium)	Agonist at the CNS GABA receptor-augment GABA function	Anxiety disorders Akathisia Agitation Alcohol withdrawal	Sleepiness Depress respiratory system
Clonazepam (Klonopin)	Agonist at the CNS GABA receptor-augment GABA function	Anxiety disorders Akathisia Agitation Panic disorders	Sleepiness Depress respiratory system
Diazepam (Valium)	Agonist at the CNS GABA receptor-augment GABA function	Anxiety disorders Akathisia Agitation Insomnia	Sleepiness Depress respiratory system
Lorazepam (Ativan)	Agonist at the CNS GABA receptor-augment GABA function	Anxiety disorders Akathisia Agitation Catatonia	Sleepiness Depress respiratory system
Oxazepam (Serax)	Agonist at the CNS GABA receptor-augment GABA function	Anxiety disorders Akathisia Agitation Alcohol withdrawal	Sleepiness Depress respiratory system
Temazepam (Restoril)	Agonist at the CNS GABA receptor-augment GABA function	Anxiety disorders Akathisia Agitation Insomnia	Sleepiness Depress respiratory system
Triazolam (Halcion)	Agonist at the CNS GABA receptor-augment GABA function	Anxiety disorders Akathisia Agitation Insomnia	Sleepiness Depress respiratory system
Buspirone (Buspar)	Agonist at the 5HT receptor	Anxiety	Dizziness Nervousness Nausea

NOTES

Psychiatric Drugs—cont'd

Drug Name	Mechanism of Action	Therapeutic Use	Side Effects
PSYCHOSTIMULANTS			
Methylphenidate (Ritalin)	Facilitate neurotransmitter release in the CNS	Attention deficit disorder Narcolepsy	Tachycardia Insomnia Anxiety Hypertension Weight loss
Dextroamphetamine (Dexedrine)	Facilitate neurotransmitter release in the CNS	Attention deficit disorder Narcolepsy	Tachycardia Insomnia Anxiety Hypertension Weight loss
Pemoline (Cylert)	Facilitate neurotransmitter release in the CNS	Attention deficit disorder Narcolepsy	Tachycardia Insomnia Anxiety Hypertension Weight loss

Question 1

Which of the following symptoms are likely to be present in a patient with anxiety disorder?

- A. Chest pain and palpitations
- B. Shortness of breath and cough
- C. Gastric reflux and diarrhea
- D. Headache and blurry vision

Question 2

Which of the following laboratory finding would most likely be due to alcohol consumption?

- A. High glucose
- B. High MCV
- C. Low GGT
- D. Low amylase

NOTES

Question 3

A patient who demonstrates a pattern of excessive attention seeking and emotionality would be diagnosed with which of the following personality disorders?

A. Histrionic
B. Dependent
C. Self-defeating
D. Passive-aggressive

Question 4

A 20-year-old presents with a 9-month history of poor social skills and social withdrawing. Also note hallucinations and delusions. After anti-psychotics which of the following is critical to the long-term management of this patient?

A. Psychosocial therapy
B. Electroshock therapy
C. Biofeedback therapy
D. Aversion therapy

Question 5

Which of the following medications is used in the treatment of attention-deficit disorder?

A. Trazodone (Desyrel)
B. Bupropion (Wellbutrin)
C. Fluoxetine (Prozac)
D. Pemoline (Cylert)

Question 6

Which of the following patients with major depressive disorder must be considered for maintenance pharmacotherapy?

A. Patient with three or more episodes of major depression.
B. Patient with diabetes and major depression.
C. Any male patient with major depression.
D. Any patient over the age of 50.

Question 7

Which of the following metabolic abnormalities is most commonly noted in patients with anorexia nervosa?

A. Hypokalemia
B. Hyponatremia
C. Respiratory alkalosis
D. Hypercalcemia

Answer 1

ANSWER **A** EXPLANATION: *DSM-IV criteria for panic attacks include palpitations, sweating, shaking, shortness or breath, chest pain, dizziness, and a feeling of unreality or fear of losing control.*

Topic: Anxiety disorders

correct ☐   incorrect ☐

NOTES

Answer 2

ANSWER **C** EXPLANATION: *Common laboratory changes in patients with alcohol dependence include elevated MCV, elevated Serum GGT, and elevated HDL.*

Topic: Alcohol abuse/dependence

correct ☐   incorrect ☐

Answer 3

ANSWER **A** EXPLANATION: *Histrionic personality disorder is characterized by excessive and superficial emotionality and the need to be the center of attention.*

Topic: Personality disorders

correct ☐   incorrect ☐

Answer 4

ANSWER **A** EXPLANATION: *Schizophrenia is most common in patients in their 20's and presents with at least a 6-month history of abnormal premorbid functioning, hallucinations, and delusions. Treatment consists of antipsychotic medications and psychosocial therapy, such as psychotherapy and skills training.*

Topic: Schizophrenia

correct ☐   incorrect ☐

Answer 5

ANSWER **D** EXPLANATION: *Treatment of attention-deficit disorder consists of psychostimulants, such as methylphenidate, dextroamphetamine, and pemoline.*

Topic: Attention-deficit disorder

correct ☐   incorrect ☐

Answer 6

ANSWER **A** EXPLANATION: *Maintenance therapy for major depressive disorders is indicated with a history of recurrent major depressive episodes. Maintenance therapy is not typically indicated in patients with comorbid disorders, or based on age or sex of the patient.*

Topic: Mood disorders

correct ☐   incorrect ☐

Answer 7

ANSWER **A** EXPLANATION: *Eating disorders can lead to a number of medical complications, including hypokalemia, metabolic acidosis or alkalosis, and anemia.*

Topic: Anorexia nervosa

correct ☐   incorrect ☐

NOTES

The Genitourinary System

10

EXAM BLUEPRINT TOPICS

Benign Conditions of the Genitourinary Tract
Benign prostatic hypertrophy
Cryptorchidism
Erectile dysfunction
Hydrocele
Varicocele
Incontinence
Nephrolithiasis
Paraphimosis/phimosis
Testicular torsion
Infectious/Inflammatory Conditions
Cystitis
Epididymitis
Orchitis
Prostatitis
Pyelonephritis
Urethritis
Neoplastic Diseases
Bladder carcinoma
Prostate carcinoma
Renal cell carcinoma
Testicular carcinoma
Wilms' tumor
Renal Diseases
Acute renal failure
Chronic renal failure
Glomerulonephritis
Nephrotic syndrome
Polycystic kidney disease
Electrolyte and Acid–Base Disorders
Hyponatremia
Hypernatremia
Hypokalemia
Hyperkalemia
Hypocalcemia
Hypercalcemia
Hypomagnesemia
Acid–base disorders

Volume depletion
Volume excess
Urinalysis

BENIGN CONDITIONS OF THE GENITOURINARY TRACT

I. Benign prostatic hypertrophy (BPH)
  a. General
    i. Process begins in the 30s and by age 80, more than 80% of men have BPH.
    ii. Risk factors are age and functioning testes.
  b. Clinical manifestations
    i. Have voiding symptoms such as hesitancy, straining, urgency, sense of incomplete voiding, weak stream, and dribbling.
    ii. On digital rectal examination, the prostate is enlarged and firm.
    iii. Neurologic examination needed to rule out neuropathic bladder, caused by peripheral neuropathy or saddle-area anesthesia.
  c. Diagnosis
    i. Prostate-specific antigen should be obtained to evaluate for possible prostate cancer.
    ii. Bladder outlet obstruction diagnosed by showing increased bladder pressure relative to uroflow with pressure-flow studies.
  d. Treatment
    i. Medical therapy
      1. Alpha-2-adrenergic blockers and 5-α-reductase inhibitors will reduce symptoms.
        (a) Side effects with alpha-2-adrenergic blockers include hypotension, dizziness, and asthenia.
        (b) Side effect with 5-α-reductase inhibitors includes sexual ejaculatory dysfunction.

NOTES

ii. Surgery
    1. Transurethral prostatectomy (TURP), resection of the prostate, is the gold standard.

II. Cryptorchidism
  a. General
    i. Unilateral or bilateral undescended testis.
    ii. In most cases, the testes descend by the third month.
    iii. Increased risk for infertility and testicular malignancy.
  b. Clinical manifestations
    i. Lack of testes on testicular examination.
  c. Diagnosis
    i. Testosterone level after human chorionic gonadotropin (HCG) stimulation to confirm presence or absence of abdominal testes.
    ii. Ultrasound or computed tomography (CT) scan can be utilized.
  d. Treatment
    i. Surgical orchidopexy by 1 year of age.

III. Erectile dysfunction
  a. General
    i. Defined as the consistent inability to maintain an erection sufficient to allow penetration and sexual intercourse.
    ii. Most cases have organic cause rather than psychogenic.
    iii. Etiologies include arterial, venous, neurogenic, or psychogenic causes.
    iv. Antihypertensives such as centrally acting sympatholytics may alter erections, and beta-blockers and spironolactone alter libido.
  b. Clinical manifestations
    i. Problems with erectile dysfunction must be separated from problems with ejaculation, libido, and orgasm.
    ii. History of systemic diseases is vital.
      1. History of hyperlipidemia, vascular disease, diabetes, and hypertension linked to erectile dysfunction.
  c. Diagnosis
    i. Laboratory testing should be obtained to rule out systemic disease.
    ii. Hormone levels such as testosterone, prolactin, follicle-stimulating hormone (FSH), and luteinizing hormone (LH) should be obtained.
    iii. Nocturnal tumescence testing should be completed to separate organic from psychogenic etiologies.
  d. Treatment
    i. Varies with etiology:
      1. Hormonal replacement
        (a) Testosterone injections given in cases of androgen deficiency.
      2. Vacuum constriction device
      3. Vasoactive therapy
        (a) Sildenafil inhibits phosphodiesterase 5, a vasoconstrictor, and allows cyclic guanosine monophosphate (cGMP) to function unopposed, and allows sustained blood flow to the penis.
          (i) Patients taking nitrates may develop hypotension.
      4. Penile prostheses
      5. Vascular reconstruction

IV. Hydrocele
  a. General
    i. Accumulation of fluid in the tunica vaginalis surrounding testes.
    ii. Typically is noncommunicating type.
      1. In noncommunicating type, the processus vaginalis was obliterated during development.
      2. Will usually disappear by 1 year of age.
      3. Communicating hydrocele may develop into an inguinal hernia.
    iii. Etiology also includes testicular torsion, epididymitis, or tumor.
  b. Clinical manifestations
    i. Mass is smooth and nontender.
  c. Diagnosis
    i. Transillumination of the scrotum confirms a fluid-filled mass.
  d. Treatment
    i. Typically resolve spontaneously.
    ii. Surgery may be needed if mass lasts past age 18 months.
    iii. All communicating hydroceles must be surgically repaired.

V. Varicocele
  a. General
    i. Abnormal dilatation of the pampiniform plexus in the scrotum.

NOTES

1. Due to incompetent valves in the spermatic vein.
    ii. Is a common cause of infertility.
    iii. Rare in boys younger than 10 years of age.
  b. Clinical manifestations
    i. Occur mainly on the left side, if on the right side and less than 10 years old, this may indicate an abdominal or renal mass.
    ii. Patient may complain of a dull ache in the testis.
    iii. On physical examination, a painless testicular mass is noted
      1. Described as a "bag of worms."
    iv. On standing, a varicocele will become more prominent.
  c. Treatment
    i. Ligation of the spermatic vein, varicocelectomy, is indicated to increase chance for fertility.
VI. Incontinence
  a. General
    i. Common in the elderly.
    ii. Occurs when urine leaks involuntary.
    iii. Classified into one of four groups.
      1. Total incontinence
        (a) Patients lose urine at all times and in all positions.
        (b) Results from loss of sphincter efficiency or abnormal connection between the urinary tract and skin (fistulas).
      2. Stress incontinence
        (a) Loss of urine with activities that increase intra-abdominal pressure (coughing, lifting).
        (b) Patients do not leak in the supine position.
        (c) Due to laxity in the pelvic floor muscles.
      3. Urge incontinence
        (a) Uncontrolled loss of urine that is preceded by a strong, unexpected urge to void.
        (b) Unrelated to position or activity.
        (c) Due to detrusor hyperreflexia or sphincter dysfunction.
        (d) Seen in inflammatory conditions or neurogenic disorders.

QUESTION

A 55-year-old male presents with worsening nocturia and urinary hesitancy. Which of the following is the next best step in the evaluation of this patient?

  A. Digital rectal examination (DRE)
  B. Prostatic specific antigen (PSA) test
  C. Transrectal ultrasound
  D. CT of the pelvis

      4. Overflow incontinence
        (a) Due to chronic urinary retention.
          (i) Seen in BPH and urethral strictures.
        (b) Results from chronically distended bladder.
  b. Clinical manifestations
    i. History most important with a voiding diary.
    ii. On physical examination, note presence of fistula, neurologic abnormalities, or distended bladder.
    iii. Rectal exam needed to determine rectal tone.
    iv. Laboratory testing should be completed to rule out urinary tract infection.
  c. Diagnosis
    i. Urodynamic evaluation should be completed.
  d. Treatment
    i. Varies with etiology.
      1. Total incontinence
        (a) Surgical reconstruction of any abnormalities.
      2. Stress incontinence
        (a) Topical estrogens
        (b) Drug therapy to increase urethral resistance.
      3. Urge incontinence
        (a) Medical therapy with antispasmodic agents, anticholinergic agents, or tricyclic antidepressants.
      4. Overflow incontinence
        (a) Urethral catheter is both diagnostic and therapeutic.
        (b) Treatment of underlying cause.

NOTES

ANSWER A EXPLANATION: *Urinary symptoms, including nocturia and hesitancy, are noted in benign prostatic hypertrophy (BPH) and prostate cancer. The first step in the evaluation of this patient is a digital rectal examination. PSA and transrectal ultrasound may be indicated to rule out possible prostate cancer.*

correct ☐   incorrect ☐

VII. Nephrolithiasis
   a. General
      i. A crystalline mass within the urinary tract.
         1. Most common are calcium oxalate.
      ii. More common in males than females, very uncommon in African Americans and Asians.

   b. Clinical manifestations
      i. Sudden onset of unbearable, colicky pain.
         1. May have nausea and vomiting associated with the pain.
      ii. Pain begins in the flank and moves anteriorly toward the groin and is referred to the testes or labia.
      iii. Hematuria is common
   c. Diagnosis
      i. Abdominal X-ray will detect most stones.
         1. Cystine and uric acid stones are not detected on X-ray.
         2. See Figure 10-1.
      ii. Helical CT scan has replaced intravenous pyelogram (IVP) as test of choice.
   d. Treatment
      i. Pain relief with opiates if needed.
      ii. Intravenous (IV) fluid hydration.

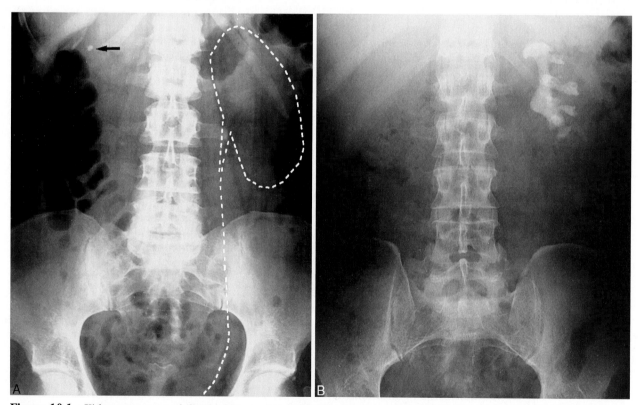

Figure 10-1 Kidney stones on abdominal X-ray. (From Mettler FA: Essentials of Radiology, 2nd ed. Philadelphia: Elsevier Saunders, 2005:221, Fig. 7-11.)

NOTES

iii. Extracorporeal shock wave lithotripsy (ESWL) is used to remove stones from 5 mm up to 2 cm.
iv. Percutaneous nephrolithotomy is used to treat stones larger than 2 cm.
v. Prevention of recurrent stones
   1. Evaluation of stone composition.
      (a) 24-hour urine for calcium, potassium, magnesium, sodium, phosphorus, citrate, oxalate, uric acid, and creatinine.
      (b) Serum studies include electrolytes, calcium, phosphorous, and parathyroid hormone.
   2. Prevention therapy
      (a) Increased fluid intake.
      (b) Diets with reduced sodium, oxalate, and protein.
      (c) Thiazide diuretics—lower calcium excretion in the urine.
VIII. Paraphimosis/phimosis
   a. General
      i. Paraphimosis is the painful swelling of the foreskin distal to a phimotic ring.
         1. Occurs if the foreskin remains retracted for a prolonged period of time.
      ii. Phimosis is the inability to retract the foreskin.
         1. Can result from repeated episodes of balanitis.
         2. Balanitis is inflammation of the glans penis as a result of poor hygiene.
            (a) In older patients, balanitis may be a presenting sign for diabetes.
   b. Treatment
      i. Applying steady, gentle pressure to the foreskin to decrease the swelling can reduce paraphimosis.
         1. Condition can reoccur; thus, dorsal slit or a circumcision should be done.
      ii. Phimosis is treated with circumcision.
IX. Testicular torsion
   a. General
      i. A urologic emergency. Diagnosis and treatment must be prompt to save the testis.
      ii. Most common cause of testicular pain in boys older than 12 years of age.

QUESTION

A 41-year-old male presents with acute onset of right flank pain. The pain is intermittent and now radiates into his right testicle. He is afebrile. Which of the following is the most likely diagnosis?

A. Incarcerated inguinal hernia
B. Appendicitis
C. Ureteral stone
D. Varicocele

   1. Torsion of the appendix of the testis is the most common cause of testicular pain in boys between ages 2 and 11 years.
   iii. Due to inadequate fixation of testis within the scrotum.
      1. Abnormal attachment is called a *bell-clapper deformity.*
   b. Clinical manifestations
      i. With acute testicular torsion, present with acute testicular pain and swelling of the scrotum.
         1. On examination, the scrotum is swollen and tender. The cremasteric reflex is absent.
      ii. With torsion of the appendix of the testis, the patient presents with gradual onset of testicular pain and scrotal erythema.
         1. On examination, palpation of the testis reveals a 3- to 5-mm tender indurated mass on the upper pole.
            (a) This mass may be visible through the scrotum and is called the *blue-dot sign.*
   c. Diagnosis
      i. Testicular flow scan or color Doppler ultrasound is required to separate testicular torsion from torsion of the appendix of the testis.
   d. Treatment
      i. Testicular torsion treated with prompt surgical exploration and detorsion.
         1. If completed within 6 hours, have excellent survival chance for testicular tissue.

NOTES

ANSWER C EXPLANATION: *Flank pain that radiates into the testicle or scrotum is noted with the presence of a urethral stone.*

correct ☐   incorrect ☐

2. After detorsion, the testis is fixed to the scrotum by scrotal orchiopexy.
   (a) This should be completed on both testes.
   ii. Torsion of the appendix of the testis will typically resolve in 3 to 10 days.
   1. No surgery is needed.
   2. Pain control is vital.

INFECTIOUS/INFLAMMATORY CONDITIONS

I. Cystitis
   a. General
      i. Infection of the bladder.
      ii. Typically due to Gram-negative rods (*Escherichia coli*) and at times Gram-positive cocci (*Enterococcus*).
      iii. Route of infection is up through the urethra.
      1. In women, symptoms appear after sexual intercourse.
   b. Clinical manifestations
      i. Present with frequency, urgency, dysuria, and suprapubic pain.
      1. Women may present with hematuria.
      ii. On physical examination, suprapubic tenderness may be noted.
   c. Diagnosis
      i. Urinalysis reveals pyuria and bacteriuria.
      ii. Urine culture is positive for bacteria.
   d. Treatment
      i. A short course of antibiotics, such as trimethoprim-sulfamethoxazole, nitrofurantoin, or fluoroquinolones.
II. Epididymitis
   a. General
      i. Most cases are infectious and divided into two groups based on age distribution.
      1. Younger than 40 years old
         (a) Typically sexually transmitted and due to *Chlamydia trachomatis* or *Neisseria gonorrhoeae*.

2. Older than 40 years old
   (a) Typically nonsexually transmitted and due to a gram-negative rod from a urinary tract infection or prostatitis.
   b. Clinical manifestations
      i. Symptoms of urethritis (pain at tip of the penis and urethral discharge) and cystitis (frequency, urgency, and dysuria) are noted.
      ii. Fever and scrotal swelling may be noted.
   c. Diagnosis
      i. Laboratory tests reveal a leukocytosis with a left shift.
      ii. Gram stain of the discharge shows increased white blood cells and/or gram-negative diplococci in patients with gonorrhoeae.
      iii. Urinalysis and culture are positive in nonsexually transmitted cases.
   d. Treatment
      i. Supportive care with bed rest and scrotal elevation.
      ii. Antibiotic therapy varies with route of transmission.
      1. Sexually transmitted treated with ceftriaxone and/or doxycycline for 10 to 21 days.
      2. Nonsexually transmitted cases treated with trimethoprim-sulfamethoxazole, erythromycin, or fluoroquinolones for 21 to 28 days.
III. Orchitis
   a. General
      i. Due to Coxsackie B or the mumps virus.
      ii. More common complication after mumps in adolescents and adults.
      iii. Trauma may also cause orchitis.
   b. Clinical manifestations
      i. Typically follows parotitis within 8 days.
      ii. Abrupt onset with fever, chills, nausea, and lower abdominal pain.
      iii. Affected testicle becomes tender and swollen.
   c. Treatment
      i. Supportive care with pain control.
      ii. About one third of affected testicles will atrophy.
      iii. Infertility is rare.

NOTES

IV. Prostatitis
   a. General
      i. Etiology varies with type of prostatitis.
         1. See Tables 10-1 and 10-2.

Table 10-1 • Causes of Prostatitis		
Type	**Definition**	**Etiology**
Acute bacterial	Acute infection of the prostate	*Escherichia coli* *Pseudomonas aeruginosa* *Serratia* *Klebsiella* *Proteus* *Enterococcus*
Chronic bacterial	Recurrent infection of the prostate	*E. coli* *P. aeruginosa* *Serratia* *Klebsiella* *Proteus* *Enterococcus*
Chronic abacterial	No sign of infection	*Mycoplasma hominis* *Ureaplasma* *Trichomonas* *Chlamydia*

QUESTION

A 25-year-old male presents with a dull ache in the left testicle. On exam, a mass is noted over the spermatic cord. The mass becomes more prominent with standing. Which of the following is the most likely diagnosis?

   A. Hydrocele
   B. Varicocele
   C. Cryptorchidism
   D. Testicular torsion

   b. Clinical manifestations
      i. Acute bacterial presents with high fever, chills, and malaise.
         1. Urinary symptoms include dysuria, frequency, and urgency.
         2. On physical examination a very tender prostate is noted on digital rectal exam.
      ii. Chronic bacterial is typically noted in elderly men and associated with recurrent urinary tract infections.
         1. Symptoms are similar to acute bacterial infection but less severe.
         2. On digital rectal examination, the prostate is normal, swollen, firm, or tender.

Table 10-2 • Comparison of Prostatitis				
	Acute Bacterial	**Chronic Bacterial**	**Nonbacterial**	**Prostatodynia**
Fever	Yes	No	No	No
Urinalysis	Positive	Negative	Negative	Negative
Expressed prostatic secretions	Contraindicated	Positive	Positive	Negative
Culture-bacterial	Positive	Positive	Negative	Negative
Treatment	Ampicillin and gentamycin	Trimethoprim-sulfamethoxazole	Erythromycin	Alpha-blocking agents

NOTES

   iii. Chronic abacterial presents with pelvic pain and urinary tract infection symptoms and pain during or after ejaculation.

  c. Diagnosis

   i. Acute bacterial is diagnosed based on clinical findings and a positive urine culture.

    1. Prostate massage is contraindicated.

   ii. Chronic bacterial and chronic abacterial are diagnosed with the two- or four-glass test.

    1. With the four-glass test, culture the initial urine stream, mid-stream, expressed prostate excretions after massage, and postmassage urine.

    2. With the two-glass test, culture urine before and after prostate massage.

  d. Treatment

   i. Acute bacterial treated with antibiotics, IV needed for severe disease.

    1. Fluoroquinolones and trimethoprim-sulfamethoxazole are indicated.

    2. Treat for 4 weeks.

   ii. Chronic bacterial infection treated with antibiotics.

    1. Fluoroquinolones and trimethoprim-sulfamethoxazole are indicated.

    2. Treat for 1 to 3 months.

    3. Alpha-blocker may be tried to improve symptoms and reduce recurrences.

   iii. Chronic nonbacterial infection is difficult to treat.

    1. Antibiotics maybe tried, but success is low.

    2. Alpha-blocker is also not indicated.

V. Pyelonephritis

 a. General

  i. An infectious inflammatory condition involving the kidney/renal pelvis.

  ii. Etiology is most commonly Gram-negative rods such as *E. coli*, *Proteus*, or *Klebsiella*.

  iii. Route of the infection is ascending from the lower urinary tract.

 b. Clinical manifestations

  i. Symptoms include fever, chills, flank pain, urgency, dysuria, and frequency.

  ii. On physical examination, vital signs reveal fever and tachycardia, and costovertebral angle tenderness is noted.

 c. Diagnosis

  i. Complete blood count reveals a leukocytosis with a left shift.

  ii. Pyuria, bacteriuria, and hematuria are noted on the urinalysis.

   1. On microscopic examination of the urine, white blood cell casts are noted.

  iii. Urine culture is positive for bacteria.

 d. Treatment

  i. Empiric antibiotic coverage with ampicillin and an aminoglycoside, pending culture results.

  ii. Treat for a total of 3 weeks.

  iii. Complications include sepsis with shock.

VI. Urethritis

 a. General

  i. Refers to inflammation of the urethra.

  ii. Most cases are acquired through sexual intercourse.

  iii. There are two types of urethritis.

   1. Gonococcal

    (a) Etiology is *N. gonorrhoeae*.

   2. Nongonococcal

    (a) Etiology is *C. trachomatis* or *Ureaplasma urealyticum*.

   3. See Table 10-3.

 b. Clinical manifestations

  i. Gonococcal

   1. Produces thick, purulent urethral discharge and burning with urination.

    (a) Almost 50% of cases may be asymptomatic.

  ii. Nongonococcal

   1. Presents with dysuria and scant urethral discharge.

NOTES

Table 10-3 • Comparison of Gonococcal and Nongonococcal Urethritis

	Gonococcal	Nongonococcal
Organism	*Neisseria gonorrhoeae*	*Chlamydia trachomatis*
Incubation period	3–10 days	7–30 days
Discharge	Profuse, purulent	Scant, watery
Diagnosis	Gram stain Culture	Immunoassay
Treatment	Ceftriaxone plus azithromycin	Azithromycin or doxycycline
Alternate treatment	Cefixime or ciprofloxacin	Erythromycin or ofloxacin

QUESTION

Which of the following clinical findings is most suggestive of acute pyelonephritis?

A. Dysuria
B. Flank pain
C. Urinary hesitancy
D. Urinary incontinence

c. Diagnosis
   i. Urethritis may be suggested if urine dipstick test for leukocyte esterase is positive and no bladder infection is present.
   ii. Gonococcal
      1. Gram stain reveals Gram-negative diplococci and many white blood cells.
      2. Culture is used to make the diagnosis.
   iii. Nongonococcal
      1. Demonstration of urethritis and exclusion of *N. gonorrhoeae* are required for diagnosis.
      2. Gram stain shows many white blood cells but no bacteria.
      3. Direct fluorescent antibody testing and enzyme immunoassay are also used to make the diagnosis.
d. Treatment
   i. Urethritis can be prevented through the use of condoms.
      1. Gonococcal
         (a) Antibiotic of choice is ceftriaxone.
         (b) If concerned about concurrent infection with *C. trachomatis*, then azithromycin or ofloxacin should also be used.

2. Nongonococcal
   (a) Azithromycin and doxycycline are the antibiotics of choice.
      (i) Erythromycin or ofloxacin can also be used.
ii. Complications
   1. Complications in males are rare, but include urethral strictures.
   2. In females, complications include pelvic inflammatory disease (PID), infertility, and ectopic pregnancy.

NEOPLASTIC DISEASES

I. Bladder carcinoma
   a. General
      i. Male-to-female ratio is 3:1.
      ii. Incidence increases with age, with the median age at diagnosis of 70 years.
      iii. Risk factors include smoking and occupational exposure to arylamine (dye, rubber, or leather workers).
   b. Clinical manifestations
      i. Present with painful hematuria, gross or microscopic.
         1. Blood remains throughout urination.
      ii. May have abdominal or flank pain.
      iii. Physical examination is typically normal.
   c. Diagnosis
      i. Flexible cystoscopy is the single most important test.
         1. Transurethral resection with cystoscopy and bladder biopsy
      ii. CT scan obtained to locate tumor and evaluate for metastatic disease.

NOTES

ANSWER **A** EXPLANATION: *Pyelonephritis presents with fever, chills, flank pain, urgency, dysuria, and frequency.*

correct ☐   incorrect ☐

 d. Treatment
  i. Transurethral resection for superficial disease.
   1. Flexible cystoscopy required every 3 months monitoring disease.
  ii. With muscle-invasive disease, radical cystoscopy with radiation or chemotherapy.

II. Prostate carcinoma
 a. General
  i. Most prostate cancers are adenocarcinoma.
  ii. Risk factors include advancing age, positive family history for prostate cancer, and African-American heritage.
  iii. No increased risk with benign prostatic hypertrophy.
 b. Clinical manifestations
  i. Patients with early-stage disease are typically asymptomatic.
  ii. Develop obstructive voiding symptoms as disease advances.
  iii. Can also develop hematuria with advanced disease.
  iv. Prostate nodule may be noted on digital rectal examination.
 c. Diagnosis
  i. Many cases diagnosed with elevated prostate-specific antigen testing.
   1. In patients with values greater than 4 ng/mL, biopsy should be done.
  ii. Diagnosis made on transrectal ultrasound with biopsy
 d. Treatment
  i. Treatment options include:
   1. Watchful waiting
   2. Androgen deprivation
   3. Radical prostatectomy
   4. Radiation therapy
  ii. Low- or intermediate-risk disease is treated with radical prostatectomy or local radiation therapy.

  iii. High-risk patients are treated with aggressive local therapy and androgen deprivation.
  iv. Patients with metastatic disease are treated with androgen deprivation after radical prostatectomy.

III. Renal cell carcinoma
 a. General
  i. Male-to-female ratio is 3:1, and incidence is highest in African Americans.
  ii. Most common cell type is clear cell.
  iii. Risk factors include obesity, hypertension, and smoking.
 b. Clinical manifestations
  i. Classic triad of flank pain, abdominal mass, and hematuria.
  ii. May also note weight loss, fatigue, and anorexia.
 c. Diagnosis
  i. Ultrasound and CT scan with biopsy needed for diagnosis.
  ii. Staging required to determine treatment and prognosis.
 d. Treatment
  i. Localized disease treated with surgical removal of tumor.
  ii. Immunomodulatory therapy with interleukin-2 effective in metastatic disease.
  iii. Poor response with radiation or chemotherapy.
  iv. Five-year survival rate is 60% to 70%.

IV. Testicular carcinoma
 a. General
  i. Primary age of onset is 15 to 35 years.
  ii. Increased risk with a history of cryptorchidism.
 b. Clinical manifestations
  i. Present with testicular pain or testicular mass.
  ii. With metastatic disease, can present with flank pain.
  iii. On physical examination, a testicular mass is noted.
 c. Diagnosis
  i. Testicular ultrasound to evaluate the mass.
  ii. Serum beta-HCG and/or alpha-fetoprotein levels are elevated.

NOTES

d. Treatment
    i. Orchiectomy with radiation therapy are used in stage 1 and II disease.
    ii. With metastatic disease, chemotherapy is added after surgery.
V. Wilms' tumor
  a. General
    i. Occurs most commonly between ages 2 and 5 years.
    ii. Frequently associated with other malformations and cytogenetic disorders.
  b. Clinical manifestations
    i. Present with increasing abdominal mass.
      1. Mass is smooth, firm, and well demarcated.
    ii. Microscopic hematuria is often noted, but gross hematuria is uncommon.
  c. Diagnosis
    i. Intrarenal mass noted on ultrasound or CT scan of the abdomen.
  d. Treatment
    i. Surgical resection of the tumor.
    ii. Chemotherapy is used in all cases.
    iii. Advanced cases also treated with radiation therapy.

RENAL DISEASES

I. Acute renal failure
  a. General
    i. Sudden reduction in kidney function.
      1. Defined as low glomerular filtration rate (GFR) and fall in urine output.
    ii. Causes of acute renal failure
      1. See Table 10-4.
  b. Clinical manifestations
    i. Symptoms develop with the development of uremia and its effects on other organ systems.
      1. Typically blood urea nitrogen (BUN) > 60 mg/dL or creatinine > 8 mg/dL.
      2. See Table 10-5.
    ii. Weight gain and edema are common.
  c. Diagnosis
    i. Typically first abnormality is elevated serum creatinine.
    ii. Microscopic examination of the urine may reveal cellular debris.

QUESTION

Which of the following increases the risk of developing testicular cancer?

  A. Benign prostatic hypertrophy
  B. Hydrocele
  C. Cystocele
  D. Cryptorchidism

---

    iii. Urine studies can be used to separate prerenal from renal.
      1. See Table 10-6.
    iv. Ultrasound of the kidney needed to rule out obstruction as possible etiology.
  d. Treatment
    i. Restore blood pressure and correct intravascular volume status.
    ii. Dialysis may be required until renal recovery.
    iii. In oliguric renal failure, a trial of loop diuretics may be tried to convert to nonoliguric failure.
    iv. Remove possible etiologic agents, such as drugs and obstruction.
II. Chronic renal failure
  a. General
    i. Slow, progressive decline in kidney function.
    ii. Creatinine clearance (CrCl) is a measure of GFR.
      1. Measurement
        (a) CrCl = {urine creatinine × volume (mL/min)/plasma creatinine}
      2. Estimated
        (a) CrCl = {(140 − sge) × weight (kg)/plasma creatinine × 72} × 0.85 (if female)
      3. Normal range
        (a) Male: 120 ± 25 mL/min
        (b) Female: 95 ± 20 mL/min
    iii. Categories
      1. Mild: GFR, 70–120 mL/min
      2. Moderate: GFR, 30–70 mL/min
      3. Severe: GFR < 30 mL/min
      4. End-stage renal disease: GFR < 10 mL/min

NOTES

ANSWER **D** EXPLANATION: *Testicular cancer risk increases with a history of cryptorchidism.*

correct ☐   incorrect ☐

5. Watch for acute exacerbations in chronic disease due to use of angiotensin-converting enzyme (ACE) inhibitors, aminoglycosides, and contrast media
6. See Table 10-7 for etiologies.
b. Clinical manifestations
   i. Symptoms develop with the development of uremia and its effects on other organ systems.
      1. Typically BUN > 60 mg/dL or creatinine > 8 mg/dL.

Table 10-5 • Symptoms of Uremia

Organ System	Symptoms
General	Fatigue and weakness
Skin	Pruritus and easy bruising
Pulmonary	Shortness of breath
Cardiovascular	Dyspnea on exertion, pericarditis
Gastrointestinal	Anorexia, nausea and vomiting
Genitourinary	Nocturia
Neurologic	Change in mental status

Table 10-4 • Causes of Acute Renal Failure

Prerenal	Renal	Postrenal
↓ Intravascular volume	Ischemic	Obstruction
Hemorrhage	Postoperative shock	Stones
Vomiting		Tumors
Diarrhea Burns		Benign prostatic hypertrophy
↑ Intravascular capacity Sepsis Vasodilators Anaphylaxis	Nephrotoxic Aminoglycosides Contrast agents	
Myocardial failure Myocardial infarction Pulmonary embolism Congestive heart failure Hepatorenal syndrome	Inflammatory Interstitial nephritis Acute glomerulonephritis Vasculitis Pregnancy related Eclampsia Abruptio placentae Renovascular disease Renal artery thrombosis	

NOTES

Table 10-6 • Urine Study Results in Acute Renal Failure

Test	Prerenal	Renal
Urine sodium	<20	>20
Urine to plasma creatinine ratio	>20	<20
Fractional sodium excretion	<1	>1

Table 10-7 • Causes of Chronic Renal Failure

Diabetes glomerulosclerosis

Hypertensive glomerulosclerosis

Glomerular disease
  Glomerulonephritis
  Systemic lupus erythematosus
  Wegener's granulomatosis

Tubulointerstitial disease
  Obstructive nephropathy
  Analgesic nephropathy
  Chronic pyelonephritis
  Myeloma kidney

Vascular disease
  Scleroderma
  Vasculitis

Cystic disease
  Polycystic kidney disease

    ii. Anemia due to decreased production of erythropoietin.
    iii. Renal osteodystrophy due to hyperparathyroidism.
      1. Increased risk for fracture and bone pain.
  c. Diagnosis
    i. Microscopic examination of the urine may reveal waxy casts.
    ii. Ultrasound of the kidney may reveal small or polycystic kidneys.

  d. Treatment
    i. Monitor progression of renal failure through measurement of serum creatinine.
    ii. Control blood pressure, blood glucose levels, and diet with protein restrictions, and avoid renal toxic drugs.
      1. ACE inhibitors slow progression of renal failure.
        (a) Monitor potassium level when starting ACE inhibitor.
    iii. Treat anemia with erythropoietin.
    iv. Calcium, vitamin D, and bicarbonate supplement to avoid bone disease.
      1. Also restrict dietary phosphate.
    v. Dialysis needed in end-stage renal disease.
      1. Kidney transplantation provides the most complete correction of end-stage disease.
    vi. Complications
      1. Hyperkalemia
      2. Acid–base disorders
      3. Hypertension
      4. Pericarditis
      5. Anemia
      6. Encephalopathy
      7. Renal osteodystrophy
III. Glomerulonephritis
  a. General
    i. Acute glomerulonephritis is an uncommon cause of acute renal failure.
    ii. Due to immune complex deposits in the kidney.
    iii. Etiologies include:
      1. Immunoglobulin A (IgA) nephropathy (Berger's disease)
      2. Postinfectious glomerulonephritis

NOTES

ANSWER B EXPLANATION: *Stress incontinence can be caused by activities that increase intra-abdominal pressure, such as coughing or lifting.*

correct ☐   incorrect ☐

3. Lupus nephritis
4. Pauci-immune glomerulonephritis
   (a) Wegener's granulomatosis
5. Goodpasture's syndrome
6. See Table 10-8 for summary.
b. Clinical manifestations
   i. Edema is noted in periorbital and scrotal regions.
   ii. Hypertension may be present.
c. Diagnosis
   i. Serologic markers
      1. Antineutrophilic cytoplasmic autoantibodies (ANCAs)
      2. Anti–glomerular basement membrane autoantibodies (anti-GMBs)
      ii. Urinalysis
         1. Dysmorphic red blood cells and red blood cell casts are common.
         2. Proteinuria is also noted.
      iii. Biopsy
   d. Treatment
      i. Correction of hypertension and fluid overload.
      ii. Corticosteroids and cytotoxic agents may be needed.
IV. Nephrotic syndrome
   a. General
      i. Seen in patients with systemic renal disease; diabetes mellitus, amyloidosis, or systemic lupus erythematosus (SLE); or idiopathic nephrotic syndrome.
      ii. Urine protein excretion greater than 3.5 g per 24 hours.
   b. Clinical manifestations
      i. Peripheral edema is the classic finding.
      ii. May note dyspnea due to pulmonary edema or abdominal fullness due to ascites.

Table 10-8 • Summary of Glomerulonephritis

Disease	Signs and Symptoms	Serologic Markers	Treatment	Notes
Poststreptococcal glomerulonephritis	Oliguric Edema	High ASO titer	Supportive	Occurs after pharyngitis and impetigo
IgA nephropathy	Gross hematuria	Elevated IgA levels	Corticosteroids	Associated with URI or flulike illness
Wegener's granulomatosis	Fever, malaise, weight loss	ANCA positive	Corticosteroids Cyclophosphamide	Respiratory tract symptoms common
Goodpasture's syndrome	Hemoptysis	Anti-GMB positive	Plasma exchange Steroids	
Lupus nephritis		ANA positive	Steroids	

ANA, antinuclear antibody; ANCA, antineutrophil cytoplasmic antibody; ASO, antistreptolysin O; GMB, anti–glomerular basement membrane autoantibodies; URI, upper respiratory infection.

NOTES

c. Diagnosis
  i. Urinalysis reveals proteinuria with little or no cellular elements noted on microscopic exam.
  ii. Serum albumin is decreased along with total protein.
  iii. As proteinuria increases, the frequency of hyperlipidemia increases.
  iv. Renal biopsy needed to classify disease.
d. Treatment
  i. Protein restriction to limit adverse effects on renal function.
  ii. Salt restriction to manage edema.
  iii. Treatment of hyperlipidemia with medications and dietary management.
  iv. Steroids needed in minimal change disease, focal segmental glomerular sclerosis, and membranous nephropathy.
  v. In diabetic nephropathy, the rate of progression of disease can be controlled by strict glycemic control.
V. Polycystic kidney disease
  a. General
    i. One of the more common hereditary disorders.
    ii. A history of urinary tract infection (UTI) and nephrolithiasis is common.
    iii. Family history is positive.
  b. Clinical manifestations
    i. Present with abdominal or flank pain and hematuria, microscopic or gross.
    ii. Hypertension is common.
    iii. On physical examination, kidneys may be palpable.
  c. Diagnosis
    i. Ultrasound of the kidney reveals more than five cysts.
    ii. Cysts also noted on CT scan.
  d. Treatment
    i. Aggressive treatment of hypertension.
    ii. Bed rest and analgesics for pain and hematuria.

ELECTROLYTE AND ACID–BASE DISORDERS

I. Hyponatremia
  a. General
    i. Defined as a serum sodium less than 130 mEq/L.

Which of the following is indicated by the presence of broad waxy casts on urinalysis?

  A. Acute glomerulonephritis
  B. Urinary tract infection
  C. Nephrotic syndrome
  D. Chronic renal failure

b. Clinical manifestations
  i. Most patients are asymptomatic.
  ii. May present with lethargy, weakness, confusion, and seizures.
c. Diagnosis
  i. Begins with serum osmolality and volume status.
  ii. Urine sodium levels needed in patients with low osmolality and hypovolemia.
  iii. See Figure 10-2.
d. Treatment
  i. Symptomatic patient
    1. Usually seen in patients with sodium < 120 mEq/L.
    2. Increase sodium by only 1 to 2 mEq/L/hour to decrease risk for demyelination of central nervous system (CNS).
    3. Treat with saline plus furosemide.
  ii. Asymptomatic patient
    1. Correct sodium at rate of 0.5 mEq/L/hour.
    2. Water restriction to about 1 L/day.
    3. Normal saline with furosemide.
    4. Demeclocycline may used, inhibits effects of antidiuretic hormone (ADH) on distal tubule.
      (a) May require a week to see onset of action.
II. Hypernatremia
  a. General
    i. An intact thirst mechanism typically prevents hypernatremia.
      1. Excess water loss will only cause hypernatremia when appropriate water intake is not possible.
      2. Etiologies
        (a) Dehydration

NOTES

ANSWER **D** EXPLANATION: *Urinalysis of the patient with chronic renal failure may reveal the presence of broad waxy casts.*

correct ☐   incorrect ☐

(b) Lactulose
(c) Mannitol therapy
(d) Diabetes insipidus
(e) Excessive sodium intake
(f) Primary aldosteronism

b. Clinical manifestations
  i. Orthostatic hypotension and oliguria are typical.,
  ii. Mental status changes such as delirium and coma are seen in severe hypernatremia.
c. Diagnosis
  i. If urine osmolality > 400 mOsm/kg, then renal water-conserving ability is intact.
    1. Due to nonrenal loses (sweating, diarrhea) or renal loses.
  ii. If urine osmolality < 250 KG/kg, then consider diabetes insipidus.
d. Treatment

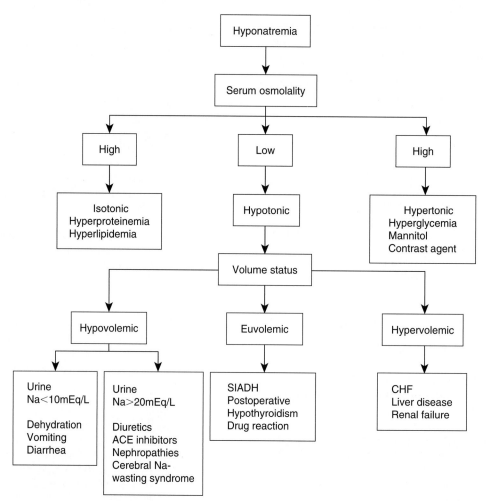

Figure 10-2 Diagnosis of hyponatremia. CHF, congestive heart failure; SIADH, syndrome of inappropriate antidiuretic hormone.

NOTES

i. Treat the underlying cause and replacement of water.
ii. Correct slowly to reduce risk for cerebral edema and neurologic impairment.
    1. Decrease sodium by 1 mEq/L/hour.
III. Hypokalemia
  a. General
    i. Normal range is 3.5 to 5.5 mEq/L.
    ii. Etiology
       1. Trauma
       2. Increased aldosterone
       3. Diuretics
       4. Hypomagnesemia
       5. Renal tubular acidosis
       6. Extrarenal loss—diarrhea, vomiting, laxative abuse
  b. Clinical manifestations
    i. In mild to moderate disease, note muscle weakness, fatigue, and muscle cramps.
    ii. In severe disease, note flaccid paralysis, hyporeflexia, tetany, and rhabdomyolysis.
  c. Diagnosis
    i. Labs reveal potassium < 3.5 mEq/L.
    ii. On electrocardiogram (EKG), note decreasing size and broadening of T waves.
       1. Increased digitalis toxicity in hypokalemia.
  d. Treatment
    i. Oral potassium supplement for mild to moderate deficiency.
    ii. IV potassium for severe deficiency.
    iii. Concurrent deficiency in magnesium may make potassium correction more difficult.
IV. Hyperkalemia
  a. General
    i. Typically associated with acidosis.
    ii. Etiologies:
       1. Hemolysis of red blood cells
       2. Thrombocytosis or leukocytosis
       3. Renal failure
       4. Drugs: heparin, spironolactone, ACE inhibitors, nonsteroidal anti-inflammatory drugs (NSAIDs)
       5. Burns
       6. Metabolic acidosis: diabetic ketoacidosis (DKA), lactic acid
       7. Excessive intake
  b. Clinical manifestations

    i. May produce muscle weakness and flaccid paralysis, abdominal distention, and diarrhea.
  c. Diagnosis
    i. Labs reveal potassium > 5.5 mEq/L.
    ii. On EKG, note peaked T waves and widening QRS.
  d. Treatment
    i. Severe hyperkalemia
       1. Concern about cardiac toxicity and EKG changes.
       2. Treatment consists of distributing potassium back into the cells via albuterol, insulin, or bicarbonate.
    ii. Nonemergent hyperkalemia
       1. Withhold potassium and give cation exchange resins.
          (a) Sodium polystyrene, ion exchange resin, can be given orally or rectally.
       2. Loop diuretics and dialysis can also be used to decrease potassium.
V. Hypocalcemia
  a. General
    i. Etiologies include:
       1. Malabsorption
       2. Vitamin D deficiency
       3. Alcoholism
       4. Diuretic therapy
       5. Hypoparathyroidism
       6. Renal failure
       7. Drugs: aminoglycosides
  b. Clinical manifestations
    i. May produce muscle spasm, tetany, seizures, and arrhythmias.
    ii. Positive Chvostek's and Trousseau's signs.

NOTES

ANSWER B EXPLANATION: *Laboratory features of nephrotic syndrome include proteinuria, hypoalbuminemia, and hyperlipidemia.*

correct ☐   incorrect ☐

c. Diagnosis
  i. On EKG, note prolonged QT interval.
  ii. Calcium level < 9.0 mg/dL.
d. Treatment
  i. Severe deficiency calcium gluconate is given IV.
  ii. In asymptomatic cases, oral calcium with vitamin D supplements is indicated.

VI. Hypercalcemia
  a. General
    i. Etiologies include:
      1. Primary hyperparathyroidism
      2. Neoplastic disease
      3. Thiazide diuretics
      4. Sarcoidosis
  b. Clinical manifestations
    i. Major symptoms include constipation and polyuria.
    ii. In severe hypercalcemia, may note stupor, coma, and azotemia.
  c. Diagnosis
    i. Symptoms occur with levels > 12 mg/dL.
    ii. EKG reveals shortened QT interval.
  d. Treatment
    i. Treat underlying cause.
    ii. Saline with furosemide is emergency treatment of choice.
    iii. In malignancy, bisphosphonates are safe and effective.

VII. Hypomagnesemia
  a. General
    i. Most of the body's magnesium is in the skeleton and soft tissue.
    ii. Most magnesium comes from green leafy vegetables.
    iii. Results from decreased intestinal absorption or increased losses in urine or stool.
      1. See Table 10-9 for etiologies.
  b. Clinical manifestations

Table 10-9 • Causes of Hypomagnesemia

Gastrointestinal
  Malabsorption
  Severe diarrhea
  Small bowel resection

Renal
  Bartter's syndrome
  Postobstructive diuresis
  Volume expansion
  Diabetic ketoacidosis
  Diuretics

Body Fluid Loss
  Burns

Other
  Alcoholism
  Thyrotoxicosis

    i. Symptoms include weakness, anorexia, cardiac arrhythmias, tetany, and seizures.
    ii. Hypokalemia often accompanies hypomagnesemia.
  c. Diagnosis
    i. Serum magnesium levels are less than 1.6 mEq/L.
  d. Treatment
    i. Mild or moderate deficiency treated with oral magnesium oxide or chloride supplement.
    ii. Severe disease treated with IV magnesium sulfate.

VIII. Acid–Base Disorders
  a. General
    i. Normal Ranges
      1. See Table 10-10.
    ii. Interpretation
      1. Acidosis versus alkalosis
        (a) If pH is less than 7.35, the patient is acidemic.
        (b) If pH is greater than 7.45, the patient is alkalemic.
      2. Determine primary process
        (a) After evaluating pH, look at P_{CO_2} and bicarbonate.

NOTES

Table 10-10 • Normal Ranges	
Test	Normal Range
pH	7.35–7.45
P_{CO_2}	35–45 mmHg
Bicarbonate	22–26 mmol/L
Sodium	135–145 mEq/L
Potassium	3.5–5.0 mEq/L
Chloride	98–108 mmol/L
P_{O_2}	80–100 mmHg

QUESTION

Chvostek's sign is seen in which of the following electrolyte disorders?

A. Hypokalemia
B. Hypocalcemia
C. Hypomagnesemia
D. Hyponatremia

(i) If pH is acidemic and P_{CO_2} is greater than 45 mmHg, the primary process is respiratory; if bicarbonate is less than 22, the primary process is metabolic.

(ii) If pH is alkalemic and the P_{CO_2} is less than 35 mmHg, the primary process is respiratory; if bicarbonate is greater than 26, the primary process is metabolic.

(b) See Table 10-11.

3. Anion gap
  (a) Difference between the major cations and anions.

(b) If elevated, suspect presence of excess organic acids or acidic foreign substances.
(c) Calculation
  (i) Anion gap = $Na^+ - (Cl^- + HCO_3^-)$
(d) Normal range is 10 to 14 mEq/L.
(e) Used to separate out different causes of metabolic acidosis.

b. Disorders
  i. Metabolic acidosis
    1. Etiology
      (a) Separated based on anion gap.
      (b) See Table 10-12.

Table 10-11 • Primary Acid–Base Disorders			
Test	Primary Disorder	Normal Range	Primary Disorder
pH	Acidemia	←7.35 to 7.45→	Alkalemia
P_{CO_2}	Respiratory acidosis	← 35 to 45 →	Respiratory alkalosis
Bicarbonate	Metabolic acidosis	← 22 to 26 →	Metabolic alkalosis

Table 10-12 • Etiology of Metabolic Acidosis	
Normal Anion Gap	Elevated Anion Gap
Gastrointestinal bicarbonate loss (diarrhea, ureteral diversions)	Lactic acidosis
Renal tubular acidosis	Diabetic ketoacidosis
Early renal failure	Uremia
Carbonic anhydrase inhibitors	Ethylene glycol intoxication
Posthypocapnia	Methanol ingestion
Hydrochloric acid administration	Salicylate intoxication

ANSWER **B** EXPLANATION: *Positive Chvostek's and Trousseau's signs are noted in hypocalcemia.*

correct ☐   incorrect ☐

2. Clinical manifestations
   (a) Dyspnea on exertion and nausea and vomiting are common.
   (b) On physical examination, labored deep respirations with use of accessory muscles may be noted.
ii. Metabolic alkalosis
   1. Etiology
      (a) Causes separated based on urine chloride.
      (b) See Table 10-13.
   2. Clinical manifestations
      (a) CNS symptoms such as confusion, obtundation, delirium, and coma can be noted.
      (b) Cardiac arrhythmias and hypotension can also be noted.
iii. Respiratory acidosis
   1. Etiology
      (a) Can be acute or chronic respiratory acidosis.
      (b) See Table 10-14.
   2. Clinical manifestations
      (a) Related to degree and duration of acidosis and presence of hypoxia.

Table 10-13 • Etiology of Metabolic Alkalosis

Low Urine Chloride	Normal or High Urine Chloride
Vomiting or nasogastric suctioning	Cushing's syndrome
Diuretic use in past	Conn's syndrome
Posthypercapnia	Exogenous steroids Bartter's syndrome Current or recent diuretic use

Table 10-14 • Etiology of Respiratory Acidosis

Acute	Chronic
Central nervous system depression (drugs, CNS event)	Chronic lung disease
Neuromuscular disorders	Chronic neuromuscular disease
Acute airway obstruction	Chronic respiratory center depression
Severe pneumonia or pulmonary edema Hemothorax, pneumothorax Ventilator dysfunction	

   (b) In acute disease, CNS symptoms such as confusion, anxiety, psychosis, and seizures may be noted.
   (c) In chronic disease, note lethargy, fatigue, and confusion.
iv. Respiratory alkalosis
   1. Etiology
      (a) Anxiety
      (b) Hypoxia
      (c) CNS disease
      (d) Drug use—salicylates
      (e) Pregnancy
      (f) Sepsis
      (g) Hepatic encephalopathy
      (h) Mechanical ventilation
   2. Clinical manifestations
      (a) May cause dizziness, perioral paresthesias, confusion, hypotension, seizures, and coma.
IX. Volume depletion
   a. General
      i. Defined as reduced total body water.
      ii. Occurs when the rate of salt and water intake is less than the combined rates of renal and extrarenal losses
      iii. Etiologies grouped into decreased fluid intake or increased fluid loss.

NOTES

1. Increased loss grouped into renal or extrarenal causes.
2. See Table 10-15.
b. Clinical manifestations
   i. Signs and symptoms vary with degree of depletion.
   ii. Orthostatic hypotension and tachycardia are common.
   iii. On physical examination, decreased skin turgor and dry mucous membranes.

QUESTION

Which of the following acid base abnormalities will develop in a patient with recurrent vomiting of gastric contents?

   A. Respiratory acidosis
   B. Respiratory alkalosis
   C. Metabolic acidosis
   D. Metabolic alkalosis

Table 10-15 • Causes of Volume Depletion.

Renal Losses	Extrarenal Losses

Hormonal deficit
  Primary diabetes insipidus
  Aldosterone insufficiency
	Hemorrhage
	Sweating and burns
	Vomiting

Renal deficit
  Renal tubular acidosis
  Bartter's syndrome
  Secondary diabetes insipidus
  Diuretic abuse
  Osmotic diuresis
  Chronic renal failure
  Interstitial nephritis
	Diarrhea
	Tube drainage

c. Diagnosis
   i. Orthostatic hypotension, with a 10-mmHg drop in diastolic pressure.
   ii. Positive response to a fluid challenge.
d. Treatment
   i. Fluid replacement with sodium-containing fluids.
   ii. Most potent fluid replacement substance is blood.
     1. Used typically in cases of hemorrhage.
X. Volume excess
  a. General
   i. Increase in total body water.
   ii. Occurs when rate of salt and water intake exceeds renal and extrarenal losses.
     1. See Table 10-16.

Table 10-16 • Causes of Volume Excess

Reduced Effective Circulating Volume	Primary Hormone Excess	Primary Renal Sodium Retention

Systemic increase in venous pressure
  Right-sided heart failure
  Constrictive pericarditis
	Primary aldosteronism	Renal failure

Local increase in venous pressure
  Left-sided heart failure
  Vena cava obstruction
	Cushing's syndrome	

Reduced oncotic pressure
  Nephrotic syndrome
  Hypoalbuminemia
	Syndrome of inappropriate antidiuretic hormone	

Cirrhosis		

NOTES

ANSWER **D** EXPLANATION: *Metabolic alkalosis is caused by vomiting, diuretic use, Cushing's syndrome, Conn syndrome, and exogenous steroids.*

correct ☐   incorrect ☐

b. Clinical manifestations
  i. Symptoms related to cause of volume excess.

Table 10-17 • Diuretics

Diuretic	Primary Effect	Side Effects
I) Proximal diuretic		
Acetazolamide	↓ Na+/H+ exchange	Hypokalemic, hyperchloremic acidosis
II) Loop diuretic		
Furosemide	↓ Na+/K+ : 2Cl− absorption	Hypokalemic alkalosis
Bumetanide		Hearing deficits
III) Early distal diuretic		
Thiazide	↓ NaCl absorption	Hypokalemic alkalosis
		Hyperglycemia
IV) Late distal diuretic		
Spironolactone	↓ Na+ absorption	Hyperkalemic acidosis
Triamterene		

Table 10-18 • Common Findings on Urinalysis

Test	Disease State
Specific gravity	Kidney function test
Protein	Functional—severe muscle exertion, pregnancy Organic—fever, hypertension, glomerulonephritis, nephrotic syndrome, infection
Glucose	Diabetes mellitus
Ketones	Diabetic ketoacidosis, starvation
Blood	Stones, infection, tumor, tuberculosis, glomerulonephritis
Nitrite	Infection
Leukocyte esterase	Infection
Microscopic	
Red blood cells	Stones, infection, tumor, tuberculosis, glomerulonephritis
White blood cells	Infection
Casts	
Red blood cell cast	Acute glomerulonephritis
White blood cell cast	Pyelonephritis
Waxy cast	Renal failure

  ii. Cases due to reduced effective circulating volume will have edema.
 c. Diagnosis
  i. Varies with underlying cause.
 d. Treatment
  i. Diuretics are the treatment of choice.
   1. See Table 10-17.
XI. Urinalysis
 a. Common findings on urinalysis.
  i. See Table 10-18.

NOTES

Question 1

Which of the following is the most common symptom of bladder cancer?

   A. Incontinence

   B. Urinary retention

   C. Hematuria

   D. Dysuria

Question 2

Which of the following is the first step in the evaluation of the patient with an increasing serum creatinine?

   A. Intravenous pyelogram

   B. Abdominal CT scan

   C. Renal ultrasound

   D. Abdominal x-ray (KUB)

Question 3

A 20-year-old presents with gradual onset of scrotal pain and swelling. The patient's temperature is 38.3 degrees C. Urinalysis reveals many white blood cells and bacteria. Which of the following is the most likely diagnosis?

   A. Testicular torsion

   B. Inguinal hernia

   C. Epididymitis

   D. Prostatitis

Question 4

A 35-year-old patient presents with nausea, hematuria, and right flank pain with radiation to the right testicle. Urinalysis reveals 50-100 red blood cells, 0-1 white blood cells, and many calcium oxalate crystals. Which of the following is the most appropriate clinical intervention?

   A. Hemiacidrin (Renacidin)

   B. IV antibiotics

   C. Extracorporeal lithotripsy and thiazide diuretics

   D. Support care with fluids and pain medications

Question 5

A 25-year-old male presents with fever and dysuria. On physical examination the prostate is very tender, enlarged, and indurated. Urinalysis reveals many white blood cells. Which of the following would be the best treatment option for this patient?

   A. Finasteride (Proscar)

   B. Ibuprofen (Motrin)

   C. Ciprofloxacin (Cipro)

   D. Phenazopyridine (Pyridium)

Question 6

How frequent should a patient perform a self-testicular examination to screen for testicular cancer?

   A. Weekly

   B. Monthly

   C. Bi-annually

   D. Yearly

NOTES

Question 7

A patient presents with the following labs:

Sodium-138 mEq/L   Glucose-230 mg/dl
Potassium-5.2 mEq/L   Creatinine-1.4 mg/dl
Chloride-100 mEq/L   BUN-45 mg/dl
Bicarb-13 mmol/L

What is the anion gap for this patient?

    A. 20
    B. 25
    C. 35
    D. 40

Answer 1

ANSWER **C** EXPLANATION: *Bladder cancer is typically noted in males with a median age of 70 years. Typical presentation is painful hematuria and possible abdominal or flank pain.*

Topic: Bladder carcinoma

correct ☐   incorrect ☐

Answer 2

ANSWER **C** EXPLANATION: *Elevation of serum creatinine may be the first findings of acute renal failure. Renal ultrasound and avoidance of renal toxic medications is the first step in the evaluation of these patients.*

Topic: Acute renal failure

correct ☐   incorrect ☐

Answer 3

ANSWER **C** EXPLANATION: *Epididymitis typically presents with fever, scrotal swelling and symptoms of urethritis. Urinalysis reveals increase number of white blood cells and bacteria.*

Topic: Epididymitis

correct ☐   incorrect ☐

Answer 4

ANSWER **D** EXPLANATION: *Nephrolithiasis presents with colicky, flank pain radiating to the testes or labia. Hematuria is common. Treatment of acute disease consists of support care with IV fluids and pain control.*

Topic: Nephrolithiasis

correct ☐   incorrect ☐

Answer 5

ANSWER **C** EXPLANATION: *Acute prostatitis presents with fever, chills, and dysuria. On physical examination the prostate is very tender. Urinalysis reveals many white blood cells. Treatment consists of antibiotics, such as fluoroquinolones, such as ciprofloxacin, or trimethoprim-sulfamethoxazole.*

Topic: Prostatitis

correct ☐   incorrect ☐

NOTES

Answer 6

ANSWER **B** EXPLANATION: *Testicular cancer screening, with self testicular examination, should be completed each month.*

Topic: Testicular carcinoma

correct ☐   **incorrect** ☐

Answer 7

ANSWER **B** EXPLANATION: *Anion gap is calculated by adding the serum chloride and bicarbonate and then subtracting this total from the serum sodium. Normal anion gap is 10-14 mEq/L.*

Topic: Acid-base disorders

correct ☐   **incorrect** ☐

NOTES

Dermatologic System

11

EXAM BLUEPRINT TOPICS

Eczematous Eruptions
Dermatitis
- Atopic
- Contact
- Diaper
- Nummular eczematous
- Perioral
- Seborrheic
- Statis

Dyshidrosis
Lichen simplex chronicus

Papulosquamous Diseases
Dermatophyte infections
- Tinea versicolor
- Tinea corporis/pedis

Drug eruptions
Lichen planus
Pityriasis rosea
Psoriasis

Desquamation
Stevens-Johnson syndrome
Toxic epidermal necrolysis
Erythema multiforme

Vesicular Bullae
Bullous pemphigoid

Acneiform Lesions
Acne vulgaris
Rosacea
Folliculitis

Verrucous Lesions
Seborrheic keratosis
Actinic keratosis

Insects/Parasites
Lice
Scabies
Spider bites

Neoplasms
Basal cell carcinoma
Melanoma
Squamous cell carcinoma

Hair and Nails
Alopecia areata
Androgenetic alopecia
Onychomycosis
Paronychia

Viral Diseases
Condyloma acuminatum (venereal warts)
Herpes simplex
Herpes zoster (shingles)
Molluscum contagiosum
Verrucae (warts)

Bacterial Infections
Cellulitis
Erysipelas
Impetigo

Other
Acanthosis nigricans
Burns
Decubitus ulcers
Hidradenitis suppurativa
Lipomas
Melasma
Urticaria (hives)
Vitiligo
Medications

ECZEMATOUS ERUPTIONS

I. Dermatitis
  a. Atopic
    i. General
      1. Pruritic inflammation of the dermis and epidermis.

NOTES

2. Often associated with a personal or family history of hay fever, asthma, allergic rhinitis, or atopic dermatitis.
   (a) 35% of infants with atopic dermatitis will develop asthma later in life.
3. Onset typically during the first few months of life.
4. Mechanism of disease is an immunoglobulin E (IgE)-mediated process.

ii. Clinical manifestations
1. In adults, a papulosquamous patchy rash is noted in the flexural regions.
2. In children, the rash is papulovesicular and affects the face and extensor surfaces.
3. The major complaint in both adults and children is pruritus and dry skin.
   (a) Triggered by contact with dust mites, pollens, detergents, soaps, sweating, stress, and scratching.
4. White dermatographism, stroking of involved skin leads to blanching, is noted in atopic dermatitis.

iii. Diagnosis
1. Based on history and clinical findings.
2. In infants, must separate atopic dermatitis from seborrheic dermatitis.
   (a) See Table 11-1.

iv. Treatment
1. Educate patients to avoid scratching and triggers.
2. Decrease pruritus with hydroxyzine and oral antihistamines.

3. Hydration of skin with hydrated petrolatum, Eucerin cream, or Lac-Hydrin.
4. Topical steroids are used to decrease inflammation.
   (a) Side effects include skin atrophy and osteoporosis.
   (b) See Table 11-9, later, for list of topical steroids.
5. Skin infections, with *Staphylococcus aureus*, are common and may require treatment with oral antibiotics, such as erythromycin, dicloxacillin, or cephalosporins.

b. Contact
   i. General
   1. Inflammatory skin reaction of the dermis and epidermis to an external agent or toxin.
      (a) If the agent directly damages the skin, it is irritant contact dermatitis.
      (b) If reaction is immunologic in nature, it is allergic contact dermatitis.
      (c) See Table 11-2.
   2. Allergic contact dermatitis is due to a delayed, cell-mediated hypersensitivity reaction.
   ii. Clinical manifestations
   1. History of exposure to irritant is major finding.
      (a) Exposures may be occupational or hobbies.

Table 11-1 • Comparison of Atopic Dermatitis and Seborrheic Dermatitis		
	Atopic Dermatitis	**Seborrheic Dermatitis**
Pruritus	Yes	No
Duration	Chronic	About 6 weeks
Family history	Positive for atopy	Negative family history
Location	Face, extensor surfaces	Axilla, diaper area

NOTES

Table 11-2 • Common Irritants and Allergens	
Irritants	**Allergens**
Soaps/detergents	Nickel
Industrial solvents	Neomycin
Plants	Fragrance
Fiberglass	Thimerosal
Wool	Formaldehyde
Cement	Plants (poison ivy/oak)
Ethylene oxide	Bacitracin

2. Irritant contact dermatitis patients will complain of burning and itching within minutes after exposure.
   (a) Skin may turn red, become edematous, and have serous fluid drainage.
3. Acute allergic contact dermatitis has sharply demarcated areas, edema, and vesicular lesions.
   (a) These lesions are frequently linear if due to plant exposure (poison ivy).
   (i) See Color Plate 3.
4. Chronic contact dermatitis can lead to dry, thick skin with lichenification.
   iii. Diagnosis
   1. Based on history and clinical findings.
   iv. Treatment
   1. Most important is removal of the irritant.
   2. Topical or systemic steroids may be needed.
      (a) See Table 11-8, later, for list of oral steroids and potency.
   3. Supportive measures include cool compresses or oatmeal baths.
c. Diaper
   i. General
   1. Includes a large group of conditions causing red, scaly rashes in the diaper region.

2. Decrease incidence with frequent diaper changes.
3. Can be due to an irritant or *Candida*.
ii. Clinical manifestations
   1. Irritant diaper dermatitis presents with red, scaly, eroded, painful plaques.
      (a) The creases are spared.
   2. *Candida* diaper dermatitis presents with bright, beefy red plaques in the inguinal or gluteal folds.
      (a) Satellite pustules are common.
iii. Diagnosis
   1. Based on history and clinical findings.
   2. Potassium hydroxide examination will reveal pseudohyphae and spores if due to *Candida*.
iv. Treatment
   1. Treatment should be directed at decreasing wetness.
   2. Barrier ointments can be used for prophylaxis.
   3. 1% Hydrocortisone can be used until inflammation is improved.
      (a) High-potency steroids should be avoided in the diaper area.
      (b) Pimecrolimus and tacrolimus, steroid-free anti-inflammatory agents, can also be used.
   4. *Candida* infections can be treated with miconazole, clotrimazole, ketoconazole, or oxiconazole.
d. Nummular eczematous
   i. General
   1. Chronic, pruritic, inflammatory dermatitis.
   2. Occur in young adulthood and old age.
   3. Common on lower legs and trunk.
ii. Clinical manifestations
   1. Present with coin-shaped plaques (4–5 cm in diameter) composed of small papules and vesicles on an erythematous base.
   2. Very pruritic.
iii. Diagnosis
   1. Based on history and clinical findings.
iv. Treatment
   1. Skin hydration with hydrated petrolatum or moisturizing cream.
   2. Topical steroids and crude coal tar may be helpful.

NOTES

e. Perioral
  i. General
    1. Occurs mainly in young women, 16 to 45 years of age.
  ii. Clinical manifestations
    1. Present with irregularly grouped, discrete erythematous papulopustules on an erythematous base.
    2. Initially perioral and last weeks to months.
      (a) Sparing of the vermilion border is noted.
  iii. Diagnosis
    1. Based on history and clinical findings.
  iv. Treatment
    1. Topical steroids should be avoided.
    2. Antibiotics are the mainstay of therapy.
      (a) Topical antibiotics include metronidazole and erythromycin.
      (b) Systemic antibiotics include minocycline, doxycycline, or tetracycline.
f. Seborrheic
  i. General
    1. A common, chronic, inflammatory papulosquamous disease.
    2. All ages are affected.
    3. Seborrheic dermatitis, diarrhea, and failure to thrive in infants are associated with a number of immunodeficiency states.
  ii. Clinical manifestations
    1. Papules are moist, transparent to pinkish orange, greasy, and scaling, with sharp margins.
    2. More common in areas with numerous sebaceous glands, such as the scalp margins, central face, and presternal area.
      (a) Classic locations include the eyebrows, base of eyelashes, nasolabial folds, and external ear canal.
    3. May itch, mainly when it involves the scalp.
    4. Cradle cap is yellow, greasy adherent scales on the vertex of the scalp in infants.
  iii. Diagnosis
    1. Based on history and clinical findings.
  iv. Treatment
    1. Daily shampooing with dandruff shampoos.
      (a) Shampoos should contain selenium sulfide or zinc pyrithione.
    2. Hydrocortisone 1% to decrease itching and redness.
    3. Topical antifungals, such as ketoconazole or ciclopirox, can be helpful in mild to moderate cases.
    4. If no response in infants think about possible zinc deficiency.
g. Stasis
  i. General
    1. Eczematous dermatitis of the legs, associated with edema, varicose veins, and hyperpigmentation.
    2. A chronic problem with relapses common.
    3. Most common on the lower legs.
  ii. Clinical manifestations
    1. Often, a history of deep vein thrombosis (DVT), surgery, or ulceration.
    2. The skin is dry, fissured, and erythematous.
    3. Pruritus, edema, and brown discoloration of the skin are common.
  iii. Diagnosis
    1. Based on history and clinical findings.
  iv. Treatment
    1. Elevation and compression of the legs will decrease edema and stasis.
    2. Cool water dressings for acute exudative inflammation.
    3. Topical or oral steroids may be required.
    4. Lubrication with bland emollients can help with dryness.
    5. Oral antihistamines may be needed for pruritus.
II. Dyshidrosis
  a. General
    i. Also called pompholyx.
    ii. Chronic, relapsing disease of unknown etiology.
  b. Clinical manifestations
    i. Presents with highly pruritic, symmetric vesicles on the palms, lateral fingers, or plantar surface of the feet.

NOTES

ii. Vesicles are 1 to 5 mm in diameter, monomorphic, deep seated, and filled with clear tapioca-like fluid.

iii. Resolve slowly over 1 to 3 weeks, leaving a red, cracked base with brown spots.

c. Diagnosis

i. Based on history and clinical findings.

d. Treatment

i. Wet dressings, with Burrow's solution, are the initial treatment.

ii. Medium or high-potency topical steroids are alternated with the wet dressings.

iii. Oral steroids may be needed in severe cases.

III. Lichen simplex chronicus

a. General

i. A localized form of lichenification, circumscribed plaques, that results from repeated rubbing and scratching.

ii. Frequently involves the wrist, ankles, anogenital skin, and back of the neck.

iii. More common in adults and can last for decades.

b. Clinical manifestations

i. Skin examination reveals sharply demarcated deeply violet-colored or red scaly plaques with thick skin lines (lichenification).

c. Diagnosis

i. Based on history and clinical findings.

ii. Must rule out tinea infection.

d. Treatment

i. Rubbing and scratching must be stopped. Occlusive dressings may be needed at night.

ii. Water soaks followed by medium- to high-potency topical steroids.

1. Low-potency steroids should be used on the face and genitals.

PAPULOSQUAMOUS DISEASES

I. Dermatophyte infections

a. Tinea versicolor

i. General

1. Infection caused by the yeast, *Pityrosporum orbiculare.*

(a) Part of normal skin flora.

QUESTION

After cleaning the backyard a patient notes severe itching and linear vesicular lesions. Which of the following is the most likely diagnosis?

A. Dyshidrosis

B. Nummular eczema

C. Contact dermatitis

D. Lichen simplex chronicus

---

2. Increased risk for infection with excess heat and humidity and oily skin.

ii. Clinical manifestations

1. Present with many small, circular, white, scaling papules on the upper trunk.

iii. Diagnosis

1. Based on history and clinical findings.

2. Potassium hydroxide examination of the scales reveals hyphae and round spores, a "spaghetti and meatballs" pattern.

iv. Treatment

1. Topical treatments include:

(a) Selenium sulfide lotion

(b) Ketoconazole shampoo

(c) Zinc pyrithione soap

(d) Miconazole, clotrimazole, or econazole

2. Oral antifungals may also be helpful.

b. Tinea corporis

i. General

1. Dermatophyte infection of the body.

(a) Dermatophytes infect and survive only in dead keratin (stratum corneum, hair, and nails).

2. More common in warm climates and epidemics occur among wrestlers.

3. There are three dermatophytes.

(a) *Microsporum*

(b) *Trichophyton*

(c) *Epidermophyton*

ii. Clinical manifestation

1. Two patterns

(a) Round annular lesions (ringworm)

(i) Begin as flat, scaly papules that slowly develop a raised border.

NOTES

(ii) Central area becomes brown or hypopigmented.
(iii) Extend in all directions.
(b) Deep inflammatory lesions
(i) Round, inflamed, elevated lesion with a red, boggy, pustular surface.
(ii) Due to infection into the hair follicle.
iii. Diagnosis
1. Potassium hydroxide examination reveals hyphae.
2. Culture may be needed to identify organism.
iv. Treatment
1. Antifungal cream for at least 1 week after resolution of the infection.
2. Oral antifungals may be needed.
(a) Griseofulvin
(b) Itraconazole
(c) Terbinafine
(d) Fluconazole
c. Tinea pedis
i. General
1. The most common area infected by dermatophytes.
2. Also known as *athlete's foot.*
3. Common in young and middle-aged adults.
4. More common in males than females.
5. Predisposing factors include shoe wearing creating a warm moist environment, locker room floors, and communal baths.
ii. Clinical manifestations
1. Three classic presentations.
(a) Interdigital
(i) Web space is dry, scaly, and fissured.
(ii) Itching is profuse.

(b) Chronic scaling of the plantar surface
(i) Entire sole is covered with fine, silvery white scales.
(ii) Itching is profuse.
(c) Acute vesicular
(i) Present with itchy sterile vesicles that are due to an allergic response to the fungus.
iii. Diagnosis
1. Potassium hydroxide examination reveals fungal elements.
iv. Treatment
1. Topical medications include butenafine, terbinafine, and sertaconazole.
2. Acute vesicular responds to Burrow's wet dressings several times a day with topical antifungal creams.
3. Oral or topical antifungal agents may be needed.
d. See Table 11-3 for summary of tinea infections.
II. Drug eruptions
a. General
i. A common complication of drug therapy.
b. Clinical manifestations
i. May present with fever, and then hours later, a diffuse maculopapular rash, hives, pruritus, or any combination may occur.

Table 11-3 • Tinea Infections	
Body Location	**Name**
Foot	Tinea pedis
Groin	Tinea cruris
Body	Tinea corporis
Face	Tinea faciei
Hand	Tinea manuum
Scalp	Tinea capitis
Beard	Tinea barbae
Nails	Onychomycosis

NOTES

c. Drug reactions
   i. Morbilliform eruptions
      1. Most frequent and very similar to viral exanthems.
      2. Due to ampicillin, isoniazid, phenytoin, quinidine, sulfonamides, and thiazides.
      3. Occur 7 to 10 days after starting the drug
      4. Maculopapular eruption, red macules, and papules become confluent and often spare the face.
      5. Itching is common.
      6. Treat with antihistamines and cooling lotions.
   ii. Urticarial drug reactions
      1. Due to an anaphylactic IgE-dependent reaction that occurs within minutes to hours of administration.
      2. Due to aspirin, penicillin, and blood products.
      3. Treat with antihistamines and cooling lotions.
         (a) Epinephrine may be needed in severe reactions.
   iii. Fixed drug eruptions
      1. Present with single or multiple, round, demarcated red plaques that appear soon after the drug exposure and reappear in the same site each time the drug is taken.

      2. Preceded by itching and burning.
      3. May occur on any part of the body, but the glans penis is the most common site.
      4. Length of time from re-exposure to onset of symptoms is 30 minutes to 6 hours.
      5. Tetracycline and cotrimoxazole frequently cause this reaction.
   iv. Drug-induced hyperpigmentation
      1. Caused by many different drugs and typically fades with time.
         (a) See Table 11-4.
   v. Chemotherapy-induced acral erythema
      1. Present with tingling of palms and soles followed in a few days by painful, well-defined symmetric swelling and erythema.

Table 11-4 • Common Drug-Induced Hyperpigmentation	
Drug	**Color Change**
Amiodarone	Dusky red on photodistributed areas
Minocycline	Blue-gray on skin and gingiva
Zidovudine	Brown discoloration on nails and lips
Antimalarial agents	Brown discoloration on shins
Hydantoin	Brown pigmentation on the face
Bleomycin	Streaking hyperpigmentation on trunk and extremities
Oral contraceptives	Brown pigmentation on the cheeks and central face

NOTES

ANSWER B EXPLANATION: *Tinea corporis infection is due the dermatophyte, Trichophyton species.*

correct ☐   incorrect ☐

    2. Commonly noted with cytosine arabinoside, fluorouracil, and doxorubicin.

    3. Treatment is supportive.

III. Lichen planus
  a. General
    i. Uncommon, inflammatory papulosquamous disorder of unknown cause.
    ii. Rare in children younger than 5 years and more common in women.
    iii. A lichen planus like reaction is noted with certain drugs, such as gold salts, beta-blockers, antimalarials, thiazide, and furosemide.
    iv. The five P's of lichen planus:
      1. Pruritic
      2. Planar
      3. Polygonal
      4. Papules
      5. Purple
  b. Clinical manifestations
    i. Itching is variable.
    ii. Lesions are 2 to 10 mm flat-topped papule with an irregular angulated border.
    iii. New lesions are purple or pink, but over time become purple.
    iv. Mainly noted on flexor surface of the wrists, shins, scalp, glans penis, and mouth.
      1. See Color Plate 4.
  c. Diagnosis
    i. Based on history and clinical findings.
  d. Treatment
    i. Antihistamines for pruritus.
    ii. Topical steroids are initial treatment for localized disease.
    iii. Intralesional triamcinolone acetonide is used for hypertrophic lesions.
    iv. Oral steroids are used in generalized skin involvement.
    v. Severe cases may require systemic retinoids or cyclosporine.

IV. Pityriasis rosea
  a. General
    i. Most cases are in patients between the ages of 10 and 40 years.
    ii. May note an upper respiratory infection (URI) within a month of onset.
    iii. Herpes simplex virus (HSV) type 7 is the suspected etiologic agent.
  b. Clinical manifestations
    i. Lesions are a salmon-colored oval plaque, 1 to 2 cm in diameter, with a fine scale at periphery, typically located first on the trunk.
      1. The first lesion is called the *herald patch*.
      2. Children may show lesions on the groin, elbows, and knees.
      3. See Color Plate 5.
    ii. Multiple smaller lesions appear later on trunk and give a Christmas tree pattern appearance.
    iii. Typically clear spontaneously in 4 to 12 weeks.
  c. Diagnosis
    i. Based on history and clinical findings.
    ii. Herald patch may be confused with tinea infection.
  d. Treatment
    i. Self-limiting and asymptomatic.
    ii. Ultraviolet B light may hasten resolution of the lesions.

V. Psoriasis
  a. General
    i. A common, chronic, inflammatory papulosquamous disease.
    ii. Due to abnormal T-lymphocyte function.
    iii. The skin, nails, and joints are affected.
    iv. Age of onset peaks during 20s and again in late 50s.
  b. Clinical manifestations
    i. Present with red, sharply defined, scaling papules that form stable round to oval plaques.
    ii. The scales are silvery white and reveal bleeding when removed.
      1. See Color Plate 6.
    iii. Typically noted on the extensor surfaces of the extremities (elbows and knees), scalp, and sacrum.
      1. Palms, soles, and face are typically spared.

NOTES

c. Diagnosis
  i. Based on history and clinical findings.
  ii. Punch biopsy shows thickening of the epidermis (acanthosis).
d. Treatment
  i. Psychosocial impact can be severe.
  ii. Three categories of treatment.
    1. Topical
     (a) Includes topical tar preparations, steroids, anthralin, and tazarotene.
    2. Phototherapy
     (a) Ultraviolet B is very effective treatment and often used with topical treatment.
    3. Systemic
     (a) Used in patients who are very uncomfortable or have lesions over more than 20% of their body.
     (b) Utilize a rotational therapy, best managed by a dermatologist.
     (c) Agents include:
      (i) Methotrexate
       (1) Side effects include nausea, fatigue, leukopenia, hepatic fibrosis, and cirrhosis.
      (ii) Cyclosporine
       (1) Side effects include hypertension and nephrotoxicity.
      (iii) Acitretin
       (1) Side effects include teratogenicity, depression, hepatitis, and increased cholesterol.
      (iv) Biologicals
       (1) Are involved with T-cell functioning.
       (2) Includes efalizumab, infliximab, and etanercept.

DESQUAMATION

I. Stevens-Johnson syndrome
  a. General
    i. Severe blistering mucocutaneous syndrome, involving at least two mucous membranes.

QUESTION

A patient presents with flat-topped, violaceous, polygonal, sharply defined papules on the flexor aspect of the wrist. Which of the following is the most likely diagnosis?

  A. Seborrheic dermatitis
  B. Pityriasis rosea
  C. Lichen planus
  D. Psoriasis

---

    ii. More common in young adults and children.
    iii. Associated with *Mycoplasma pneumoniae* infection and drugs, such as phenytoin, phenobarbital, sulfonamides, and aminopenicillins.
  b. Clinical manifestations
    i. Acutely have erythematous papules, dusky-appearing vesicles, and target lesions.
    ii. Lesions typically noted on the trunk and face.
    iii. Oral, genital, and perianal mucosa develop bullae and erosions.
    iv. Lesions may become eroded and infected.
    v. Patients often note skin to be tender and burning.
  c. Diagnosis
    i. Based on history and clinical findings.
    ii. Skin biopsy shows full thickness epidermal necrosis with mostly normal dermis.
  d. Treatment
    i. Uncomplicated cases resolve typically within 1 month.
    ii. Treatment focuses on removing offending agent and maintaining nutritional and fluid requirements.
    iii. Children have a slightly better prognosis than adults.
II. Toxic epidermal necrolysis
  a. General
    i. Rare, life-threatening disease with widespread blistering and sloughing of skin.
    ii. Typically related to drug ingestion, recent immunization, viral infection, mycoplasma infection, streptococcal infection, or syphilis.

NOTES

ANSWER **C** EXPLANATION: *Lichen planus presents on the flexor surfaces of the wrists and shins, scalp, and mouth, as flat-topped papule lesions, 2-10 mm in size. The five P's of lichen planus include pruritic, planar, polygonal, papules, and purple.*

correct ☐   incorrect ☐

1. Drugs include:
   (a) Sulfonamides
   (b) Antimalarials
   (c) Anticonvulsants
   (d) Nonsteroidal anti-inflammatory drugs (NSAIDs)
   (e) Allopurinol
b. Clinical manifestations
   i. Present with a diffuse red sunburn-like skin with scattered target lesions and bullae.
   ii. Bullae join together and result in widespread skin sloughing.
   iii. Gentle pressure easily produces epidermal detachment leaving a tender glistening raw surface.
c. Diagnosis
   i. Based on history and clinical findings.
   ii. Skin biopsy reveals a full-thickness necrotic epidermis.
d. Treatment
   i. Overall mortality rate is 30% to 50%.
   ii. Treatment focuses on pain control, removal of possible offending agent, maintaining fluid balance, and local wound care.
III. Erythema multiforme
   a. General
      i. Common, acute inflammatory disease.
      ii. Associated with HSV, *Mycoplasma pneumoniae*, and URIs.
   b. Clinical manifestations
      i. Characterized by many different lesions, including target-shaped skin lesions, erythematous macules and papules, urticarial-like lesions, vesicles, and bullae.
         1. See Color Plate 7.
      ii. Target lesions are dusky red, round papules and macules that may itch.

1. Are 1 to 3 cm in size with a central dark red area surrounded by a pale edematous area.
      iii. Appear on the palms, soles, backs of hands and feet, and extensor surfaces of the forearms and legs.
   c. Diagnosis
      i. Based on history and clinical findings.
   d. Treatment
      i. Typically resolves in 1 month.
      ii. Most patients do not require treatment.
      iii. Widespread disease does respond to systemic steroids.

VESICULAR BULLAE

I. Bullous pemphigoid
   a. General
      i. An uncommon, autoimmune blistering disease that primarily affects the elderly (>60 years of age).
      ii. Due to IgG autoantibodies directed against hemidesmosomal proteins.
   b. Clinical manifestations
      i. Begin with localized areas of erythema or pruritic papules that form plaques.
         1. Generally noted in the skin folds and flexural areas.
         2. Rare on the head and face.
      ii. Plaques turn dark red in 1 to 3 weeks as the vesicles and bullae rapidly appear.
      iii. Bullae are tense and rupture in 1 week, leaving an eroded base that heals rapidly.
      iv. Itching is moderate to severe.
   c. Diagnosis
      i. Based on history and clinical findings.
      ii. Skin biopsy shows subepidermal bulla with infiltration of eosinophils.
   d. Treatment
      i. Goal of treatment is to stop blistering, decrease itching, and protect against secondary infection.
      ii. Oral steroids are the best treatment until blistering stops.
      iii. Topical steroids may be used in limited disease.

NOTES

ACNEIFORM LESIONS

I. Acne vulgaris
   a. General
      i. One of the most common skin disorders.
      ii. Common between ages 10 and 15 years and lasts 5 to 10 years.
      iii. Disease due to plugged sebaceous pores, increased sebum production, and increased *Propionibacterium acnes.*
   b. Clinical manifestations
      i. Two types of lesions.
         1. Inflammatory
            (a) Consist of papules (<5 mm in diameter), pustules (central core of purulent material), and nodules/cysts (>5 mm in diameter).
         2. Noninflammatory
            (a) Consist of open (blackheads) and closed (whiteheads) comedones.
         3. See Color Plate 8.
      ii. Disease severity based on number of lesions.
         1. See Table 11-5.
   c. Diagnosis
      i. Based on history and clinical findings.
   d. Treatment
      i. Treatment is continual, not curative.
         1. Therapy should take into account medical and psychosocial issues.
         2. Response may not be noted for weeks.
      ii. Treatment varies with type of lesions and severity of disease.
         1. Comedones
            (a) Use agents that cause mild drying and peeling. Includes:

Table 11-5 • **Acne Severity Grading**		
Severity	**Papules/Pustules**	**Nodules**
Mild	Few to several	None
Moderate	Several to many	Few to several
Severe	Many and/or extensive	Many

               (i) Benzoyl peroxide
                  (1) Side effects include allergic contact dermatitis.
               (ii) Retinoids
                  (1) Include azelaic acid, tretinoin (Retin-A), and tazarotene
                  (2) Side effects include facial dryness and erythema.
                  (3) Response to treatment in 1 to 4 weeks.
         2. Papules and pustules
            (a) Agents used above for comedones are used along with the following:
               (i) Topical antibiotics
                  (1) Clindamycin
                  (2) Erythromycin
               (ii) Oral antibiotics
                  (1) Tetracycline
                  (2) Erythromycin
                  (3) Doxycycline
                  (4) Minocycline
               (iii) Antibiotics must be taken for weeks to be effective.
         3. Nodules and cysts
            (a) Isotretinoin (Accutane) is very effective.
               (i) Related to vitamin A.
               (ii) A potent teratogen and induces an elevation in triglycerides.
               (iii) Therapy is typically 16 to 20 weeks in length.

QUESTION

A 30-year-old presents with a number of salmon-red oval, slightly raised plaques on the trunk and proximal upper extremities. The patient states the rash started with a single lesion and then spread. The patient is on phenytoin for a seizure disorder. Which of the following is the most likely diagnosis?

   A. Tinea corporis
   B. Erythema migrans
   C. Pityriasis rosea
   D. Drug eruption

NOTES

ANSWER **C** EXPLANATION: *Pityriasis rosea presents as salmon-colored, oval plaques about 1-2 cm in diameter. A fine scale is noted at the periphery. Lesions are first noted on the trunk.*

correct ☐   incorrect ☐

    (b) Triamcinolone, a steroid, can be injected into the cysts.
    (c) Oral prednisone is used in severe acne.
  iii. Hormonal treatment
    1. Includes:
      (a) Oral contraceptives
      (b) Spironolactone
      (c) Corticosteroids

II. Rosacea
  a. General
    i. A chronic inflammatory acneiform disorder.
    ii. Typically affecting middle-aged and older adults.
    iii. Cause is unknown, but is not a type of acne.
      1. No comedones are noted.
  b. Clinical manifestations
    i. Intermittent flushing erythema and recurrent appearance of papules, pustules, and telangiectases.
    ii. Noted mainly on cheeks, nose, brow, and chin.
    iii. Patients may note burning and itching.
    iv. Can progress to rhinophymata, a bulbous appearance of the nose due to sebaceous hyperplasia.
  c. Diagnosis
    i. Based on history and clinical findings.
  d. Treatment
    i. Antibiotics treatment includes oral tetracycline and topical metronidazole.
    ii. Maintenance therapy with tetracycline is a necessity.
    iii. Hot drinks should be avoided because they lead to flushing.

III. Folliculitis
  a. General
    i. Inflammation in the hair follicle.
    ii. A number of different types.
      1. Mechanical: results from persistent trauma.
      2. Bacterial
        (a) Can be spread by trauma, scratching, and shaving.
        (b) Most common cause is *S. aureus* infection.
          (i) *Pseudomonas* is indicated in hot-tub folliculitis.
      3. Fungal
  b. Clinical manifestations
    i. Present with dome-shaped pustules with erythematous halos in the follicle.
    ii. Lesions may be tender.
    iii. Typically no systemic symptoms.
  c. Diagnosis
    i. Based on history and clinical findings.
  d. Treatment
    i. Heat, friction, and occlusion must be eliminated.
    ii. Mupirocin (Bactroban) can be used for superficial disease.
    iii. Oral antistaphylococcal antibiotics are indicated for extensive or spreading disease.
      1. Antibiotics include oxacillin, dicloxacillin, and cefuroxime.

VERRUCOUS LESIONS

I. Seborrheic keratosis
  a. General
    i. Common, benign, persistent epidermal lesion.
    ii. Often confused with cutaneous malignancies.
    iii. Typically noted after 30 years of age.
  b. Clinical manifestations
    i. Most lesions are 0.2 to 3 cm in diameter. Lesions may be flat or raised and may be smooth, velvety, or verrucous.
      1. A well-circumscribed border with a stuck on appearance.
      2. Surface crumbles when picked.
    ii. Color varies; white, pink, brown, and black may be noted.
    iii. Presence of horn cysts on the surface assist in the diagnosis.

NOTES

iv. Can arise on any part of the body, except lips, palms, and soles.
  1. Common on areola of both males and females.
  c. Diagnosis
    i. Based on history and clinical findings.
    ii. Sudden onset of numerous lesions may be associated with internal malignancy.
  d. Treatment
    i. Cryosurgery is used for flat or lightly raised lesions.
    ii. Cautery and curettage are used for thicker lesions.
II. Actinic keratosis
  a. General
    i. Common, persistent, keratotic lesion with malignant potential.
    ii. Formation due to years of sun exposure.
    iii. Lesions more common after 40 years of age.
    iv. About 10% to 20% of lesions progress to squamous cell carcinoma.
  b. Clinical manifestations
    i. Lesions typically found on sun-exposed areas of elderly patients.
    ii. Lesions found mainly on the face, neck, head, and hands, and typically 3 to 6 mm in size.
    iii. Present as poorly defined area of redness or telangiectasia.
      1. Lesions become more defined and develop a thin, yellow, or transparent scale.
      2. See Color Plate 9.
  c. Diagnosis
    i. Based on clinical findings and biopsy results.
  d. Treatment
    i. Must have annual follow-up and avoid sun.
    ii. Single lesions can be treated with cryotherapy (liquid nitrogen).
    iii. Topical 5-fluorouracil can be used to decrease the number of superficial lesions.

INSECTS/PARASITES

I. Lice
  a. General
    i. Lice are flat, wingless insects that infest the hair of the scalp, body, and pubic region.

      1. *Pediculus humanus* var. *capitis* infects the head.
      2. *Pediculus corporis* causes body lice.
      3. *Phthirus pubis* infects the pubic hair.
    ii. Attached to the skin, feed off human blood, and lay nits on the hair shaft.
      1. Nits are the white, hard, oval lice eggs.
    iii. Transmission via close personal contact and hats or brushes.
    iv. Girls affected more often than boys.
  b. Clinical manifestations
    i. Lice are 3 to 4 mm in length and can be seen on the scalp and hair shafts.
    ii. Nits are small white eggs attached to the hair shaft.
    iii. Lice feces can be seen on the skin as small, rust-colored flecks.
    iv. Pruritus is common.
    v. Posterior cervical adenopathy may be noted.
  c. Diagnosis
    i. Based on identification of the lice or nits.
  d. Treatment
    i. Topical treatments
      1. Permethrin (Elimite)
      2. Lindane (Kwell)
      3. Malathion (Ovide)
        (a) Not recommended for children.
      4. All should be repeated in 1 week.
      5. Family must also be treated.
    ii. Oral treatments
      1. Ivermectin
        (a) Repeat in 10 days.
    iii. Nit removal
      1. Essential and requires a special nit comb.

NOTES

ANSWER **D** EXPLANATION: *Isotretinoin is a potent teratogen and induces elevations in serum triglycerides.*

correct ☐   incorrect ☐

II. Scabies
  a. General
    i. Caused by *Sarcoptes scabiei* var. *hominis*.
      1. The mite is ⅓-mm long and has a flattened, oval body with eight legs.
    ii. Very contagious.
  b. Clinical manifestations
    i. Patient presents with severe itching that is worse at night.
    ii. Classic lesion is a burrow that is linear, curved or S-shaped, slightly elevated vesicle or papule.
      1. Found in the finger webs, wrists, sides of hand and feet, penis, buttocks, and scrotum.
    iii. Rash appears about 2 to 6 weeks after exposure.
  c. Diagnosis
    i. Based on clinical findings.
  d. Treatment
    i. Permethrin (Elimite) or lindane (Kwell) can be applied to the skin from the neck down and repeated in 1 week.
    ii. Oral ivermectin can be used in most patients and should be repeated in 2 weeks.
    iii. All clothes and bedding should be washed in hot water.
III. Spider bites
  a. General
    i. Bites are common, but of the 50 species of spiders in the United States, only the black widow and brown recluse spider produce severe reactions.
    ii. Black widow spider is 3 to 4 cm in length and has a red hourglass-shaped marking on the ventral surface of the abdomen.
      1. Disease due the envenomation of a neurotoxin.
      2. Typically encountered near woodpiles, logs, barns, or in shoes.
    iii. Brown recluse spider is 1.5 cm in length, is yellow, tan, or brown, and has a dark-brown violin-shaped marking on its thorax.
      1. Typically noted in south central United States and found in woodpiles, attics, garages, and basements.
  b. Clinical manifestations
    i. Black widow spider bite typically reveals mild erythema or swelling at the bite site.
      1. Red-brown fang marks may be noted.
      2. Severe reactions present with cramping abdominal pain, hypertension, muscle complaints, irritability, and agitation.
    ii. Brown recluse spider bite presents with local pain and burning due to vasospasm.
      1. A local hivelike reaction followed by cyanosis and expanding necrosis.
      2. Systemic symptoms, fever, chills, vomiting, weakness, and muscle and joint pain may be noted.
  c. Diagnosis
    i. Based on clinical findings and having a high degree of suspicion.
  d. Treatment
    i. Black widow spider bites are treated with ice to restrict spread of venom.
      1. Antivenom can be given for acute symptoms.
    ii. Brown recluse spider is treated with supportive care.
      1. With severe necrosis, local wound care and antibiotics are needed.

NEOPLASMS

I. Basal cell carcinoma
  a. General
    i. Most common cutaneous malignancy.
      1. More common after age 40 years.
    ii. Locally invasive, slow growing, and rarely metastasizes.
    iii. Risk factors include sun exposure and prior ionizing radiation.
  b. Clinical manifestations
    i. Lesions most common on face, scalp, ears, and neck.

NOTES

    ii. Lesion is pearly-white, dome-shaped papule with overlying telangiectasias.
      1. See Color Plate 10.
   iii. Lesions frequently ulcerate, bleed, and develop a crusted center.
   iv. Lesion color varies from brown, black, or blue.
  c. Diagnosis
    i. Based on clinical findings and biopsy.
  d. Treatment
    i. Goal is elimination of the tumor.
   ii. Options for treatment include:
      1. Electrosurgery (electrodesiccation and curettage)
        (a) Five-year cure rate is 92% for primary tumors.
      2. Office excision
        (a) Five-year cure rate is 90% for primary tumors.
      3. Mohs' surgery
        (a) Five-year cure rate is 99% for primary tumors.
      4. Radiation therapy
        (a) Five-year cure rate is 90% for primary tumors.

II. Melanoma
  a. General
    i. Malignancy of the melanocytes.
   ii. Most common cancer in women aged 25 to 29 years.
   iii. Risk factors
      1. Fair skin
      2. Presence of atypical nevi
      3. Personal history of melanoma
      4. Positive family history of atypical nevi or melanoma
      5. History of severe blistering sunburn
      6. Congenital nevi
  b. Clinical manifestations
    i. Most common early symptom is itching; later develop tenderness, bleeding, and ulceration.
   ii. Early signs include increase in size, change in color or shape of the lesion.
   iii. Appearance of melanoma varies considerably.
      1. See Color Plate 11.
      2. See Table 11-6.

Table 11-6 • ABCDs of Malignant Melanoma
Asymmetry
Border irregularity
Color variation
Diameter > 6 cm

  c. Diagnosis
    i. Diagnosis made by biopsy.
      1. Shave biopsy is not indicated.
   ii. Prognosis varies with certain conditions.
      1. Prognosis is better with:
        (a) Thin melanoma
        (b) Melanoma on the extremity
        (c) Localized disease
        (d) Female and younger patients
  d. Treatment
    i. Survival rates and treatment options vary with the stage of the disease.
   ii. Frequent follow-up is required.
   iii. Treatment
      1. Stage I treated with surgical intervention.
      2. Stages II and III are treated with surgical intervention and adjuvant treatment with high-dose interferon-2-alpha.
   iv. Five-year survival rates
      1. Stage I: 90% to 95%
      2. Stage II: 45% to 80%
      3. Stage III: 25% to 70%
      4. Stage IV: 5% to 20%

III. Squamous cell carcinoma
  a. General
    i. Arise from keratinocytes of the skin or mucosal surface.
   ii. Most commonly noted on the hands, neck, and head of elderly people.
   iii. Risk factors include:
      1. Ultraviolet light exposure
      2. Chemicals (hydrocarbons and arsenic)
      3. Tobacco
      4. Chronic infections
      5. Human papillomavirus

NOTES

b. Clinical manifestations
   i. Typically found on sun-damaged skin.
   ii. Early lesions have the appearance of actinic keratosis.
   iii. Lesion has a red, poorly defined base with an adherent yellow-white scale.
      1. See Color Plate 12.
   iv. Over time, the lesions become larger and more raised, and develop a firm, red nodule with a necrotic center.
   v. Regional lymph nodes must be examined.
c. Diagnosis
   i. Made by skin biopsy.
   ii. Risk factors for metastasis include:
      1. Tumor greater than 2 cm in diameter
      2. Decreased degree of differentiation
      3. Recurrent lesions
      4. Tumor arising from a scar or chronic wound
      5. Location
         (a) Increased risk with lesions on the ear or lip.
d. Treatment
   i. Long-term prognosis for nonmetastatic, adequately treated cancer is excellent.
   ii. Treatment of primary lesions is wide local excision.
      1. Mohs' surgery is an option if tissue sparing is important.
   iii. Radiation is a treatment option.

HAIR AND NAILS

I. Alopecia areata
   a. General
      i. Nonscarring hair loss, of rapid onset in a sharply defined area.
      ii. Cause is unknown.
      iii. Most common in children and young adults.
      iv. Associated with thyroid disease, pernicious anemia, Addison's disease, systemic lupus erythematosus (SLE), ulcerative colitis, and diabetes mellitus.
   b. Clinical manifestations
      i. Pattern of hair loss is patchy.
         1. Areas of hair loss are typically 1 to 4 cm in size.
      ii. Skin is very smooth or may have short stubs of hair.
      iii. Nail dystrophy may be noted.
   c. Diagnosis
      i. Based on history and clinical findings.
   d. Treatment
      i. Most hair regrows, and treatment is not needed.
      ii. If treatment is needed, intradermal triamcinolone or topical anthralin or minoxidil may be effective.
II. Androgenetic alopecia
   a. General
      i. Premature loss of hair on the central scalp.
      ii. A physiologic reaction due to androgens in genetically predisposed men.
      iii. Typically begins after puberty and is fully expressed by the time the patient is in his or her 40s.
   b. Clinical manifestations
      i. Early, the hair follicles are transformed into vellus-like follicles.
      ii. Later, the follicles disappear, and scale becomes shiny and smooth.
      iii. Thinning begins in the temporal region and then progresses into a M-shaped recession.
      iv. Later, total hair loss is noted in the central scalp.
   c. Diagnosis
      i. Based on history and clinical findings.
   d. Treatment
      i. Topical minoxidil (Rogaine)
         1. Regrowth takes 8 to 12 months.
         2. Side effects include increased cardiac output and left ventricular mass, dizziness, and tachycardia.
      ii. Oral finasteride (Propecia)
         1. Works by blocking 5-alpha-reductase.
         2. Side effects include decreased libido and erectile dysfunction.
      iii. Hair transplantation
III. Onychomycosis
   a. General
      i. Fungal infection (tinea) of the nail plate.
      ii. Trauma predisposes to infection.
   b. Clinical manifestations
      i. Four clinical patterns.

NOTES

1. Distal subungual
   (a) Distal plate is yellow or white, and the nail rises and separates from the underlying bed.
2. White superficial
   (a) Nail is soft, dry, and powdery.
   (b) Nail plate is not thick and remains adherent to the bed.
3. Proximal subungual
   (a) Surface of the nail plate remains intact, but hyperkeratotic debris causes the nail to separate.
4. *Candida*
   (a) Nail plate is thick and turns yellow to brown.

  c. Diagnosis
   i. Made by potassium hydroxide examination.
   ii. Confirmed by fungal culture.
  d. Treatment
   i. Systemic antifungal agents are more effective than topical agents.
   ii. Antifungal agents include:
      1. Lamisil
      2. Sporanox
      3. Fluconazole

IV. Paronychia
  a. General
   i. Bacterial or fungal infection of the proximal and lateral nail fold.
   ii. Acute and chronic disease
      1. Acute infection is due to trauma and manipulation.
         (a) *Pseudomonas* may infect the space between nail plate and nail bed.
      2. Chronic infection is due to contact irritant exposure.
  b. Clinical manifestations
   i. Present with pain and swelling.
   ii. In acute infection, pus accumulates behind the cuticle or deeper in the lateral nail folds.
   iii. In chronic infection, many or all fingers are involved.
      1. Tenderness, erythema, and mild swelling may be noted.
      2. Nail plate is distorted but uninfected.
  c. Diagnosis
   i. Based on clinical findings.
  d. Treatment

QUESTION

Which of the following is the most common type of skin cancer?

  A. Squamous cell carcinoma
  B. Merkel cell carcinoma
  C. Basal cell carcinoma
  D. Melanoma

---

  i. Acute infection is treated with antistaphylococcal antibiotics.
  ii. Chronic infection is treated with group V topical steroids and agents such as miconazole or fluconazole.

VIRAL DISEASES

I. Condyloma acuminatum (venereal warts)
  a. General
   i. Infection of the genital or anal skin by human papillomavirus.
   ii. Warts spread rapidly over moist areas.
  b. Clinical manifestations
   i. The lesions are asymptomatic.
   ii. Lesion appearance varies from person to person.
   iii. Lesions may be pale pink to white, rough, barely raised papules, or have projections on a broad base.
   iv. Lesion surface may be smooth, velvety and moist, and lacks the hyperkeratosis.
   v. Lesions may coalesce and form a large, cauliflower-like mass.
  c. Diagnosis
   i. Based on clinical findings.
  d. Treatment
   i. Liquid nitrogen cryotherapy can be performed.
      1. Treatment may be painful.
   ii. Electrocautery and curettage can be used for a few isolated lesions.
   iii. Podofilox can be used for external genital warts.
      1. Adverse effects include pain, burning, and inflammation.

NOTES

ANSWER C EXPLANATION: *Basal cell carcinoma is the most common type of skin cancer. Risk factors include sun exposure and ionizing radiation.*

correct ❑   incorrect ❑

iv. Condoms may reduce transmission to partners.
v. Increased risk for cervical cancer is related to human papillomavirus infection.

II. Herpes simplex
   a. General
      i. Direct contact with infected secretions is the major transmission mode.
         1. Humans are the only natural reservoir.
      ii. Cause both acute and latent infection.
         1. Acute infection consists of development of multinucleated giant cells.
         2. Latent infection can be triggered by fever, trauma, and exposure to ultraviolet light.
   b. Clinical manifestations
      i. HSV type 1
         1. Grouped or single vesicular lesions that become pustular and form single or multiple ulcers.
            (a) Umbilicated vesicles are classic for herpesvirus infection.
         2. Symptoms occur 3 to 7 days after exposure.
         3. Can involve any mucosal surface.
         4. Lesions are very painful and last for 5 to 10 days.
         5. May become latent within sensory nerve root ganglion.
         6. Recurrences, average 4 per year, are typically unilateral and last about 7 days.
         7. Herpes Whitlow is HSV infection involving the finger or nail area.
         8. Herpes gladiatorum is cutaneous herpes in athletes involved in contact sports.
      ii. HSV type 2
         1. Cause of genital herpes.
         2. Incubation period is 5 days from sexual contact to onset of lesions.
         3. Lesions are small erythematous papules that form into vesicles and then pustules.
         4. With primary disease, the lesions are painful, multiple, and extensive.
            (a) May have systemic symptoms such as fever, headache, and myalgias.
         5. Recurrent disease is typically shorter in duration and typically localized to the genital region, without systemic symptoms.
            (a) Prodromal paresthesias may be noted 12 to 24 hours before the appearance of the lesions.
   c. Diagnosis
      i. Can be made by cell culture, Tzanck smear, antibody detection, and polymerase chain reaction (PCR).
         1. Tzanck smear shows multinucleated giant cells.
         2. PCR is the test of choice for diagnosis of HSV encephalitis.
   d. Treatment
      i. Use of acyclovir, valacyclovir, or famciclovir is indicated.
         1. Topical agents can be used.
         2. Intravenous (IV) acyclovir is needed in HSV encephalitis.
      ii. Prophylactic measures include avoidance of contact with HSV-positive secretions and daily antivirals to suppress recurrences.
      iii. Because of high mortality and morbidity with neonatal HSV infection, cesarean birth should be used to prevent transmission to infant from actively infected mother.

III. Herpes zoster (shingles)
   a. General
      i. Viral infection of the skin involving a single or multiple dermatomes.
      ii. Results from reactivation of the varicella virus after an earlier episode of chickenpox.
      iii. Increased likelihood of unknown malignancy in patients with zoster.
   b. Clinical manifestations
      i. Systemic symptoms include headache, photophobia, and malaise.
      ii. Fever is uncommon.
      iii. Pain and burning may precede rash by 3 to 5 days.

NOTES

iv. Lesions begin as red swollen plaques. Vesicles arise in clusters from the red plaques.
  1. See Color Plate 13.
v. Vesicles umbilicate or rupture before forming crusts.
  1. Crusts fall off in 2 to 3 weeks.
vi. Ophthalmic zoster
  1. Involves any branch of the ophthalmic nerve.
  2. Vesicles on the side or tip of the nose are associated with corneal involvement.
  3. Should be treated by an ophthalmologist.
c. Diagnosis
  i. Based on history and clinical findings.
  ii. Tzanck smear may be positive.
d. Treatment
  i. Treatment
    1. Topical therapy (wet dressings) or oral steroids decrease the acute pain and improve rash resolution.
      (a) Have no effect on postherpetic neuralgia.
    2. Oral antiviral agents decrease acute pain, inflammation, and viral shedding.
      (a) Most effective if started within first 48 hours.
      (b) Agents include acyclovir, valacyclovir, or famciclovir.
      (c) Topical antivirals play no role in treatment of herpes zoster.
  ii. Complications
    1. Postherpetic neuralgia
      (a) Pain persists more than 30 days after the rash.
      (b) Pain is severe and intractable.
      (c) Treatment
        (i) Amitriptyline can be used for prevention.
        (ii) Treatment of acute symptoms consists of oral analgesics, topical lidocaine patch, tricyclic antidepressants, gabapentin, steroids, or topical capsaicin cream.
        (iii) Consult with a pain management specialist may be needed.

QUESTION

A patient presents with pain and swelling of the distal fourth digit. Pus is noted behind the cuticle. Which of the following is the most likely diagnosis?

A. Paronychia

B. Onychomycosis

C. Tinea manuum

D. Psoriasis

IV. Molluscum contagiosum
  a. General
    i. Localized, self-limiting viral infection of the skin.
    ii. Spread by autoinoculation.
      1. Autoinoculation around the eyes is common in children.
    iii. Peak incidence, ages 3 to 9 and 16 to 24 years.
  b. Clinical manifestations
    i. Most lesions are asymptomatic.
    ii. Lesions are 1- to 2-mm shiny, white to flesh-colored, dome-shaped papules.
      1. A small central umbilication is noted.
      2. See Color Plate 14.
    iii. Over weeks, the lesion increases in size to 2 to 5 mm.
    iv. Most lesions are noted on the upper trunk, extremities, and face.
    v. Untreated lesions persist for 6 to 9 months.
  c. Diagnosis
    i. Based on history and clinical findings.
  d. Treatment
    i. May resolve spontaneously in 6 to 9 months.
    ii. Skin-to-skin contact should be avoided.
    iii. Curettage can be used to remove the central infectious core.
    iv. Cryosurgery can be used without scarring.
    v. Topical agents include cantharidin solution, imiquimod cream, and tretinoin cream.
V. Verrucae (warts)
  a. General
    i. Benign epidermal proliferations caused by human papillomavirus.

NOTES

ANSWER **A** EXPLANATION: *Paronychia is a bacterial or fungal infection of the proximal and lateral nail fold. Present with pain, swelling, and accumulation of pus behind the cuticle or lateral nail folds.*

correct ☐   incorrect ☐

    ii. Transmission is by simple contact.
      1. Local spread by autoinoculation.
    iii. Peak incidence is age 12 to 16 years.
    iv. Incubation period is 1 to 6 months.
  b. Clinical manifestations
    i. Flesh-colored papules evolve into dome-shaped, gray to brown, hyperkeratotic, rough papules.
    ii. Common sites include the hands, periungual skin, elbows, knees, and plantar surfaces.
  c. Diagnosis
    i. Based on clinical findings.
    ii. Biopsy may be needed to rule out squamous cell carcinoma.
  d. Treatment
    i. May spontaneously resolve within 2 years.
    ii. Over-the-counter preps (salicylic acid) are safe and effective.
    iii. Cryotherapy, liquid nitrogen can be effective.
      1. Pain and blistering may be noted after treatment.

BACTERIAL INFECTIONS

I. Cellulitis
  a. General
    i. Infection of the dermis and subcutaneous tissue.
    ii. Increased risk in patients with diabetes mellitus, cirrhosis, renal failure, malnutrition, cancer, or history of IV drug abuse.
  b. Clinical manifestations
    i. Present with fever, erythema, edema, and pain.
    ii. On examination, an expanding red, swollen, tender, or painful plaque with an indefinite border.
    iii. Regional lymphadenopathy may occur.
  c. Diagnosis
    i. Laboratory tests reveal a leukocytosis.
    ii. Most often caused by group A streptococcus and *S. aureus*.
      1. Other agents include:
        (a) *Erysipelothrix rhusiopathiae*: fish handlers
        (b) *Aeromonas hydrophilia*: swimming in fresh water
        (c) *Vibrio* species: swimming in salt water
        (d) *Pasteurella multocida*: animal bite or scratch
  d. Treatment
    i. Empiric antibiotic therapy should be directed against staphylococcal and streptococcal organisms.
      1. Antibiotic choices include:
        (a) Penicillinase-resistant penicillin (dicloxacillin)
        (b) Amoxicillin/clavulanate
        (c) First-generation cephalosporin
        (d) Azithromycin or clarithromycin
II. Erysipelas
  a. General
    i. Acute, inflammatory cellulitis in which lymphatic involvement is prominent.
    ii. Involves the dermis and upper subcutaneous tissue.
    iii. Most common pathogen is group A streptococci.
  b. Clinical manifestations
    i. Onset is sudden with prodromal symptoms of malaise, high fever, chills, and myalgias.
    ii. Adenopathy and lymphangitis may also occur.
    iii. One or more red, tender, and firm spots that rapidly increase in size.
      1. Form a tense and deeply erythematous, hot, sharply demarcated elevated shiny patch.
    iv. Most commonly located on the lower leg.
    v. Red, painful streaks of lymphangitis may be noted extending toward regional lymph nodes.
  c. Diagnosis
    i. Based on clinical findings.
    ii. White blood cell count is elevated.

NOTES

d. Treatment
    i. Antibiotic options include penicillin V, amoxicillin, azithromycin, or clarithromycin.

III. Impetigo
  a. General
    i. Self-limiting, common, contagious, superficial skin infection.
    ii. Produced by *Streptococcus pyogenes* or *S. aureus.*
    iii. May develop after a minor injury.
    iv. Predisposing conditions include warm, moist climates and poor hygiene.
  b. Clinical manifestations
    i. Lesions most commonly noted on the face.
    ii. Two forms: bullous and nonbullous
      1. Bullous
        (a) Start clear and become cloudy.
        (b) Collapse leading to a lesion with a thin, flat honey-crusted center with a rim.
      2. Nonbullous
        (a) Vesicles or pustules rupture, leaving a red, moist base.
        (b) A honey-yellow crust is also present on the lesion.
      3. See Color Plate 15.
  c. Diagnosis
    i. Based on clinical findings.
  d. Treatment
    i. Mupirocin ointment or cream (Bactroban) is used for limited, localized infection.
    ii. Severe infections are treated with oral antibiotics.
      1. Dicloxacillin
      2. Cephalexin
      3. Azithromycin
      4. Clarithromycin

OTHER

I. Acanthosis nigricans
  a. General
    i. Thickened, velvety hyperpigmentation of the flexural skin.
    ii. Associated with obesity and diabetes.
    iii. Can be caused by medications, such as estrogen or nicotinic acid.

QUESTION

Which of the following is used to treat verrucae?

  A. Acyclovir (Zovirax)
  B. Penicillin
  C. Salicylic acid
  D. Tretinoin cream (Retin-A)

---

  b. Clinical manifestations
    i. Complain of an asymptomatic, dirty appearance to the skin folds.
    ii. Skin shows symmetric, velvety brown thickening.
      1. Skin surface is rough.
    iii. Most commonly noted on the neck or axillae.
  c. Diagnosis
    i. Based on clinical findings.
  d. Treatment
    i. Lac-Hydrin is used to soften the skin.

II. Burns
  a. General
    i. Classified into six groups based on mechanism of injury.
      1. Scalds
        (a) Child abuse accounts for a large number of immersion scald burns.
      2. Contact burns
      3. Fire
      4. Chemical
      5. Electrical
      6. Radiation
    ii. Highest incidence of burns occurs during the first few years of life and between ages of 20 and 29 years.
  b. Clinical manifestations
    i. Skin is the largest organ of the body.
      1. Three major layers.
        (a) Epidermis—outermost layer and composed of stratified epithelium.
          (i) Acts as a barrier.
        (b) Dermis—composed of connective tissue and ground substance.
          (i) Serves as support and participates in collagen synthesis.

NOTES

ANSWER C Explanation: *Verrucae is treated with salicylic acid or cryotherapy. They may disappear spontaneously in two years.*

correct ☐   incorrect ☐

(c) Subcutaneous tissue—third layer and composed of areolar and fatty connective tissue.
    (i) Thickness varies and contains sweat glands, skin appendages, and hair follicles.

ii. Depth of burns classified according to degrees.
  1. First-degree
    (a) Minor epithelial damage of epidermis
    (b) Redness, tenderness, and pain are present
    (c) No blistering is present, and two-point discrimination is intact.
    (d) Healing takes several days and occurs without scarring.
    (e) Most common causes are flash burns and sunburn.
  2. Second-degree
    (a) Superficial partial-thickness burn
      (i) Involves epidermis and superficial dermis layers.
      (ii) Skin appears pink, moist, and soft, and thin-walled blisters are present.
      (iii) Skin is very tender to touch.
      (iv) Heals in 2 to 3 weeks, typically without scarring.
    (b) Deep partial-thickness burn
      (i) Involves the epidermis and extends into the lower (reticular) dermis layer.
      (ii) Skin appears red and blanched white with thick-walled blisters.
      (iii) Heal in 3 to 6 weeks; scarring is possible with the develop-ment of contractions across joints.
    (c) Second-degree burns typically due to splash scalds.
  3. Third-degree

    (a) Full-thickness burn that destroys epidermis and dermis.
    (b) Skin is white or leathery with underlying clotted vessels and is numb.
    (c) Skin grafting is needed unless burn is small (<1 cm in diameter).
    (d) Caused by immersion scalds, flame burns, chemical and high-voltage electrical injuries.
  4. Fourth-degree
    (a) Full-thickness destruction of skin, subcutaneous tissue, fascia, muscle, bone, and other structures.
    (b) Treatment requires débridement and reconstruction of tissues.
    (c) Result from prolonged exposure to causes of third-degree burns.
c. Diagnosis
  i. Burn wound assessment
    1. Rule of Nines
      (a) Adult body surface area (BSA)
        (i) 9% head and neck
        (ii) 9% each upper extremity
        (iii) 18% anterior portion of trunk
        (iv) 18% posterior portion of trunk
        (v) 18% each lower extremity
        (vi) 1% to perineum and genitalia
      (b) Children BSA
        (i) 18% head and neck
        (ii) 9% each upper extremity
        (iii) 18% anterior portion of trunk
        (iv) 18% posterior portion of trunk
        (v) 14% each lower extremity
        (vi) 1% to perineum and genitalia
      (c) See Figure 11-1 for the Rule of Nines.
  ii. Carboxyhemoglobin
    1. Carbon monoxide level should be obtained.
    2. Treat with 100% oxygen until level less than 10%.
      (a) Hyperbaric oxygen may be needed if presence of metabolic acidosis, history of neurologic deficits, pregnancy, cardiac abnormalities, or extremes of age.
  iii. Cyanide

NOTES

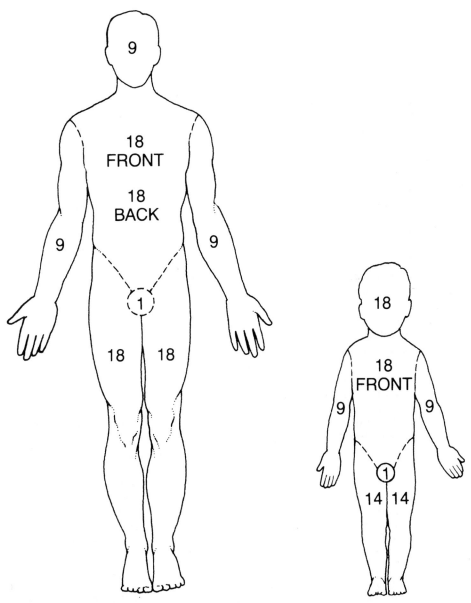

Figure 11-1   Rule of Nines for estimating percentage of burn area. (From Roberts JR, Hedges JR, Vroucher D, et al: Clinical Procedures in Emergency Medicine, 4th ed. Philadelphia: WB Saunders 2004:751, Fig. 39-1.)

NOTES

1. Inhalation injury may lead to cyanide poisoning.
2. Treat with nitrite-thiosulfate antidote.

d. Treatment
   i. Early response to burn incidents has a great influence on the magnitude of injury.
   ii. Prehospital care
      1. Evaluate for signs of inhalation injury
         (a) Includes dyspnea, burns on mouth and nose, singed nasal hairs, sooty sputum, and cough.
         (b) Treat with humidified oxygen, non-rebreathing mask at 10 to 12 L/min.
      2. All burned clothing and skin should be washed with cool water.
         (a) Inhibits lactate production and acidosis.
         (b) Limits vascular permeability.
         (c) Decreases dermal ischemia.
   iii. Hospital care
      1. Fluid resuscitation
         (a) Tremendous fluid loss.
         (b) Adequate fluid resuscitation is evidenced by normal urine output.
            (i) 1 mL/kg/hour in those younger than 2 years old.
            (ii) 0.5 mL/kg/hour in older children.
            (iii) 30 to 40 mL/hour in adults.
         (c) Parkland formula for fluid resuscitation
            (i) Uses lactated Ringer's solution.
            (ii) Total volume given is 4 mL/kg/% body surface area burned during the first 24 hours.
               (1) One half of total is given the first 8 hours, and the rest given over the next 16 hours.
               (2) Percent body surface area burned includes only second- and third-degree burns.
         (d) Galveston formula for fluid resuscitation
            (i) Used in children.

(ii) Uses 5% dextrose in lactated Ringers.
(iii) Total volume given is 5000 mL/m^2 of body surface area burned plus 2000 mL/m^2 during the first 24 hours.
   (1) One half of total is given the first 8 hours, and the rest given over the next 16 hours.
   (2) Dextrose is added to prevent hypoglycemia.
2. Pain management
   (a) Requirement for pain medications is inversely related to depth of burn injury.
      (i) Full-thickness burns are painless, due to sensory nerve damage.
   (b) Morphine is the medication of choice.
3. Escharotomy
   (a) Full-thickness circumferential burn of an extremity may result in vascular compromise.
   (b) May note loss of pulses and increase in tissue compartment pressures.
   (c) Escharotomy prevents ischemic injury.

III. Decubitus ulcers
   a. General
      i. Due to prolonged pressure on areas of the skin, resulting in tissue damage.
      ii. Typically occur on bony prominences, such as the hip, sacrum, or lateral malleolus.
      iii. Requires three forces: pressure, shear, and friction.
      iv. Predisposing conditions include:
         1. Paraplegia/quadriplegia
         2. Diabetes mellitus
         3. Peripheral vascular disease
         4. Peripheral neuropathy
         5. Immobility
   b. Clinical manifestations
      i. Detection requires complete skin examination.
      ii. Present with painless open sores.

NOTES

iii. Vary in size and depth.
iv. May note presence of tissue damage, necrotic tissue, and exudate.
v. Varying stages of ulcers.
  1. See Table 11-7.
c. Diagnosis
  i. Based on clinical findings.
d. Treatment
  i. Management involves prevention, early recognition, and aggressive treatment.
  ii. Stages I and II are best treated with local care and pain management.
  iii. Stages III and IV often require surgical intervention.
    1. Debridement of necrotic tissue and wound care with wet-to-dry dressings is often required.
  iv. Antibiotics are required if complications of sepsis or osteomyelitis are suspected.
  v. The key is prevention.
IV. Hidradenitis suppurativa
  a. General
    i. Chronic, suppurative, and scarring disease of the skin and subcutaneous tissue.
    ii. Occurs most commonly in the axillae, anogenital region, and female breast.
      1. More common in obese patients.
      2. Cigarette smoking is a major triggering factor.
    iii. A disease of the follicle.
  b. Clinical manifestations

Table 11-7 • Stages of Decubitus Ulcers

Stage	Description
I	Erythema of intact skin
II	Partial-thickness skin loss of epidermis and dermis
III	Full-thickness skin loss Does not extend through fascia
IV	Full-thickness skin loss with extensive destruction Damage through the fascia, often involving the muscle and bone Sinus tracts are common

QUESTION

A 40-year-old presents with second and third degree burns to the upper right extremity and anterior trunk. What is the percent of body surface area covered by the burns?

A. 18
B. 27
C. 36
D. 45

i. Classic finding is a double comedone, a blackhead with two or more surface openings that communicate under the skin.
ii. Disease will progress with development of deep, dermal inflammation and development of large, painful abscesses.
iii. Disease onset typically in second and third decades of life.
c. Diagnosis
  i. Based on history and clinical findings.
d. Treatment
  i. Large cysts should be incised and drained.
  ii. Small cysts can be injected with triamcinolone acetonide.
  iii. Antibiotics are the mainstay of therapy.
    1. Long-term therapy with tetracycline, erythromycin, doxycycline, or minocycline.
  iv. Isotretinoin may be effective in selected area.
V. Lipomas
  a. General
    i. Subcutaneous tumors of adipose tissue.
  b. Clinical manifestations
    i. Typically located on the trunk, neck, and proximal limbs.
    ii. Soft, symmetric, and easily movable over deeper structures.
    iii. May be single or multiple and vary in size.
  c. Diagnosis
    i. Based on clinical findings.
  d. Treatment
    i. If a cosmetic defect is evident, lipomas may be surgically removed.

NOTES

ANSWER **B** EXPLANATION: *Using the rule of nines, burns to the upper right extremity (9%) and anterior trunk (18%) is equal to a body surface area of 27%.*

correct ☐   incorrect ☐

VI. Melasma
  a. General
    i. Acquired brown pigmentation of the face and neck.
    ii. More common in women with darker skin tones.
    iii. Occurs during the second and third trimester of pregnancy or on oral contraceptives.
  b. Clinical manifestations
    i. More common on the forehead, malar eminences, upper lip, and chin.
    ii. Symmetric macular eruption of brown hyperpigmentation is noted.
  c. Diagnosis
    i. Based on clinical findings.
  d. Treatment
    i. Will fade after pregnancy or stopping oral contraceptives.
    ii. Avoid sun exposure; sunscreens are recommended.
    iii. Bleaching creams can be used.
VII. Urticaria (hives)
  a. General
    i. Divided into acute, chronic, and physical.
    ii. Acute
      1. Last less than 6 weeks.
      2. More common in atopic individuals.
      3. Due to histamine release mediated by IgE.
    iii. Chronic
      1. Last longer than 6 weeks.
      2. Patients should be evaluated for the five I's:
        (a) Ingestants: foods, additives, antibiotics
        (b) Inhalants: dust, pollen
        (c) Injectants: drugs, stings, bites
        (d) Infections: bacterial, viral, fungal, parasitic
        (e) Internal disease: chronic infections, SLE, thyroid disease
    iv. Physical
      1. Brief attack of urticaria induced by physical stimuli.
      2. Most attacks last 1 to 6 hours.
      3. Types
        (a) Dermatographism: produced by rubbing or stroking of skin.
        (b) Pressure: due to pressure from walking, standing, or wearing tight garments.
        (c) Cholinergic: due to overheating from exercise.
        (d) Cold: due to sudden drop in air temperature or exposure to cold water.
        (e) Solar: due to exposure to ultraviolet light.
  b. Clinical manifestations
    i. Pruritus is very common.
    ii. Plaques are pink, red, or flesh colored, nonpitting, and edematous.
    iii. Vary in size from a few millimeters to several centimeters.
    iv. Linear lesions suggest physical urticaria.
    v. As old lesions resolve, new lesions appear.
  c. Diagnosis
    i. Based on clinical findings.
  d. Treatment
    i. All suspected triggers should be avoided.
    ii. Antihistamines are used initially.
      1. Histamine-1 blockers such as hydroxyzine work best.
      2. Nonsedating histamine-1 blockers, such as loratadine and cetirizine, do not work as well.
    iii. Prednisone is used in cases not controlled by antihistamines.
      1. Prednisone may not be helpful in chronic urticaria.
    iv. Epinephrine is used in extensive, severe cases.
VIII. Vitiligo
  a. General
    i. A depigmenting disease due to destruction of melanocytes.
    ii. Typically note first episode after an emotional stress, illness, or skin trauma.

NOTES

b. Clinical manifestations
   i. There are two types.
      1. Type A
         (a) Fairly symmetric pattern of white, depigmented, 0.5- to 5.0-cm macules and patches.
         (b) Common locations include dorsal hands, fingers, face, body folds, axillae, and genitalia.
      2. Type B
         (a) Limited to one segment of the body.
c. Diagnosis
   i. Biopsy of lesion shows absence of melanocytes.
d. Treatment
   i. Broad-spectrum sunscreens are needed.
   ii. Limited disease can be treated with topical steroids.
   iii. Concealing agents can hide lesions.

IX. Medications
   a. Oral corticosteroids
      i. See Table 11-8.
   b. Topical steroids

Table 11-8 • Oral Corticosteroids Comparison

Generic Name	Equivalent Dose (mg)
Cortisone	25
Cortisol	20
Prednisolone	5
Prednisone	
Triamcinolone	4
Methylprednisolone	4
Dexamethasone	0.75
Betamethasone	0.60

      i. See Table 11-9.

Table 11-9 • Topical Steroids

Group	Generic	Percentage
I (Super)	Clobetasol propionate	0.05
	Halobetasol propionate	0.05
II (High)	Betamethasone dipropionate	0.05
	Halcinonide	0.1
	Fluocinonide	0.05
III (Medium)	Betamethasone dipropionate	0.05
	Triamcinolone acetonide	0.5
	Amcinonide	0.1
IV (Medium)	Triamcinolone acetonide	0.1
	Mometasone furoate	0.1
	Hydrocortisone	0.2
V (Medium)	Triamcinolone acetonide	0.1
	Desonide	0.05
	Hydrocortisone butyrate	0.1
	Fluocinolone acetonide	0.025
	Hydrocortisone valerate	0.2

(continued)

NOTES

Table 11-9 • Topical Steroids—cont'd		
Group	**Generic**	**Percentage**
VI (Low)	Prednicarbate	0.05
	Triamcinolone acetonide	0.025
	Fluocinolone acetonide	0.01
VII (Low)	Hydrocortisone acetate	1.0
	Hydrocortisone	1.0

Question 1

Which of the following best describes the rash of pityriasis rosea?

A. Salmon colored oval plaques
B. Purple colored flat papules
C. Clear fluid filled vesicles
D. Red, raised scales

Question 2

A 16-year-old wrestler presents with three, round, scaly papules that have raised borders. Which of the following laboratory tests would assist in making the correct diagnosis?

A. Tzank smear
B. Gram stain
C. KOH prep
D. Wright's stain

Question 3

On physical examination of a 21-year-old male the physician assistant notes a cluster of verrucous lesions on the corona of the penis. Which of the following is the most likely diagnosis?

A. Condyloma acuminata
B. Candidiasis balanitis
C. Syphilitic chancre
D. Herpes genitalis

Question 4

Which of the following is the best treatment option for a patient with stage I melanoma?

A. Radiation therapy
B. Surgical excision
C. SQ vincristine
D. IV alpha interferon

NOTES

Question 5

A 20-year-old patient presents with sever itching between their fingers. On physical examination linear elevated vesicles are noted on the finger webs. Which of the following is the treatment of choice for this patient?

    A. Minocycline (Minocin)
    B. Fluconazole (Diflucan)
    C. Mebendazole (Vermox)
    D. Permethrin (Elimite)

Question 6

Which of the following laboratory tests must be monitored in patients on isotretinoin (Accutane)?

    A. Serum potassium
    B. Serum triglycerides
    C. Serum calcium
    D. Serum carotene

Question 7

Stevens-Johnson syndrome is most commonly linked to exposure of which of the following medications?

    A. Levofloxacin (Levaquin)
    B. Glucophage (Metformin)
    C. Phenytoin (Dilantin)
    D. Amiodarone (Cordarone)

Answer 1

ANSWER **A** EXPLANATION: *Pityriasis rosea lesions are described as salmon colored oval plaques, a-2 cm in diameter, with fine scales at the periphery. Multiple smaller lesions on the trunk give a Christmas tree pattern.*

Topic: Pityriasis rosea

correct ❑   incorrect ❑

Answer 2

ANSWER **C** EXPLANATION: *Tinea corporis, dermatophyte infection of the body, is common among wrestlers, and present as flat, scaly papules that develop a raised border with the center becoming brown or hypopigmented. Diagnosis is made by noting the presence of hyphae on KOH prep.*

Topic: Tinea corporis

correct ❑   incorrect ❑

Answer 3

ANSWER **A** EXPLANATION: *Condyloma acuminatum, or venereal warts, presentation varies from pale to white, rough barely raised papules to large raised lesions on a broad base.*

Topic: Condyloma acuminatum

correct ❑   incorrect ❑

NOTES

Answer 4

ANSWER **B** EXPLANATION: *Melanoma, malignancy of the melanocytes, treatment varies with the stage. Stage I is treated with surgical excision and stage II-IV are treated with both surgical intervention and high-dose interferon.*

Topic: Melanoma

correct ❑   incorrect ❑

Answer 6

ANSWER **B** EXPLANATION: *Isotretinoin (Accutane) is used to treat acne. Isotretinoin is a potent teratogen and induces elevated triglycerides. Triglyceride level should be monitored.*

Topic: Acne vulgaris

correct ❑   incorrect ❑

Answer 5

ANSWER **D** EXPLANATION: *Scabies, caused by Sarcoptes scabiei, presents with sever itching that is worse at night. The classic lesion is a burrow that is linear, curved, or S-shaped, slightly elevated vesicle or papule. Typically found in the finger webs, wrists, penis, buttocks, and scrotum.*

Topic: Scabies

correct ❑   incorrect ❑

Answer 7

ANSWER **C** EXPLANATION: *Stevens-Johnson syndrome, a desquamation syndrome, is associated with Mycoplasma pneumoniae infection and medications, such as phenytoin, phenobarbital, sulfonamides, and aminopenicillins.*

Topic: Stevens-Johnson syndrome

correct ❑   incorrect ❑

NOTES

The Hematologic System

12

EXAM BLUEPRINT TOPICS

Anemia
Iron deficiency anemia
Thalassemia
Sideroblastic anemia
Vitamin B_{12} deficiency
Folate deficiency
Anemia of chronic disease
Hemolytic anemia
Aplastic anemia
Malignancies
Acute lymphocytic leukemia (ALL)
Chronic lymphocytic leukemia (CLL)
Acute myelogenous leukemia (AML)
Chronic myelogenous leukemia (CML)
Hairy cell leukemia
Lymphoma
Multiple myeloma
Coagulation Disorders
Factor VIII disorder
Factor IX disorder
Factor XI disorder
Thrombocytopenia
  • Idiopathic thrombocytopenic purpura (ITP)
  • Thrombotic thrombocytopenic purpura (TTP)
  • Von Willebrand's disease
  • Disseminated intravascular coagulation

ANEMIA

I. Definition
  a. Any condition resulting from a significant decrease in the total erythrocyte mass.
  b. A hemoglobin of less than 12 g/dL in females and less than 14 g/dL in males or a hematocrit of less than 36% in females and less than 42% in males.

II. Erythropoiesis
  a. Definition
    i. A series of events during which the hematopoietic cells mature into functional blood cells.
  b. Controlled by many different factors, including erythropoietin, granulocyte colony-stimulating factor, granulocyte-macrophage colony-stimulating factor, and cytokines such as interleukin-3 and interleukin-5.
  c. Normal red blood cell
    i. Biconcave disk with a life span of about 120 days.
  d. Reticulocyte
    i. A cell that remains after the nucleus is lost from an orthochromic normoblast.
    ii. Contains RNA and other cellular remnants that stain blue with methylene blue stain.
    iii. Reticulocyte index or corrected reticulocyte count
      1. Used to correct for degree of anemia.
      2. Formula (see Fig. 12-1)
    iv. Normal range, 1% to 2% or an absolute reticulocyte count of 50,000 to 60,000/μL.
    v. Interpretation
      1. Elevated reticulocyte count and index in anemia secondary to increased destruction of red blood cells.
      2. Decreased reticulocyte count and index in anemia secondary to decreased production of red blood cells.

III. Clinical signs and symptoms of anemia
  a. Due to decreased oxygen transport
    • Fatigue
    • Dyspnea
    • Angina
  b. Due to decreased blood volume
    • Pallor
    • Postural hypotension

NOTES

$$\text{Observed reticulocyte count (\%)} \times \frac{\text{Patient's Hematocrit}}{\text{Normal Hematocrit}} = \text{Reticulocyte Index}$$

Figure 12-1 Formula for reticulocyte index.

- Syncope
- Headache
- Tinnitus
 c. Due to increased cardiac output
   - Tachycardia
   - Systolic ejection heart murmur
   - Lightheadedness
 d. Due to hemolysis of red blood cells
   - Jaundice
   - Splenomegaly
IV. Classification
 a. Cytochromic classification
   i. Microcytic (mean corpuscular volume [MCV] < 80 fL)
      1. Iron deficiency anemia
      2. Thalassemia
      3. Anemia of chronic disease
      4. Lead poisoning
      5. Sideroblastic anemia
   ii. Normocytic (MCV = 80–100 fL)
      1. Anemia of chronic disease
      2. Hemolytic anemia
      3. Anemia of acute hemorrhage
      4. Aplastic anemia
   iii. Macrocytic (MCV > 100 fL)
      1. Vitamin B_{12} deficiency
      2. Folate deficiency
V. Normal ranges
 a. See Table 12-1.
VI. Anemia flowchart (see Fig. 12-2)
VII. Iron deficiency anemia
 a. Normal iron metabolism
   i. Daily intake and loss are small, unless increased blood loss with bleeding or hemolysis of red blood cells.
   ii. Absorption occurs mainly in the duodenum and upper jejunum.
   iii. Transported by transferrin and stored as ferritin.
 b. Etiologies
   i. Blood loss
      1. Gastrointestinal (GI), menstruation, pulmonary, or urinary sources.
      2. Evaluate for GI blood loss in males with iron deficiency.
   ii. Increased iron demand
      1. Due to pregnancy, lactation, and rapid growth and development.

Table 12-1 • Normal Ranges	Male	Female
White blood cell count	5,000–10,000/µL	5,000–10,000/µL
Red blood cell count	$4.5–5.9 \times 10^6$/µL	$4.1–5.1 \times 10^6$/µL
Hemoglobin	14–16 g/dL	12–14 g/dL
Hematocrit	42%–52%	36%–48%
Mean corpuscular volume (MCV)	80–100 fL	80–100 fL
Mean corpuscular hemoglobin (MCH)	28–33 pg	28–33 pg
Mean corpuscular hemoglobin concentration (MCHC)	32–36 g/dL	32–36 g/dL
Platelet count	150,000–450,000/µL	150,000–450,000/µL

NOTES

iii. Malabsorption
  1. Due to gastrectomy, pancreatic insufficiency, sprue, or short bowel syndrome.
iv. Poor dietary intake
v. Hemolysis
c. Signs and symptoms
  i. See signs and symptoms above.
  ii. Pica syndrome
  iii. Angular stomatitis and atrophy of tongue mucosa secondary to impaired epithelial function.
  iv. Spooning or curling of nails (koilonychia).
d. Laboratory features
  i. Cell morphology
    1. Typically microcytic, hypochromic.

QUESTION

Which of the following is a possible etiology for a macrocytic anemia?

A. Iron deficiency
B. Sickle cell anemia
C. Vitamin B12 deficiency
D. Hereditary spherocytosis

      (a) Will vary with degree of iron deficiency
      (b) See Color Plate 16.
  ii. Iron studies
    1. See Table 12-2.

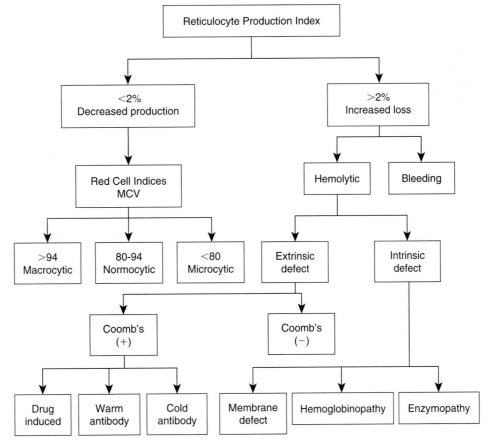

Figure 12-2 Anemia flowchart.

NOTES

ANSWER C Explanation: *Both vitamin B12 and folate deficiency are causes of macrocytic anemia. Iron deficiency is microcytic and sickle cell and hereditary spherocytosis are normocytic.*

correct ☐   incorrect ☐

e. Therapy
  i. Identify and correct underlying cause.
  ii. Transfusion
    1. Reserved for those with cardio-vascular instability, with continued blood loss, or in need of immediate intervention.
  iii. Iron therapy
    1. Oral
      (a) Treat with 300 mg of elemental iron per day.
        (i) Ferrous sulfate 325 mg, PO tid
      (b) Complications include GI distress, such as abdominal pain, nausea, vomiting, or constipation.
      (c) Monitor response to therapy with noting increased reticulocyte count in 7 to 10 days and increase in hemoglobin/hematocrit in 2 to 3 weeks.
      (d) If patient fails to respond to treatment, evaluate for possible patient noncompliance, incorrect diagnosis (thalassemia), poor absorption, erythropoietin deficiency, or other concurrent anemia.
    2. Parenteral
      (a) Used in those unable to tolerate oral therapy.
      (b) Major complication is anaphylaxis.

VIII. Thalassemia
  a. Etiology
    i. A group of hereditary disorders in which there is a defect in the synthesis of one or more of the globin polypeptide chains in hemoglobin.
      1. Mature adult hemoglobin is a tetramer of two alpha-chains and two beta-chains.
      2. If ratio is not right, hemoglobin may precipitate out in the red blood cell.
    ii. Leads to absent or decreased synthesis of the affected globin chain and development of nonfunctioning hemoglobin.
    iii. Primarily affects people of Mediterranean, African, or Asian ancestry.
      1. Especially common where malaria is endemic.
  b. Types
    i. Alpha-thalassemia
      1. Defect in the alpha-chain synthesis, results in excess of beta-chains.
      2. Four types
        (a) Silent carrier
          (i) Deletion of one alpha gene.

Table 12-2 • Comparison of Iron Studies in Various Disorders

	Total Serum Iron (µg/dL)	Total Iron Binding Capacity (µg/dL)	Percentage Saturation	Ferritin (µg/L)	Bone Marrow Iron Stores
Normal	50–150	300–360	30–50	50–200	Normal
Iron deficiency anemia	<30	>360	<10	<15	Decreased
Inflammation	<50	<300	10–20	Normal	Normal
Thalassemia	Normal	Normal	30–80	50–300	Normal
Sideroblastic anemia	Normal to high	Normal	30–80	50–300	Increased

NOTES

(b) Alpha-thalassemia trait
  (i) Deletion of two alpha genes.
  (ii) Mild anemia
(c) Hemoglobin H
  (i) Deletion of three alpha genes.
  (ii) Severe anemia with signs of hemolysis
(d) Hydrops fetalis
  (i) Deletion of all four alpha genes.
  (ii) Leads to death in utero

ii. Beta-thalassemia
1. Defect in the beta-chain synthesis, results in excess alpha-chains.
2. Two types
  (a) Beta-thalassemia minor
    (i) Microcytic anemia
  (b) Beta-thalassemia major (Cooley's anemia)
    (i) Severe anemia with bone changes
    (ii) Copper-colored skin
    (iii) Jaundice and hepatosplenomegaly

c. Laboratory features
  i. Microcytic, hypochromic red blood cells
    1. Target and teardrop cells are common on microscopic evaluation of the blood.
  ii. MCV is low, typically less than 75 fL.
  iii. Normal iron studies
  iv. Hemoglobin electrophoresis is diagnostic.

d. Therapy
  i. Transfuse as needed.
    1. Watch for iron overload with multiple transfusions.
  ii. Commonly misdiagnosed as iron deficiency anemia and treated with iron supplements.
    1. Can lead to iron overload.
  iii. Splenectomy may be needed in beta-thalassemia major and hemoglobin H disease.
  iv. Genetic counseling should be done with all patients diagnosed with thalassemia.

IX. Sideroblastic anemia
  a. Etiology
    i. Due to a mitochondrial defect that prevents the incorporation of iron into hemoglobin.

ii. Iron then accumulates in the mitochondria around the red blood cell nucleus forming a ringed sideroblast.

b. Classification
  i. Acquired
    1. Secondary to prolonged exposure to toxins or drugs
      (a) Seen with ethanol, lead, and isoniazid.
    2. Seen typically in patients older than 65 years
  ii. Hereditary
    1. X-linked recessive
    2. Seen in both men and women, typically diagnosed during first three decades of life.
  iii. Idiopathic
    1. A type of myelodysplastic syndrome.

c. Laboratory features
  i. Blood smear
    1. Dimorphic cell population, microcytic, hypochromia with normocytic or macrocytic cells.
  ii. Mild anemia with increased serum iron and ferritin. Total iron-binding capacity (TIBC) is normal or decreased, and transferrin is decreased.
  iii. Low reticulocyte count.
  iv. Bone marrow
    1. Ringed sideroblasts noted on bone marrow exam when stained with Prussian blue stain.

d. Therapy
  i. Treat the underlying cause.

NOTES

    ii. Red blood cell transfusions for severe anemia.
      1. May require an iron-chelating agent (desferrioxamine) after numerous transfusions to avoid iron overload.

X. Vitamin B_{12} deficiency
  a. Normal vitamin B_{12} metabolism
    i. Vitamin B_{12} needed for normal nuclear maturation and DNA synthesis. Leads to slow cell division.
    ii. Obtained only through dietary sources, such as meats, cheese, milk, and eggs.
    iii. Absorbed in terminal ileum and stored in the liver.
      1. Liver stores will last for years.
  b. Etiologies
    i. Decreased intake of vitamin B_{12}
      1. Seen in strict vegetarians.
    ii. Impaired absorption of vitamin B_{12}
      1. Lack of intrinsic factor or autoimmune destruction of parietal cells (pernicious anemia).
        (a) Pernicious anemia also associated with other autoimmune disorders such as Graves' disease, thyroiditis, and adrenal insufficiency.
      2. Malabsorption in patients with sprue or inflammatory bowel disease.
      3. Competitive absorption problem due to bacterial overgrowth or fish tapeworm (*Diphyllobothrium latum*)
    iii. Increased requirement for vitamin B_{12}
      1. Uncommon because of large stores of vitamin B_{12}, but can be seen in pregnancy and patients with neoplastic disorders.
    iv. Impaired utilization of vitamin B_{12}
  c. Signs and symptoms
    i. See anemia signs and symptoms above (section III)

    ii. Red, beefy tongue.
    iii. May have neurologic signs and symptoms such as:
      1. Loss of memory
      2. Paresthesia and numbness in the extremities.
        (a) This is the earliest neurologic sign.
      3. Diminished position or vibratory sense.
      4. Weakness and ataxia
  d. Laboratory features
    i. Red blood cells macrocytic (MCV >110 fL) and oval in shape.
      1. See Color Plate 17.
    ii. White blood cells are hypersegmented with more than five lobes.
    iii. Platelets are large and decreased in number.
    iv. Low reticulocyte count.
    v. Decreased serum vitamin B_{12} levels (<200 pg/mL).
      1. Values less than 100 indicate significant deficiency.
    vi. Schilling's test
      1. Interpretation
        (a) See Table 12-3.
    vii. Anti-intrinsic factor antibody or antiparietal cell antibodies may be present in pernicious anemia.
  e. Therapy
    i. Treat underlying cause.
    ii. Parenteral vitamin B_{12} for life.
    iii. Monitor response by checking for increase in reticulocyte count in 7 days.
    iv. Neurologic symptoms may not resolve.

Table 12-3 • Interpretation of Schilling Test

Condition	^{57}Co-labeled vitamin B_{12} without intrinsic factor	^{57}Co-labeled vitamin B_{12} with intrinsic factor
Normal	≥8%	≥8%
Pernicious anemia	Decreased	Corrected
Vitamin B_{12} malabsorption	Decreased	Not corrected

NOTES

v. Pernicious anemia patients at increased risk for gastric cancer.

XI. Folate deficiency
  a. Normal folate metabolism
    i. Folate is needed for synthesis of nuclear proteins.
      1. Vitamin B_{12} is a required cofactor for folate metabolism.
    ii. Obtained through dietary sources, such as green leafy vegetables, liver, and eggs.
    iii. Absorbed in proximal jejunum and stored in the liver.
      1. Liver stores last only a few months.
  b. Etiologies
    i. Decreased intake of folate
      1. Seen in patients with poor diets and alcoholism.
    ii. Impaired absorption of folate
      1. Due to intestinal bypass surgery, malabsorption syndromes, and phenytoin (Dilantin) use.
    iii. Increased requirement for folate
      1. Seen in pregnancy, children, hyperthyroidism, and neoplasia.
    iv. Impaired utilization
      1. Seen with folate antagonists such as trimethoprim-sulfamethoxazole (Bactrim).
      2. Alcohol impairs utilization of folate in the bone marrow.
  c. Signs and symptoms
    i. Same signs and symptoms as vitamin B_{12} deficiency **EXCEPT** no neurologic abnormalities.
    ii. Also note diarrhea, cheilosis, and glossitis.
  d. Laboratory features
    i. Macrocytic (MCV >100 fL) red blood cells.
    ii. Hypersegmented neutrophils.
    iii. Platelets are large and decreased in number.
    iv. Low reticulocyte count.
    v. Serum and red blood cell folate levels are low (≤4 ng/mL).
  e. Therapy
    i. Treat with replacement therapy.
      1. Folate, 1–5 mg/day PO.
    ii. Monitor response by checking for increase in reticulocyte count in 7 days.

QUESTION

Which of the following is decreased in pernicious anemia?

  A. Intrinsic factor
  B. Pyruvate kinase
  C. Hemoglobin F
  D. Iron

XII. Anemia of chronic disease
  a. Etiology
    i. Most common cause of anemia in the hospitalized or chronically ill patient.
    ii. Seen in patients with chronic:
      1. Infection
      2. Inflammatory disease
      3. Malignancy
      4. Renal disease
  b. Signs and symptoms
    i. Same as anemia listed above (see section III).
    ii. Will also have the signs and symptoms of the underlying cause.
  c. Laboratory features
    i. Red blood cells are normocytic, normochromic or microcytic, hypochromic.
    ii. Decreased reticulocyte count.
    iii. Increased erythrocyte sedimentation rate (ESR).
    iv. Decreased serum iron but normal or increased serum ferritin.
  d. Therapy
    i. Treat underlying cause.
    ii. Erythropoietin may be helpful.
XIII. Hemolytic anemia
  a. General
    i. Only a hemolytic process or acute blood loss will cause the hemoglobin to drop greater than 1 g per week.
    ii. The red blood cell has three components that may be involved in a hemolytic process.
      1. Metabolic machinery (enzymes)
      2. Hemoglobin
      3. Red cell membrane
    iii. Reticulocyte count is elevated in hemolytic anemia.

NOTES

ANSWER **A** EXPLANATION: *Pernicious anemia is due to lack of intrinsic factor.*

correct ❑   incorrect ❑

b. Etiology
   i. Acquired hemolytic anemia
   ii. Congential hemolytic anemia
      1. Membrane abnormalities
      2. Hemoglobinopathies
      3. Enzyme deficiency
c. Signs and symptoms
   i. Splenomegaly and jaundice are common on physical exam.
   ii. Laboratory features
      1. In general may note:
         (a) Increased lactate dehydrogenase (LDH)
         (b) Hemoglobinuria
         (c) Increased indirect bilirubin
         (d) Decreased haptoglobin in intravascular hemolysis.
            (i) Haptoglobin is a protein that binds free hemoglobin in the bloodstream.
         (e) Blood smear may show spherocytes, schistocytes, or helmet cells.
      2. Coombs' test
         (a) Direct
            (i) Detects antibody on red blood cell surface
               (1) Used in the evaluation of acquired hemolytic anemia.
               (2) Detects anti–immunoglobulin (IgG or IgM) or anticomplement (C3).
         (b) Indirect
            (i) Detects antibody in the plasma.
            (ii) Used in the cross-matching of blood products.
d. Specific hemolytic disorders
   i. Acquired hemolytic anemia
      1. Distinguished by results of the Coombs' test.
      2. Coombs' negative
         (a) Hypersplenism

(i) Have increased removal of cellular elements by the spleen.
(ii) Causes:
   (1) Primary (idiopathic)
   (2) Secondary
      [a] Acute/chronic infections
         [i] Malaria, tuberculosis, hepatitis
      [b] Chronic inflammatory disease
         [i] Systemic lupus erythematosus (SLE), sarcoidosis
      [c] Congestive splenomegaly
      [d] Myeloproliferative disorders
      [e] Leukemia/lymphoma
(iii) Diagnosed by demonstrating shortened red cell survival and splenic sequestration.
(iv) Treat underlying cause or splenectomy.
(b) Microangiopathic
   (i) Mechanical disruption of the red blood cells.
   (ii) Must see schistocytes on peripheral blood smear.
   (iii) Seen with disseminated intravascular coagulation (DIC), thrombotic thrombocytopenic purpura (TTP), hemolytic-uremic syndrome (HUS), and traumatic cardiac hemolysis with artifical heart valves.
(c) Chemical
   (i) Seen with lead poisoning and fresh-water drowning.
(d) Physical
   (i) Seen with burns over greater than 20% of body.
(e) Infectious
   (i) Common with malaria, viral infections such as parvovirus B19, and *Clostridium welchii* infection.

NOTES

3. Coombs' positive
    (a) Drug-induced
        (i) Three mechanisms
            (1) Hapten type
                [a] Coombs' positive for anti-IgG
            (2) Immune complex
                [a] Coombs' positive for C3.
            (3) Autoantibody
                [a] Coombs' positive for anti-IgG.
                [b] May last for months even after stopping medications.
        (ii) See Table 12-4.
        (iii) Treatment
            (1) Stop drugs
            (2) Autoantibody type may need treatment with steroids.
    (b) Warm autoantibody
        (i) Usually IgG antibody.
        (ii) Primary (idiopathic) or secondary due to tumor infection or autoimmune disorder (SLE).
        (iii) Treat with steroids and splenectomy.
    (c) Cold autoantibody
        (i) Usually IgM antibody.
        (ii) Causes intravascular hemolysis.
        (iii) Cold agglutinins secondary to viral or mycoplasmal infection.
            (1) May have elevated mean corpuscular hemoglobin concentration (MCHC; >36 g/dL).
        (iv) Poor response to steroids

Table 12-4 • Summary of Drug-Induced Hemolytic Anemias

Mechanism	Hapten	Immune Complex	Autoantibody
Example	Penicillin	Quinidine	Methyldopa
Coombs' test	Positive	Positive	Positive
Anti-IgG	Positive	Rarely positive	Positive
Anti-C3d	Rarely positive	Positive	Negative
Drugs	Cephalothin Ampicillin Methicillin	Hydrochlorothiazide Antihistamines Rifampin Isoniazid Sulfonamides Insulin Tylenol	L-Dopa Ibuprofen Diclofenac Interferon-alpha

NOTES

ANSWER C EXPLANATION: *Evaluation of the thalassemias includes hemoglobin electrophoresis to detect the presence of abnormal hemoglobins.*

correct ❏   incorrect ❏

ii. Congenital hemolytic anemia
  1. Membrane abnormalities
    (a) Hereditary spherocytosis
      (i) Autosomal dominant disorder
      (ii) Most common congenital hemolytic anemia in the white population.
      (iii) Features include splenomegaly and numerous spherocytes on peripheral smear.
      (iv) Will have a positive osmotic fragility test.
      (v) Treatment includes splenectomy if indicated and folic acid to decrease risk for folate deficiency.
    (b) Hereditary elliptocytosis
      (i) Autosomal dominant disorder.
      (ii) Present with 40% to 60% elliptocytes on peripheral smear.
      (iii) Treatment, if needed, is splenectomy.
  2. Enzyme deficiency
    (a) Glucose-6-phosphate dehydrogenase (G6PD) deficiency
      (i) Sex-linked disorder
        (1) Commonly of African or Mediterranean descent.
      (ii) Defect in hexose-monophosphate shunt.
      (iii) Hemolysis is intravascular (red blood cell lysis secondary to stress) and extravascular (red blood cells age prematurely).
      (iv) Due to stress-induced hemolysis secondary to sulfonamides, antimalarials, vitamin K, infection, or fava beans.
      (v) Labs include hemoglobinuria, decreased G6PD activity level, and may note Heinz bodies on peripheral smear.
        (1) Heinz bodies are due to oxidation of hemoglobin.
      (vi) Treatment
        (1) Avoid medications that stress red blood cells.
        (2) Folate supplements.
    (b) Pyruvate kinase deficiency
      (i) Very rare disorder, commonly seen in children.
      (ii) Defect in Embden-Meyerhof pathway.
      (iii) Present with anemia, jaundice, and splenomegaly.
      (iv) Diagnose by checking enzyme activity.
      (v) Treatment
        (1) Transfusion as needed.
        (2) Folate supplement.
  3. Hemoglobinopathies
    (a) Sickle cell anemia
      (i) Inherited disorder resulting in production of defective hemoglobin.
        (1) Decreased solubility in deoxygenated form; this leads to sickling.
      (ii) Defect in position 6 on the beta-chain.
      (iii) Very common in African-American population (0.3%)
        (1) Homozygotes have sickle cell disease.
      (iv) Signs and symptoms
        (1) Anemia: pallor and fatigue
        (2) Hemolysis: jaundice and gallstones.
        (3) Dactylitis
        (4) Leg ulcers
        (5) Priapism
        (6) Pulmonary, cerebral, and splenic emboli
        (7) Retinal artery obstruction leading to blindness.
        (8) Sickle cell crisis

NOTES

[a] Skeletal pain
[b] Fever
[c] Anemia
[d] Jaundice
[e] Note: Look for infection as source of sickle cell crisis.
(v) Laboratory features
(1) Microcytic hypochromic or normocytic anemia
(2) Elevated reticulocyte count
(3) Sickle cells noted on peripheral blood smear.
[a] See Color Plate 18.
(4) Elevated bilirubin
(5) Hemoglobin electrophoresis
[a] Diagnostic with 100% HbS in sickle cell disease.
(vi) Treatment
(1) Avoid triggers
(2) Good nutrition
(3) Folic acid supplements
(4) Vaccines: *Haemophilus* and pneumococcal.
(5) Hydroxyurea as an antisickling agent.
(6) Crisis
[a] Pain control
[b] Transfusions
[c] Antibiotics for infection
(vii) Outcomes
(1) Survival depends on number of crises per year.
(b) Sickle cell trait
(i) Heterozygotes are carriers of sickle cell trait.
(ii) May have mild anemia and typically asymptomatic.
(iii) Laboratory features
(1) Hemoglobin electrophoresis
[a] 50% HbS in sickle cell carriers.
(c) Hemoglobin SC disease
(i) Patient has milder symptoms than with sickle cell disease.

QUESTION

Which of the following can lead to a microangiopathic hemolytic anemia?

A. Hypersplenism
B. Lead poisoning
C. Mycoplasma infection
D. Hemolytic-uremic syndrome

(ii) Retinopathy and splenomegaly are noted.
(iii) Hemoglobin C crystals and marked target cells on peripheral smear.
(d) Hemoglobin C disease
(i) Mild to moderate anemia.
(ii) Note hemoglobin crystals and target cells on peripheral smear.
(iii) Diagnose with hemoglobin electrophoresis.
XIV. Aplastic anemia
a. General
i. Pancytopenia with bone marrow hypocellularity.
b. Etiologies
i. Acquired
1. Idiopathic
2. Radiation
3. Chemicals such as benzene
4. Drugs such as chemotherapy agents, chloramphenicol, heavy metals, and insecticides.
5. Viruses such as hepatitis and parvovirus B19.
6. Immune diseases
7. Paroxysmal nocturnal hemoglobinuria
(a) Rare acquired disorder.
(b) Clinical features include variable hemoglobinuria and pancytopenia.
(c) Laboratory features include increased reticulocytes and negative direct Coombs' test.
(d) Ham's test or sucrose lysis test is positive.

NOTES

ANSWER D EXPLANATION: *Microangiopathic hemolytic anemia can be due to disseminated intravascular coagulation, thrombotic thrombocytopenia purpura, hemolytic-uremic syndrome, and artifical heart valves.*

correct ☐   incorrect ☐

    ii. Inherited
       1. Fanconi's anemia
       2. Preleukemia
  c. Signs and symptoms
    i. Bleeding is common early in this disease.
    ii. Symptoms of anemia (see section III).
    iii. Patients typically look and feel well despite the pancytopenia.
  d. Laboratory features
    i. Bone marrow is hypocellular and fatty.
  e. Treatment
    i. Bone marrow transplantation
    ii. Immunosuppression

MALIGNANCIES

I. Acute lymphocytic leukemia (ALL)
  a. General
    i. Most common leukemia in childhood, uncommon in adults.
    ii. Immature lymphoblasts are produced with no further differentiation.
  b. Etiologies
    i. Radiation exposure linked to development of ALL.
  c. Signs and symptoms
    i. Abrupt onset of fatigue, malaise, bone pain, sweats, bleeding, and easy bruising.
    ii. Physical examination reveals pallor, petechiae, and ecchymoses.
  d. Laboratory features
    i. Pancytopenia develops secondary to marrow replacement by tumor cells.
    ii. Elevated white cell count in two thirds of patients.
    iii. Elevated uric acid and lactate dehydrogenase (LDH).
    iv. Increased blasts noted in bone marrow.
       1. 30% to 100% blasts.

    v. May have a t(9; 22) translocation (Philadelphia chromosome)
       1. Presence of this translocation indicates a poorer prognosis.
    vi. French American British (FAB) classification divides ALL into three types: L1, L2, and L3.
  e. Therapy
    i. Remission induction
       1. Chemotherapy
    ii. Postremission therapy
       1. Consolidation chemotherapy
    iii. Central nervous system (CNS) prophylaxis required
       1. Intrathecal methotrexate or brain radiation.
    iv. Bone marrow transplantation

II. Chronic lymphocytic leukemia (CLL)
  a. General
    i. An indolent lymphoproliferative disorder characterized by lymphocytosis, lymphadenopathy, and splenomegaly.
    ii. Most commonly seen in elderly men.
  b. Etiology
    i. Cause of CLL is unknown.
  c. Signs and symptoms
    i. Most patients are asymptomatic.
    ii. May present with fatigue, lethargy, weight loss, and decreased exercise tolerance.
    iii. Physical examination reveals enlarged lymph nodes, mainly cervical, and splenomegaly is rare until late in the disease.
  d. Laboratory features
    i. An absolute lymphocytosis in the peripheral blood.
       1. Absolute lymphocyte count greater than 15,000/μL.
       2. Smudge cells present.
    ii. Anemia and thrombocytopenia may be present.
  e. Therapy
    i. Chemotherapy
       1. Chlorambucil is first-line agent.
    ii. Radiation therapy
       1. Used for localized lymphadenopathy and splenomegaly that do not respond to chemotherapy.
    iii. Monoclonal antibodies
    iv. Bone marrow transplantation

NOTES

III. Acute myelogenous leukemia (AML)
  a. General
      i. Group of heterogenous disorders characterized by uncontrolled proliferation of primitive hematopoietic cells.
      ii. Increased incidence with age.
      iii. FAB classification
          1. M0, MI, M2, and M3 show increasing degree of differentiation of myeloid leukemic cells.
          2. M4 and M5 have features of monocytic cells.
          3. M6 has features of the erythroid cells.
          4. M7 is acute megakaryocyte leukemia.
  b. Etiologies
      i. Strong link to toxin exposure, such as benzene and carbon tetrachloride, and alkylating agents, such as melphalan and nitrosoureas.
      ii. Increased risk with ionizing radiation.
      iii. Increased risk with trisomy 21 (Down's syndrome).
  c. Signs and symptoms
      i. Abrupt onset of fatigue, malaise, bone pain, sweats, bleeding, easy bruisability, or signs of infection.
      ii. Physical examination reveals pallor, petechiae, and ecchymoses.
  d. Laboratory features
      i. 30% to 100% blasts noted in bone marrow.
          1. Auer rods present in blasts are virtually pathognomonic for AML.
      ii. Anemia and thrombocytopenia are present.
  e. Therapy
      i. Remission induction
          1. Chemotherapy with daunomycin and cytarabine.
          2. Watch for severe myelosuppression and infection.
      ii. Postremission therapy
          1. Intensive consolidation chemotherapy
          2. No CNS prophylaxis is needed.
      iii. Bone marrow transplantation
IV. Chronic myelogenous leukemia (CML)
  a. General
      i. A chronic myeloproliferative disorder characterized by excessive growth and development of differentiated cells.
      ii. Incidence of CML increases with age.
  b. Etiology
      i. No etiologic agent has been identified.
  c. Signs and symptoms
      i. Symptoms include fatigue, weight loss, night sweats, and malaise.
      ii. Physical examination reveals marked splenomegaly.
      iii. Lymphadenopathy is rare.
  d. Laboratory features
      i. Elevated white blood cell count with presence of complete cell line from blasts to mature neutrophils.
          1. Basophilia may be present.
      ii. Philadelphia (Ph[1]) chromosome is present in 95% of CML cases.
      iii. Increased uric acid noted in most patients.
          1. May lead to a gouty arthritis after treatment.
      iv. Low leukocyte alkaline phosphatase (LAP) score.
          1. This will assist in separating CML from leukemoid reaction.
  e. Therapy
      i. Based on age and phase of disease.
      ii. Hydroxyurea as a debulking agent to decrease white blood cell count.
      iii. Nontransplantation therapy
          1. Interferon-alpha
          2. Imatinib mesylate
      iv. Transplantation therapy
          1. Allogenic stem cell transplantation
V. Hairy cell leukemia
  a. General
      i. A chronic B-cell disorder.
      ii. More common in elderly people, with males affected more than females.
  b. Signs and symptoms
      i. May have hepatosplenomegaly.
      ii. Peripheral lymphadenopathy is rare.
  c. Laboratory features
      i. Pancytopenia is present.
      ii. Lymphocytes have hairlike, cytoplasmic projections.
  d. Therapy
      i. Splenectomy
      ii. 2-Chlorodeoxyadenosine (2-CDA) produces remission in 90% of cases.
VI. Lymphoma
  a. Hodgkin's lymphoma
      i. General

NOTES

1. Malignant disorder of the lymphatic system that mainly affects the lymph nodes.
2. Onset of disease has a bimodal distribution.
   (a) First peak in second and third decades of life.
   (b) Second peak after age 50 years.
3. More common in males and less common in African Americans.
4. Have contiguous spread from lymph node to lymph node, with a central distribution of affected nodes.

ii. Etiology
1. May be a link to Epstein-Barr virus.

iii. Signs and symptoms
1. Localized lymphadenopathy is common.
   (a) Lymph nodes are firm, freely mobile, and nontender.
2. Chronic pruritus may be seen.
3. May have a disulfiram-like reaction with alcohol ingestion.
4. May have fever, weight loss, and night sweats (B symptoms).
   (a) Presence of B symptoms is poor prognostic indicator.

iv. Laboratory features
1. Noting Reed-Sternberg cells in lymph node tissue makes diagnosis.
   (a) Reed-Sternberg cells are large, binucleated cells with prominent nucleoli.
2. Mild to moderate anemia may be present.
3. ESR is elevated.

v. Therapy
1. Staging of disease is very important for treatment and prognosis.
   (a) Staging should include lymph node biopsy, chest X-ray, computed tomography (CT) scan of chest and abdomen, complete blood count, ESR, and chemistry profile including liver function tests.
2. Treatment includes radiation therapy for localized disease and chemotherapy for advanced disease.
   (a) 85% curable with treatment.

b. Non-Hodgkin's lymphoma

i. General
1. Solid tumor of the immune system.
2. 90% are B cell in origin.

ii. Etiology
1. Unknown, although immune system abnormalities, infectious agents, and environmental and occupational exposure have been implicated.

iii. Signs and symptoms
1. Symptoms include chest pain, cough, superior vena cava syndrome, abdominal and back pain, and spinal cord compression.
   (a) Due to lymphadenopathy in the mediastinum or retroperitoneum.
2. May also present with fever, weight loss, and night sweats.
3. Most common presentation is lymphadenopathy.
   (a) Noted in the cervical, axillary, or inguinal region.
   (b) Nodes are firm and nontender, with size greater than 1 cm.

iv. Laboratory features
1. Biopsy results vary depending on type of non-Hodgkin's lymphoma.

v. Therapy
1. Surgical excision
2. Radiation therapy
3. Chemotherapy

VII. Multiple myeloma
a. General
   i. Neoplastic proliferation of a single clone of plasma cells (B cells).
   ii. Seen more commonly in patients older than 65 years.
   iii. Twice the incidence in African Americans compared with whites.
b. Etiology
   i. Cause is unclear, may be linked to organic solvents, herbicides, and insecticides.
c. Signs and symptoms
   i. Symptoms include bone pain (mainly in the back and chest), weakness, and fatigue.
   ii. May also develop symptoms due to development of acute infection, renal insufficiency, and hypercalcemia.
d. Laboratory features

NOTES

i. Normocytic, normochromic anemia
ii. Serum protein electrophoresis shows a peak or localized band.
   1. IgG M protein is most common.
   2. Light chain (Bence Jones protein).
iii. Increase in number of plasma cells.
iv. X-ray of bones reveals punched-out lytic lesions.
   1. Compression and pathologic fractures are common.
   2. See Figure 12-3.
v. Diagnostic criteria
   1. Bone marrow greater than 10% plasma cells or a plasmacytoma and one of the following:
      (a) M protein in the serum (usually > 3 g/dL).
      (b) M protein in the urine
      (c) Lytic bone lesions
e. Therapy
   i. Chemotherapy with melphalan and prednisone.
   ii. Autologous stem cell transplantation.
   iii. Patients are very prone to infection.
      1. Vaccinations and antibiotics may be required.

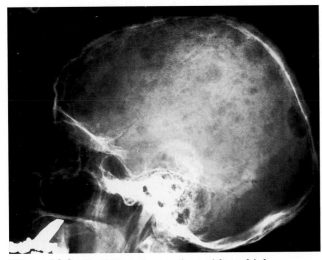

Figure 12-3 Skull X-ray in a patient with multiple myeloma. (From Mettler F. Essentials of Radiology, 2nd ed. Philadelphia: Elsevier Saunders, 2005:17, Fig. 2-3.)

QUESTION

Which of the following leukemia is a B-cell disorder that is more common in the elderly and on peripheral blood smear white blood cells are noted with long projections?

    A. Refractory anemia with excess blasts
    B. Chronic lymphocytic leukemia
    C. Acute lymphocytic leukemia
    D. Hairy cell leukemia

COAGULATION DISORDERS

I. Hemostasis
   a. See Figure 12-4 for coagulation cascade.
II. Factor VIII disorder
   a. General
      i. Hemophilia A is a deficiency in factor VIII (antihemophilic factor).
      ii. Sex-linked recessive disorder.
      iii. Seen in 1 per 5000 male births.
   b. Signs and symptoms
      i. Severity of signs and symptoms vary with circulating levels of the factor.
      ii. Delayed bleeding after trauma or surgery.
         1. Due to inability to stabilize platelet plug.
         2. May present with excessive bleeding at circumcision.
      iii. Hemarthroses are spontaneous or following trauma.
      iv. Retroperitoneal hematomas.
      v. CNS bleeds may occur without trauma.
   c. Laboratory features
      i. Prolonged partial thromboplastin time (PTT)
      ii. Prothrombin time (PT), platelet count, and bleeding time are normal.
      iii. Decreased activity level of factor VIII.
   d. Therapy
      i. Prevent trauma
      ii. Avoid aspirin and other antiplatelet medications.
      iii. Supplement coagulation factor
         1. Factor VIII concentrate

NOTES

ANSWER **D** EXPLANATION: *Hairy cell leukemia is a B-cell disorder and most common in the elderly. On peripheral blood smear the white blood cells have hair-like projections.*

correct ☐   incorrect ☐

2. Fresh frozen plasma or cryoprecipitate
    iv. Genetic counseling to family.
III. Factor IX disorder
  a. General
    i. Hemophilia B is a deficiency in factor IX (antihemophilic factor B or Christmas factor).
    ii. Sex-linked recessive disorder.
    iii. Seen in 1 per 30,000 male births.
  b. Signs and symptoms
    i. Signs and symptoms are no different than those seen in factor VIII deficiency.
    ii. Severity of signs and symptoms vary with circulating levels of the factor.
    iii. Delayed bleeding after trauma or surgery.
      1. Due to inability to stabilize platelet plug.

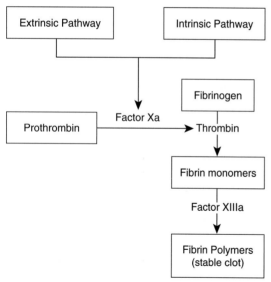

Figure 12-4 Coagulation cascade.

2. May present with excessive bleeding at circumcision.
    iv. Hemarthrosis are spontaneous or following trauma.
    v. Retroperitoneal hematomas.
    vi. CNS bleeds may occur without trauma.
  c. Laboratory features
    i. Prolonged PTT
    ii. Prothrombin time (PT), platelet count, and bleeding time are normal.
    iii. Decreased activity level of factor IX.
  d. Therapy
    i. Prevent trauma
    ii. Avoid aspirin and other antiplatelet medications.
    iii. Supplement coagulation factor
      1. Factor IX concentrate
      2. Fresh frozen plasma or cryoprecipitate
    iv. Genetic counseling to family.
IV. Factor XI disorder
  a. General
    i. Rare disorder but more common in Ashkenazi Jews.
    ii. Autosomal disorder, either recessive or dominant patterns noted.
    iii. Factor XI is a component of the contact phase of the coagulation system.
  b. Etiology
    i. Bleeding is not as severe as with factor VIII or IX deficiency.
  c. Signs and symptoms
    i. Spontaneous bleeding and hemarthroses are uncommon.
    ii. Patients undergoing basic surgery, such as tonsillectomy or dental extraction, are at high risk for bleeding unless replacement therapy is given.
  d. Laboratory features
    i. Prolonged PTT, normal PT, and decreased factor XI activity
  e. Therapy
    i. Fresh frozen plasma is the mainstay of treatment.
V. Thrombocytopenia
  a. Idiopathic thrombocytopenic purpura (ITP)
    i. General
      1. Autoimmune bleeding disorder in which patients develop antibodies against their own platelets.

ii. Etiology
   1. Childhood ITP is usually acute and follows a viral infection.
   2. In adults, onset is more gradual, without a preceding illness, and is chronic in course.
iii. Signs and symptoms
   1. No splenomegaly.
   2. Superficial bleeding of the skin, mucous membranes, and genitourinary tract.
iv. Laboratory features
   1. Decreased platelet count.
   2. Rule out pseudothrombocytopenia.
     (a) Pseudothrombocytopenia due to:
      • Artifact of automated cell counting
      • Platelet satellitism
   3. Check coagulation studies to rule out disseminated intravascular coagulation.
v. Therapy
   1. Acute disease is self-limited.
   2. Chronic disease will need high-dose steroids and possible splenectomy.
   3. Stop all drugs that may be worsening thrombocytopenia.
     (a) Drugs include trimethoprim-sulfamethoxazole, quinine, penicillins, furosemide, phenytoin, cimetidine, and many others.
b. Thrombotic thrombocytopenic purpura (TTP)
  i. General
   1. Characterized by severe thrombocytopenia, microangiopathic hemolytic anemia, and neurologic abnormalities.
   2. HUS, commonly seen in infants and children, is very similar to TTP.
     (a) Typically present with GI signs and symptoms, abdominal pain, and diarrhea.
     (b) Microangiopathic hemolytic anemia.
     (c) Thrombocytopenia is mild to moderate.
     (d) No neurologic abnormalities.
     (e) Acute renal failure is common.
     (f) Severe hypertension is seen.
  ii. Etiology
   1. Unknown etiology.

QUESTION

A 70-year-old male presents with anemia and a history of recurrent bacterial infections. Blood smear shows rouleaux and an elevated total protein is noted on the chemistry panel. Which of the following is the next best test in the evaluation of this patient?

A. Bone marrow biopsy
B. Serum protein electrophoresis
C. Flow cytometry studies
D. Cryoglobulin level

---

iii. Signs and symptoms
   1. Fever.
   2. Neurologic abnormalities, including headache, aphasia, or stupor.
iv. Laboratory features
   1. Thrombocytopenia
   2. Schistocytes on peripheral blood smear.
   3. Increased reticulocyte count.
   4. Increased LDH.
   5. Normal PT, PTT, and fibrinogen levels.
v. Therapy
   1. Large-volume plasmapheresis
c. Von Willebrand's disease
  i. General
   1. Von Willebrand protein normally binds to factor VIII, delivering it to sites of coagulation and preventing its clearance from the circulation.
   2. A platelet function disorder.
  ii. Etiology
   1. Absence of von Willebrand's factor (VWF) results in failure to form a primary platelet plug.
   2. Types
     (a) Type I: Autosomal dominant with a deficiency of VWF.
     (b) Type II: Autosomal dominant with defective VWF.
     (c) Type III: Autosomal recessive with complete absence of VWF.
iii. Signs and symptoms

NOTES

ANSWER **B** EXPLANATION: *Multiple myeloma, a plasma cell disorder, presents with an elevated serum total protein and rouleaux on the peripheral blood smear. Multiple myeloma is common in the elderly and patients have a history of recurrent bacterial infection, due to defective humoral immune system.*

correct ☐   incorrect ☐

    1. Symptoms include easy bruising and mucosal surface bleeding.
       (a) Symptoms may worsen with aspirin or nonsteroidal anti-inflammatory drug (NSAID) ingestion.
    2. Menorrhagia
    3. Hemarthrosis and retroperitoneal bleeding is rare, except in type III.
  iv. Laboratory features
    1. Prolonged bleeding time
    2. Prolonged PTT
       (a) Due to factor VIII deficiency.
  v. Therapy
    1. Administer factor VIII concentrates
    2. DDAVP a synthetic analog of antidiuretic hormone (ADH)

       (a) Induces the release of VWF.
  d. Disseminated intravascular coagulation
    i. General
      1. Condition in which coagulation factors are activated and degraded simultaneously.
      2. Patient will present with both bleeding and thrombosis.
    ii. Etiology
      1. Triggered by endothelial cell injury or release of tissue factors that activates the coagulation cascade.
       (a) See Figure 12-5.
      2. Can be caused by:
       (a) Obstetric complications
         (i) Amniotic fluid embolism
         (ii) Retained dead fetus
         (iii) Abruptio placentae
       (b) Transfusion reactions
       (c) Malignancy
         (i) Pancreatic carcinoma
         (ii) Adenocarcinoma
         (iii) Acute promyelocytic leukemia
       (d) Trauma
         (i) Brain injury
         (ii) Crush injury
         (iii) Burns

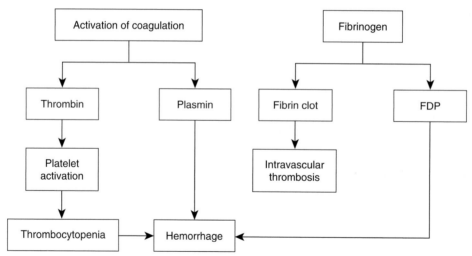

Figure 12-5 Pathogenesis of disseminated intravascular coagulation.

NOTES

(e) Infection or sepsis
 (i) Gram-negative bacteria
(f) Acute pancreatitis
(g) Adult respiratory distress syndrome (ARDS)
iii. Signs and symptoms
 1. Bleeding is the most common clinical finding.
  (a) Bleeding from skin and mucous membranes.
 2. May develop small purpuric to large ecchymoses.
 3. Thrombotic events include gangrenous digits and nose, and hemorrhagic necrosis of the skin.

iv. Laboratory features
 1. Prolonged PT, PTT, and thrombin time.
 2. Thrombocytopenia due to platelet consumption.
 3. Elevated fibrin degradation products (FDP) or D-dimer due to fibrinolysis that is occurring.
v. Therapy
 1. Must treat underlying cause of the DIC.
 2. Control major symptoms
  (a) For bleeding, give fresh frozen plasma and platelets.
  (b) For thrombosis, give intravenous (IV) heparin.

Question 1

A 67-year-old male presents with melena and weight loss. CBC reveals hemoglobin of 8.9 g/dl, hematocrit 27%, and an MCV 74 fl. Which related cardiac sign is most likely to be noted on physical examination?

A. Bradycardia
B. II/VI systolic murmur
C. Mid-systolic click
D. S4 gallop

Question 2

A 60-year-old presents with fatigue. On examination his tongue is red and fissured and decreased vibratory sensation is noted in the lower extremities. CBC reveals the following:

WBC- 8.1 x 10^9/L
Hgb- 10.1 g/dl
Hct- 31%
MCV- 124 fl
MCH- 40.4 pg
MCHC- 32.5%
Platelet- 160,000/μL

Examination of the blood smear reveals anisocytosis, poikilocytosis, and hypersegmented neutrophils. Which of the following tests would be helpful in the evaluation of this patient?

A. Direct Coombs test
B. Serum vitamin B12 level
C. Serum ferritin level
D. Erythrocyte sedimentation rate

NOTES

Question 3

A patient presents with thrombocytopenia, schisto-cytes, fever, and headache. Which of the following is the most likely diagnosis?

A. Von Willebrand's disease
B. Idiopathic thrombocytopenia purpura
C. Disseminated intravascular coagulation
D. Thrombotic thrombocytopenic purpura

Question 4

A 52-year-old male presents with a painless 3cm mass in his neck. He has also noted night sweats. Which of the following is the next best step in the evaluation of this patient?

A. Complete blood count
B. Erythrocyte sedimentation rate
C. Bone marrow biopsy
D. Lymph node biopsy

Question 5

A patient currently taking coumadin presents with spontaneous nosebleeds. Laboratory tests reveal a pro-time of 45 seconds and INR 6.9. Which of the following is the treatment of choice for this patient?

A. Heparin
B. Salicylate
C. Vitamin K
D. Protamine sulfate

Question 6

Which of the following tests is most useful in monitoring effective response to treatment in patients with iron deficiency anemia?

A. Hemoglobin level
B. Hematocrit level
C. Reticulocyte count
D. Iron level

Question 7

Which of the following coagulation factors is deficient in hemophilia B?

A. VI
B. VII
C. VIII
D. IX

Answer 1

ANSWER **B** EXPLANATION: *Clinical signs of anemia include tachycardia and a systolic ejection heart murmur, due to increased cardiac output. Pallor and postural hypotension may be noted due to decreased blood volume.*

Topic: Anemia

correct ☐   incorrect ☐

Answer 2

ANSWER **B** EXPLANATION: *Vitamin B12 deficiency presents with red, beefy tongue and neurologic complaints, such as paresthesia and numbness of the extremities. CBC results reveal an elevated MCV, thrombocytopenia, and hypersegmented neutrophils. Diagnosis is made by measuring serum vitamin B12 levels.*

Topic: Vitamin B12 deficiency

correct ☐   incorrect ☐

Answer 3

ANSWER **D** EXPLANATION: *Thrombotic thrombocytopenic purpura (ITP) presents with severe thrombocytopenia, microangiopathic hemolytic anemia (have presence of schistocytes), and neurologic abnormalities.*

Topic: Thrombotic thrombocytopenic purpura

correct ☐   incorrect ☐

Answer 4

ANSWER **D** EXPLANATION: *Hodgkin's lymphoma is common after age 50 and presents with a non-tender, firm lymph node; may also note B-symptoms, such as fever, weight loss, and night sweats. Evaluation of this patient consists of lymph node biopsy.*

Topic: Hodgkin's lymphoma

correct ☐   incorrect ☐

Answer 5

ANSWER **C** EXPLANATION: *Overdose of coumadin is treated with vitamin K or fresh frozen plasma. Protamine sulfate is used to treat overdose of heparin.*

Topic: Coagulation disorders

correct ☐   incorrect ☐

Answer 6

ANSWER **C** EXPLANATION: *Iron deficiency anemia is treated with ferrous sulfate and response to therapy can be measured by elevation in reticulocyte count in 7-10 days after starting treatment.*

Topic: Iron deficiency anemia

correct ☐   incorrect ☐

Answer 7

ANSWER **D** EXPLANATION: *Hemophilia B (Christmas disease) is due to a deficiency of factor IX and hemophilia A is due to deficiency of factor VIII.*

Topic: Factor IX disorders

correct ☐   incorrect ☐

NOTES

Infectious Disease

13

EXAM BLUEPRINT TOPICS

Fungal Disease
Candidiasis
Cryptococcosis
Histoplasmosis
Pneumocystis
Bacterial Disease
Botulism
Chlamydia
Cholera
Diphtheria
Gonococcal infections
Salmonellosis
Shigellosis
Tetanus
Mycobacterial Disease
Tuberculosis
Atypical mycobacterial disease
Parasitic Disease
Amebiasis
Ascariasis
Giardiasis
Hookworms
Malaria
Pinworms
Tapeworms
Toxoplasmosis
Spirochetal Disease
Lyme disease
Rocky Mountain spotted fever
Syphilis
Viral Disease
Cytomegalovirus infections
Epstein-Barr virus infections
Erythema infectiosum
Herpes simplex
Human immunodeficiency virus (HIV) infection
Human papillomavirus infections

Influenzae
Mumps
Rabies
Roseola
Rubella
Rubeola (Measles)
Varicella-zoster virus infections
Other

GENERAL INFORMATION

I. Gram stain
  a. See Table 13-1 for summary of bacterial Gram stain results.

FUNGAL DISEASE

I. Candidiasis
  a. General
    i. Candidiasis is the most common opportunistic fungal infection.
    ii. Most common organism is *Candida albicans* but also includes *Candida glabrata, Candida parapsilosis,* and *Candida tropicalis.*
    iii. *Candida* species reproduce by budding.
    iv. Infections range from mucous membrane infection to life-threatening disseminated disease.
  b. Epidemiology
    i. *Candida* species are normal flora in the gastrointestinal and genitourinary tract and the skin.
  c. Clinical manifestations
    i. Oropharyngeal (thrush) and esophageal infections
      1. White plaques on the buccal mucosa, palate, oropharynx, or tongue.

NOTES

Table 13-1 • Common Gram Stain Results

Gram-Positive Cocci	Gram-Positive Rods	Gram-Negative Cocci	Gram-Negative Rods
Staphylococcus	*Corynebacterium*	*Neisseria*	*Escherichia*
Streptococcus	*Listeria*		*Klebsiella*
Peptostreptococcus	*Erysipelothrix*		*Enterobacter*
	Lactobacillus		*Serratia*
	Bacillus		*Pseudomonas*
	Propionibacterium		*Proteus*
			Salmonella
			Shigella
			Moraxella
			Haemophilus

2. Scraping lesions reveals an erythematous, non-ulcerated mucosa.
3. Suspect immune dysfunction (human immunodeficiency virus [HIV]) in an otherwise healthy person.

  ii. Vulvovaginitis
1. Common infection in women of childbearing age.
2. Risk factors include increased estrogen levels, diabetes mellitus, therapy with corticosteroids or antibiotics, and HIV infection.
3. Symptoms include vaginal discomfort, curd-like discharge, and pruritus.
4. Vaginal walls are erythematous and show white plaques.
5. Labia are erythematous and swollen.

  iii. Cutaneous infection
1. Occurs mainly in the intertriginous areas or under large breasts or pannus.
2. Lesions are erythematous with a distinct border and there are multiple satellite lesions.

  iv. Disseminated infection
1. Most common is candidemia.
   (a) Risk factors include broad-spectrum antibiotics, central intravenous catheters, renal failure, and corticosteroid therapy.
2. Can also cause endocarditis and hepatosplenic infection.

  d. Diagnosis
   i. KOH prep or Gram stain reveals budding yeast and pseudohyphae.
   ii. Germ tube–positive.
   iii. Disseminated disease diagnosed by culture of blood or other sterile body fluid.
1. Imaging studies, such as computed tomography (CT) scan, are also required to determine extent of disease.

  e. Treatment
   i. Thrush treated with clotrimazole troches.
   ii. Esophagitis treated with fluconazole or itraconazole.
   iii. Vaginitis treated with miconazole or clotrimazole.
   iv. Disseminated disease treated with amphotericin B or fluconazole.
1. Amphotericin B is nephrotoxic.

II. Cryptococcosis
  a. General
   i. Organism causing infection is yeast called *Cryptococcus neoformans.*
   ii. Infection occurs most often in patients who are immunosuppressed.

NOTES

iii. Meningitis is the most common clinical presentation but can have pulmonary infection.

b. Epidemiology
   i. Infections linked to pigeon excreta.
   ii. Increased risk of infection with CD4 count <50.

c. Pathogenesis
   i. Organism is inhaled causing pulmonary infection first.
   ii. If host defenses not adequate then infection can disseminate.

d. Clinical manifestations
   i. Central nervous system (CNS) infection
      1. Headache, nuchal rigidity, lethargy, confusion, photophobia, papilledema, nausea, and vomiting.
      2. Fever is noted in half of cases.
   ii. Pulmonary infection
      1. Typically have underlying chronic obstructive pulmonary disease.
      2. Fever, cough, and dyspnea.

e. Diagnosis
   i. Culture
   ii. Mucicarmine stain or India ink prep-positive
   iii. Latex agglutination testing
   iv. Cerebral spinal fluid (CSF) reveals elevated white blood cells (WBCs) (rarely >500/μL) with a predominance of lymphocytes, elevated total protein, and decreased glucose.

f. Treatment
   i. Amphotericin B plus flucytosine for 6 weeks for CNS infection.
   ii. Fluconazole or itraconazole for pulmonary infection.

III. Histoplasmosis
   a. General
      i. Caused by *Histoplasmosis capsulatum*.
         1. A dimorphic fungus, a mold at temperatures <35° C and yeast at 35° C–37° C.
   b. Epidemiology
      i. Endemic in the Mississippi and Ohio River valleys.
      ii. Increased number of organisms in bird or bat guano in caves, soil, and abandoned buildings.

QUESTION

Which of the following is used to treat vulvovaginitis due to Candida albicans?

A. Amphotericin B
B. Ceftriaxone (Rocephin)
C. Miconazole (Monistat)
D. Rifampin (Rifadin)

---

c. Pathogenesis
   i. Inhale organism and develop localized pulmonary infection.
   ii. Phagocytized organisms survive and travel within the macrophages to hilar and mediastinal lymph nodes.
   iii. Severity of infection based on organism load and immune response.

d. Clinical manifestations
   i. Acute pulmonary
      1. Symptoms include fever, chills, fatigue, nonproductive cough, and myalgias.
      2. Patchy lobar or multilobe infiltrate noted on chest X-ray.
   ii. Chronic pulmonary
      1. Progressive and fatal.
      2. Seen in older patients with history of chronic obstructive pulmonary disease.
      3. Symptoms include fever, fatigue, anorexia, weight loss, productive cough with purulent sputum, and hemoptysis.
      4. Chest X-ray reveals upper lobe infiltrates with multiple cavities.
   iii. Disseminated
      1. Occurs mainly in immunocompromised patients, such as HIV (CD4 counts <200/μL), post-transplant, or corticosteroid therapy.
      2. Symptoms include fever, chills, anorexia, weight loss, hypotension, dyspnea, and hepatosplenomegaly.
      3. Blood test reveals pancytopenia and diffuse pulmonary infiltrates revealed on chest X-ray.

NOTES

ANSWER C EXPLANATION: *Vulvovaginitis, due to candida albicans, is treated with miconazole or clotrimazole. Amphotericin B is used to treat systemic candidiasis.*

correct ☐   incorrect ☐

e. Diagnosis
   i. Culture
     1. Can take 6 weeks to grow.
   ii. Biopsy stained with methenamine silver.
   iii. Wright's stain of peripheral blood.
   iv. Complement fixation (CF) or immunodiffusion (ID) testing.

     1. M precipitin band on ID testing.
   v. Enzyme immunoassay on urine or serum for disseminated disease.
f. Treatment
   i. Itraconazole for mild to moderate disease.
   ii. Amphotericin B for severe disease.
   iii. Treatment typically not used for acute pulmonary histoplasmosis unless patient immunocompromised.
   iv. All disseminated disease is treated.
IV. Pneumocystis
  a. General
   i. Most frequent case-defining infection in acquired immunodeficiency syndrome (AIDS).

Table 13-2 • Summary of Systemic Fungal Organisms

	Histoplasmosis	Blastomycosis	Coccidioidomycosis	Candidiasis	Cryptococcus	Aspergillosis
Type	Dimorphic	Dimorphic	Dimorphic	Yeast	Yeast	Fungus
Epidemiology	Mississippi and Ohio River valleys. Soil, caves, and old buildings.	North central and south central U.S. Soil or decaying wood.	Southwestern U.S. Soil	Normal flora on GI, GU, and skin	Western U.S. Pigeon excreta	Ubiquitous: water and soil
Route of infection	Inhalation	Inhalation	Inhalation	Direct or blood	Inhalation	Inhalation
Disease	Pulmonary Disseminated	Pulmonary Disseminated	Pulmonary Disseminated	Vulvovaginitis Esophagitis Cutaneous Oropharyngeal	CNS Pulmonary	Pulmonary
Diagnosis	Culture Special stains CF and ID Enzyme assay	Culture Stains	Culture Stains CF	Gram stain KOH prep Culture	Culture Latex agglutination	Culture
Treatment	Itraconazole Amphotericin B	Itraconazole Amphotericin B	Ketoconazole Fluconazole Itraconazole Amphotericin B	Clotrimazole Miconazole Fluconazole	Amphotericin B Flucytosine	Amphotericin B Itraconazole

GI, gastrointestinal; GU, genitourinary; CNS, central nervous system; CF, complement fixation; ID, immunodiffusion.

NOTES

ii. Disease caused by *Pneumocystis carinii*.
  1. Eukaryotic microbe with fungal characteristics.
b. Epidemiology
  i. Exposed early in life and organism remains latent.
  ii. Activated during severe immune system depression.
c. Clinical manifestations
  i. Symptoms include hacking, nonproductive cough, fever, and dyspnea.
  ii. Lung examination is typically normal, but may have rales and wheezing.
d. Diagnosis
  i. Hypoxemia is most useful marker and predictor of outcome.
  ii. Bronchoalveolar lavage with special stains.
  iii. Chest X-ray typically reveals interstitial infiltrates beginning in the perihilar region and spreading lower, in a butterfly pattern.
  iv. Increased uptake on Gallium scan.
  v. Elevated lactate dehydrogenase (LDH) levels.
  vi. CD4 counts typically <200 cells/mm^3.
e. Treatment
  i. Acute disease
    1. Trimethoprim-sulfamethoxazole
    2. Parenteral pentamidine
    3. Clindamycin plus primaquine
  ii. Prophylactic treatment
    1. Needed for all patients at high risk.
      (a) Prior *Pneumocystis* infection
      (b) CD4 count <200 cells/mm^3.
    2. Trimethoprim-sulfamethoxazole
      (a) Dapsone
      (b) Aerosolized pentamidine

BACTERIAL DISEASE

I. Botulism
  a. General
    i. Absorbed from gut, lung, or wound.
      1. Does not penetrate intact skin.
    ii. Severe neuroparalytic disease
    iii. Caused by botulism toxin produced by *Clostridium botulinum.*

QUESTION

Histoplasmosis is endemic in which part of the United States?

A. Western
B. Southwest
C. Hudson river valley
D. Ohio river valley

  1. A Gram-positive spore forming obligate anaerobe.
  2. Found in soil, marine environments, and agricultural products.
  iv. Toxin works by binding to receptors and blocks acetylcholine.
b. Clinical forms
  i. Food-borne botulism
    1. Most common form.
    2. Due to ingestion of preformed toxin in inadequately prepared food (home-canned foods are common).
    3. Occurs in outbreaks.
  ii. Wound botulism
    1. Unusual form of botulism.
    2. Traumatic wounds with soil contamination.
  iii. Infant botulism
    1. Due to production of neurotoxin in the gastrointestinal tract, after colonization of *C. botulinum* from the soil or honey.
    2. Typical age is 1–9 months.
    3. Symptoms of "floppy baby syndrome" include:
      (a) Lethargy
      (b) Diminished suck
      (c) Constipation
      (d) Weakness
      (e) Diminished spontaneous activity with loss of head control
  iv. Inhalation botulism
c. Clinical manifestations
  i. Bulbar musculature affected first causing diplopia, dysphonia, dysarthria, and dysphagia.
  ii. Decreased salivation, ileus, and urinary retention due to involvement of the cholinergic autonomic nervous system.

NOTES

   iii. Neurologic
     1. Bilateral cranial nerve VI palsy
     2. Ptosis
     3. Dilated pupils
     4. Decreased gag reflex
     5. Descending involvement of motor neurons to peripheral muscles, which can lead to respiratory failure.
   iv. Nausea and vomiting
   v. Afebrile
  d. Diagnosis
   i. Analysis of food, serum, stool, and gastric contents for toxin.
   ii. Stool or food culture.
  e. Treatment
   i. Supportive care.
   ii. Passive immunization with botulinum antitoxin.
   iii. Antibiotic treatment needed only in wound botulism.
   iv. Prevention
     1. Destroy spores with heat or irradiation.
     2. Inhibit germination by reducing pH, refrigerating, freezing, or drying.
     3. No honey to infants under age 1.

II. *Chlamydia*
  a. General
   i. Obligate intracellular bacteria.
   ii. Organisms:
     1. *Chlamydia trachomatis*
     2. *Chlamydia pneumoniae*
     3. *Chlamydia psittaci*
  b. Diseases
   i. Trachoma
     1. Most common cause of preventable blindness.
     2. A chronic follicular conjunctivitis.
     3. Treated with topical ocular application of tetracycline and erythromycin for 21–60 days.
   ii. Urethritis/Cervicitis

     1. Causes 30%–40% of cases of nongonococcal urethritis.
     2. Present with mild clear or cloudy urethral discharge, urethral discomfort, and mild dysuria.
     3. Treat with tetracycline or azithromycin.
   iii. Epididymitis/Salpingitis
     1. Spread from urethra to epididymis or fallopian tubes.
     2. Present with unilateral testicular pain, scrotal erythema and tenderness, or swelling over the epididymis. In women present with low abdominal pain and dyspareunia.
     3. Treat with tetracycline or azithromycin.
   iv. Atypical pneumonia
     1. Present with nonproductive cough, sore throat, and hoarseness.
     2. Crackles are heard on lung exam.
     3. Chest X-ray reveals a pneumonitis.
     4. Treat with tetracycline or erythromycin.
   v. Psittacosis
     1. Systemic infection of the reticuloendothelial system.
     2. Abrupt febrile illness with shaking chills and fever, headache, myalgias, arthralgias, and nonproductive cough.
     3. Chest X-ray reveals single or multiple localized bronchopneumonic patches.
     4. Treat with tetracycline or doxycycline.
  c. See Table 13-3 for summary of diseases caused by *Chlamydia*.

III. Cholera
  a. Acute watery "rice water" diarrhea caused by an exotoxin produced by *Vibrio cholerae*.
  b. Present with diarrhea after travel to a cholera-endemic area.
  c. Spreads via contaminated water and food.
  d. Signs and symptoms are due to the severe water loss.
  e. Diagnosis made by stool culture and serology.
  f. Treatment:
   i. Rehydration via oral route with WHO/UNICEF solution, Pedialyte, or rice solution.
   ii. Adjunctive antibiotics may be indicated with tetracycline, fluoroquinolones, and macrolides.

NOTES

IV. Diphtheria
  a. Tonsillopharyngitis and/or laryngitis due to *Corynebacterium diphtheriae.*
  b. Humans are the only natural reservoir, and infection spreads in close-contact settings through respiratory droplets.
  c. After an incubation period of 1–7 days the illness begins with a sore throat, malaise, and fever.
  d. Whitish exudate appears on the tonsils and later becomes a grayish membrane.
    i. Membrane is very adherent and bleeds easily on attempted removal.
  e. May develop myocarditis, conduction disturbances, and neurologic impairment.
  f. Fatality rate is 5%–10%.
  g. Treatment:
    i. Equine diphtheria antitoxin.
    ii. Parenteral penicillin to limit local infection and prevent transmission.
    iii. Prophylactic antibiotics for close contacts.
  h. Prevention:
    i. Immunization with diphtheria toxoid. See immunization schedule.
V. Gonococcal infections
  a. Sexually transmitted disease due to infection with *Neisseria gonorrhoeae*, Gram-negative diplococci.
  b. Diseases
    i. Urethritis
    ii. Endocervicitis
    iii. Neonatal conjunctivitis (ophthalmia neonatorum)

  c. Clinical manifestations
    i. Urethritis
      1. Dysuria and purulent urethral discharge
    ii. Endocervical
      1. Vaginal discharge and abnormal vaginal bleeding
      2. On exam cervicitis with mucopurulent discharge present
      3. Easily induced bleeding with gentle swabbing of the cervix
    iii. Conjunctivitis
      1. Mucopurulent discharge on conjunctivae.
      2. Treat with topical antibiotics or 1% silver nitrate.
  d. Diagnosis
    i. Gram stain showing intracellular Gram-negative diplococci.
      1. Gram stain insensitive in females.
    ii. Culture

QUESTION

An HIV positive patient presents with fever and cough. Chest x-ray reveals bilateral interstitial infiltrates. Which of the following is the most likely diagnosis?

  A. Tuberculosis
  B. Pneumocystis pneumonia
  C. Non-Hodgkin's lymphoma
  D. Histoplasmosis

Table 13-3 • Diseases Caused by *Chlamydia*

Organism	Disease	Host	Transmission
C. trachomatis	Trachoma	Children	Fomites/flies
	Urethritis/Cervicitis	Sexually active people	Direct sexual contact
	Epididymitis/Salpingitis	Sexually active people	Direct sexual contact
C. psittaci	Atypical pneumonia	Birds	Aerosol
C. pneumoniae	Atypical pneumonia	Humans	Respiratory droplets

NOTES

ANSWER **B** EXPLANATION: *Pneumocystis pneumonia, is common in HIV positive patients, and presents with cough and fever. Chest x-ray may be normal or reveal bilateral interstitial infiltrates.*

correct ☐   incorrect ☐

e. Treatment
   i. See Table 13-4 for treatment of gonococcal infections.
   ii. Treat sexual partner.
   iii. Consider HIV and syphilis testing.
f. Disseminated gonococcal disease
   i. Present with polyarticular tenosynovitis, dermatitis, and/or septic arthritis.
g. Pelvic inflammatory disease
   i. Due to infection with *Chlamydia* or gonorrhea.
   ii. Present with low abdominal pain, fever, malaise, and anorexia.
   iii. On exam note lower abdominal tenderness, cervical motion tenderness, bilateral adnexal tenderness, and signs of cervicitis or vaginal infection.
   iv. Fallopian scarring may occur and result in infertility or ectopic pregnancy.

Table 13-4 • Treatment of Endocervical and Urethral Infections

Treatment of Choice (Initial Single Dose Treatment)	Alternative Treatments
Ceftriaxone 125 mg IM	Ceftizoxime 500 mg IM
Cefpodoxime 400 mg PO	Cefotaxime 500 mg IM
Ciprofloxacin 500 mg PO	Gatifloxacin 400 mg PO
Ofloxacin 400 mg PO	Azithromycin 1 g PO
Levofloxacin 250 mg PO	

Follow-up Therapy
Azithromycin 1 g PO single dose or Doxycycline 100 mg PO BID for 7 days

Note: The fluoroquinolones should not be used in patients who acquired disease in areas where fluoroquinolone-resistance is high. This includes Asia, Pacific Islands, Hawaii, and California.

v. Treatment
   1. IV therapy of cefoxitin or cefotetan plus doxycycline; or clindamycin plus gentamicin.
   2. Oral therapy includes ofloxacin or levofloxacin plus metronidazole; or single dose of ceftriaxone plus doxycycline with or without metronidazole.
   3. Treatment should be for 14 days total.
VI. Salmonellosis
  a. Typhoid fever
    i. Caused by *Salmonella typhi*.
    ii. Transmitted via fecal-oral route through contaminated water or food.
    iii. Signs and symptoms
      1. At onset have fever, chills, malaise, dry cough, anorexia, and headache that build in intensity and abdominal tenderness.
      2. Followed by erythematous macules or papules (rose spots) that appear on the shoulders, thorax, and abdomen during the second week of infection.
      3. Intestinal bleeding or perforation may occur.
    iv. Diagnosis
      1. Normal or low WBC count with increased bands.
      2. Blood cultures.
      3. Widal test for agglutinating antibodies against the O and H antigens of *S. typhi*.
    v. Treatment
      1. Fluoroquinolones
      2. Chloramphenicol, amoxicillin, or trimethoprim-sulfamethoxazole.
  b. Other *Salmonella* infections
    i. Most common causes include *S. enteritidis* and *S. typhimurium*.
    ii. Infection in humans occurs from consuming food products contaminated with the organisms.
      1. Sources include poultry, reptiles, and amphibians.
    iii. Clinical manifestations
      1. Asymptomatic carrier
      2. Enterocolitis
      3. Present with crampy abdominal pain and diarrhea.
      4. Fever
      5. WBCs present in the stool with mucus.
      6. Enteric fever

NOTES

7. Similar to typhoid fever.
8. Prolonged sustained fever, relative bradycardia, splenomegaly, rose spots, and leukopenia.
9. Bacteremia
10. Fever and chills lasting for days.
11. Increased incidence in patients with diseases associated with hemolysis, such as sickle cell disease.
iv. Diagnosis
1. Stool culture
2. Serologic studies are not helpful.
v. Treatment
1. Enterocolitis
   (a) Antibiotic therapy is typically not needed.
2. Bacteremia and enteric fever.
   (a) Fluoroquinolones or third-generation cephalosporins.

VII. Shigellosis
a. General
   i. Infection due to *Shigella* that results in colitis affecting mainly the rectosigmoid colon.
   ii. Transmitted by fecal-oral route and via person-to-person through contaminated hands.
   iii. A small inoculum is needed to cause disease and the organism is secreted in the stool for up to 6 weeks.
b. Clinical manifestations
   i. Initial presentation is a nonspecific prodrome followed by intestinal symptoms (cramps, loose stools, and watery diarrhea).
   ii. Followed by passage of blood and mucus in the stool, tenesmus and rectal pain.
   iii. Abdominal pain is located in the left lower quadrant.
c. Treatment
   i. Always requires antibiotics.
   ii. Ciprofloxacin in adults and trimethoprim-sulfamethoxazole, ampicillin, or azithromycin in children.
   iii. Do not give agents that decrease intestinal motility, which may worsen symptoms.
d. Post-dysenteric syndromes
   i. Arthritis
   ii. Reiter's triad of arthritis, urethritis, and conjunctivitis.

QUESTION

A patient presents with fever, hoarseness, and sore throat. On exam, a tenacious grey membrane covering the pharynx is noted. Which of the following is the most likely diagnosis?

A. Streptococcal pharyngitis
B. Vincent's angina
C. Oral candidiasis
D. Diphtheria

VIII. Tetanus
a. General
   i. A neurologic syndrome due to a neurotoxin produced by *Clostridium tetani*.
   ii. Found in the soil.
b. Clinical manifestations: Generalized tetanus
   i. Incubation period 7–21 days.
   ii. Most common complaint is trismus (lockjaw).
   iii. Other features include irritability, diaphoresis, dysphagia with hydrophobia, and back muscle spasms.
c. Diagnosis
   i. Based on clinical findings.
   ii. History of immunization makes tetanus unlikely.
d. Treatment
   i. Supportive care and appropriate wound care if indicated.
   ii. Benzodiazepines to control muscle spasm.
   iii. Passive immunization with human tetanus immunoglobulin (TIG) 500 units IM.
   iv. Active immunization.
   v. Antibiotic therapy: metronidazole or penicillin.
e. Prevention
   i. Active immunization with DPaT (diphtheria and tetanus toxoids and pertussis absorbed).
      1. Given at 2 months, 4 months, 6 months, 15 months, and 4–6 years.
   ii. Td (tetanus and diphtheria toxoids) every 10 years in adults.
   iii. Appropriate wound management.

NOTES

ANSWER **D** EXPLANATION: *Diphtheria presents with fever, hoarseness, and pharyngitis. On examination, a grey pseudomembrane is noted covering the pharynx.*

correct ☐   incorrect ☐

MYCOBACTERIAL DISEASE

I. Tuberculosis
   a. General
      i. Disease caused by *Mycobacterium tuberculosis*, acid-fast bacillus.
      ii. Humans are only natural reservoir.
      iii. Spread by aerosolized respiratory secretions.
   b. Clinical manifestations
      i. Pulmonary disease
         1. Cough with hemoptysis, fever and sweating are common.
         2. Other complaints include malaise, fatigue, weight loss, chest pain, and dyspnea.
      ii. Extrapulmonary disease can occur at the following sites:
         1. Lymphatic
         2. Pleural
         3. Genitourinary
         4. Bone or joint
         5. Disseminated
         6. Meninges and CNS
         7. Gastrointestinal
         8. Pericardial
   c. Diagnosis
      i. Chest X-ray reveals lesions in the upper lung fields.
         1. See Figure 13-1.
      ii. Sputum smears and cultures
         1. Acid-fast or modified acid-fast smears.
         2. Culture is the gold standard.
   d. Treatment
      i. All patients with communicable tuberculosis must be treated or quarantined.
      ii. Active tuberculosis patients should receive multiple agents.

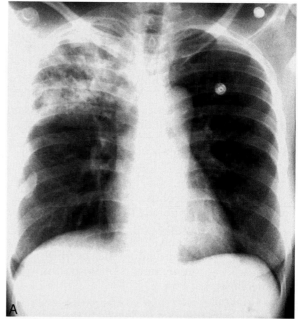
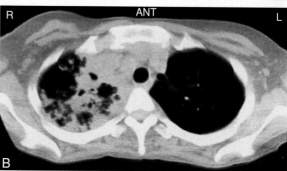

Figure 13-1   Chest X-ray: Tuberculosis. (From Mettler FA: (2005). Essentials of Radiology, 2nd ed. Philadelphia, Elsevier Saunders, 2005, p. 84. Fig. 3-49A.)

      iii. Multiple treatment regimens are available. Drugs include:
         1. Isoniazid
         2. Rifampin
         3. Rifabutin
         4. Pyrazinamide
         5. Ethambutol
         6. Streptomycin
   e. Prevention
      i. Treatment of latent infection:
         1. Isoniazid for 9 months

NOTES

2. Rifampin for 4 months
II. Atypical mycobacterial disease
  a. *Mycobacterium avium-intracellulare*
    i. Pulmonary infection typically occurs in patients with underlying lung disease.
    ii. Disseminated disease noted in patients with advanced HIV.
    iii. Symptoms include fever, weight loss, anorexia, abdominal pain, and diarrhea.
    iv. Diagnosis made by culture of the organism from the blood, bone marrow, or tissue.
      1. Treatment
        (a) Azithromycin or clarithromycin, rifabutin or rifampin, and ethambutol.
        (b) Prophylaxis treatment with azithromycin or clarithromycin when CD4 count <50 cells/µL.

PARASITIC DISEASE

I. Amebiasis
  a. General
    i. Prevalence is high in many developing countries.
      1. Typically in areas with poor sanitation.
    ii. Caused by *Entamoeba histolytica.*
    iii. May led to liver abscess formation.
  b. Clinical manifestations
    i. Many patients are asymptomatic.
    ii. May present with bloody mucous containing diarrhea, pain, urgency, and tenesmus.
    iii. Left lower quadrant tenderness is common in acute colitis.
    iv. If liver abscess then note fever, right upper quadrant pain with radiation to right shoulder or back.
      1. Diarrhea is not common in patients with liver abscess.
  c. Diagnosis
    i. Fecal leukocytes are often absent.
    ii. Diagnosis made with identification of trophozoites or cysts in stool or involved tissue.
      1. See Figure 13-2.

QUESTION

Sputum from a patient with hemoptysis and fever is positive for acid-fast bacilli. What is the most likely diagnosis?

  A. Tuberculosis
  B. Blastomycosis
  C. Aspergillosis
  D. Psittacosis

    iii. Hepatic ultrasound for evaluation of liver abscess.
    iv. Serology studies may be helpful.
  d. Treatment
    i. Antibiotic of choice is metronidazole, targets trophozoites.
      1. Paromomycin needed after metronidazole to treat the cyst form.
    ii. Possible drainage for liver abscess
II. Ascariasis
  a. General
    i. Very common helminthic infection throughout the world.
      1. Noted mainly in southeastern United States.

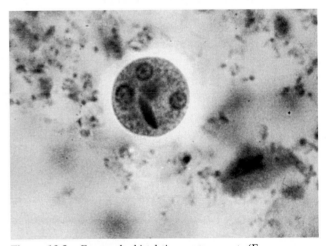

Figure 13-2 *Entamoeba histolytica,* mature cyst. (From Mandell: Principle and Practice of Infectious Diseases, 5th ed. 2000, p. 2799, Fig. 262-3.)

NOTES

ANSWER A EXPLANATION: *Tuberculosis presents with fever, cough, night sweats, and hemoptysis. The organism, Mycobacterium tuberculosis, is acid-fast positive*

correct ☐   incorrect ☐

---

  ii. Caused by *Ascaris lumbricoides.*
  iii. Found in contaminated soil.
  iv. Once ingested, larvae emerge in the small intestine and migrate to the lung and then back to the intestine.
 b. Clinical manifestations
  i. Typically asymptomatic.
  ii. With heavy exposure may have cough, dyspnea, or asthma with eosinophilia.
  iii. With intestinal infection symptoms include abdominal pain, distention, nausea, anorexia, and intermittent diarrhea.
  iv. With heavy worm load may develop intestinal obstruction or obstruction of the biliary system.
 c. Diagnosis
  i. Abdominal X-ray reveals a "whirlpool" pattern of intraluminal worms.
  ii. Diagnose by noting large, brown, tri-layered eggs in the stool.
 d. Treatment
  i. Treat with mebendazole or albendazole.

  ii. Remove patient from contaminated site.
III. Giardiasis
 a. General
  i. Caused by *Giardia lamblia*, a flagellated protozoan.
  ii. Acquired from lake or stream water, contaminated food, and personal contact (day care centers).
  iii. Most commonly identified cause of waterborne outbreaks of diarrhea.
 b. Clinical manifestations
  i. Incubation period is 1–2 weeks.
  ii. Symptoms include bloating, cramping, and flatulence followed by foul-smelling diarrhea.
   1. May develop a malabsorption syndrome.
  iii. Fever is uncommon after the first few days of the disease.
 c. Diagnosis
  i. Examine stool for presence of cysts.
   1. See Figure 13-3.
  ii. Enzyme immunoassay antigen tests
 d. Treatment
  i. Drugs of choice are metronidazole and albendazole.
   1. Paromomycin is used in pregnant women.
  ii. Cysts resist chlorination, but are killed by boiling or by filtration.

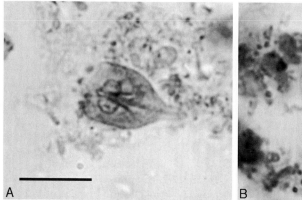
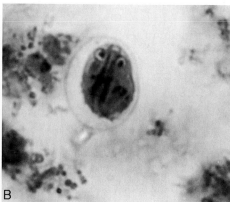

Figure 13-3 *Giardia lamblia,* trophozoite, and cyst. (From Mandell GL: Principle and Practice of Infectious Diseases, 5th ed. Churchill Livingstone. 2005, p. 3199, Fig. 277-1.)

NOTES

IV. Hookworms
  a. General
    i. Worldwide disease, occurs occasionally in southeastern United States.
    ii. Caused by one of two nematodes, *Ancylostoma duodenale* or *Necator americanus.*
    iii. Infection acquired by skin exposure to larvae in soil contaminated by human feces.
      1. Once in the skin the larvae move to the lung and break into alveoli.
      2. Larvae are coughed up and then swallowed and take up residence in the jejunum.
      3. This cycle takes approximately 4 weeks.
  b. Clinical manifestations
    i. Present with a pruritic rash (ground itch) at the site of entry.
    ii. The pulmonary phase is typically asymptomatic, but may have cough, patchy infiltrates, and eosinophilia.
    iii. Intestinal phase symptoms are related to worm burden and may include abdominal pain, nausea, and bloating.
    iv. Anemia may develop later due to blood loss.
  c. Diagnosis
    i. Made by noting eggs in stool sample.
  d. Treatment
    i. Drugs of choice include albendazole or mebendazole.
    ii. Iron replacement may also be indicated.
    iii. Improve sanitation.
V. Malaria
  a. General
    i. Any fever in a traveler is malaria until proven otherwise.
    ii. Four *Plasmodium* species cause human malaria.
      1. *P. falciparum*
      2. *P. vivax*
      3. *P. ovale*
      4. *P. malariae*
    iii. Life cycle
      1. Female anopheline mosquito bites and infects human with sporozoites.
      2. Evolve from sporozoites to schizonts to merozoites in the liver.

---

      3. Merozoites are released from the liver and invade the red blood cells, where they multiply.
  b. Clinical manifestations
    i. Fever manifested by three-phases:
      1. Cold stage: chills lasting up to several hours.
      2. Hot stage: high fever lasting several hours.
        (a) May be cyclic.
          (i) *P. vivax* and *ovale* every 48 hours.
          (ii) *P. malariae* every 72 hours.
          (iii) *P. falciparum* has continuous fevers.
        (b) Fever corresponds to lysis of red blood cells.
      3. Drenching sweats
    ii. May also present with headache, backache, abdominal pain, nausea and vomiting, hypotension, and altered mental status during hot stage.
    iii. *P. falciparum* may be complicated by coma (cerebral malaria) or renal failure with hemoglobinuria (blackwater fever).
  c. Diagnosis
    i. Must have high degree of suspicion.
    ii. Examination of thick and thin blood smears for parasite.
  d. Treatment
    i. Control of the vector very important.
    ii. Chemoprophylaxis with chloroquine in chloroquine-sensitive areas.

NOTES

     1. In areas with high chloroquine resistance use mefloquine, doxycycline, or chloroquine plus proguanil.
  iii. Treatment of malaria
     1. *P. falciparum:*
       (a) Quine sulfate plus doxycycline
     2. *P. falciparum,* severe disease:
       (a) Quinidine gluconate (IV) and switch to oral when possible.
     3. *P. vivax* or *ovale,* confirmed:
       (a) Chloroquine plus primaquine (screen for G-6-PD deficiency).
     4. *P. malariae,* confirmed:
       (a) Chloroquine
  iv. See www.cdc.gov for latest treatment guidelines.

VI. Pinworms
  a. General
    i. Most prevalent helminthic infection in the United States.
    ii. Typically affects children in day care centers, institutionalized individuals, and people living in crowed places.
    iii. Caused by *Enterobius vermicularis.*
     1. Adult worms take up residence in the cecum.
     2. Females migrate to the perianal region at night where they lay eggs.
     3. Eggs are infectious for up to 20 days.
  b. Clinical manifestations
    i. Most common complaint is perianal or perineal itching and insomnia.
    ii. Infection transmitted by patient's hands.
    iii. May affect multiple family members.
  c. Diagnosis
    i. Cellophane tape test.
    ii. Diagnosis made by noted ovoid eggs under the microscope.
  d. Treatment

    i. Treat with mebendazole or albendazole as a single dose, repeated in 2 weeks.
    ii. Encourage personal and family hygiene.
VII. Tapeworms
  a. See Table 13-5 for summary of tapeworm infections.
VIII. Toxoplasmosis
  a. General
    i. Caused by *Toxoplasma gondii,* a protozoan.
    ii. A zoonosis, with the definitive host being cats.
    iii. Two routes of infection:
     1. Oral ingestion of undercooked or raw meat.
     2. Transplacental transmission to fetus.
    iv. An opportunistic pathogen in people with HIV.
  b. Clinical manifestations
    i. Primary infection is unrecognized in most cases or presents as a self-limited and nonspecific illness.
     1. May have lymphadenopathy and fatigue without fever.
    ii. Immunocompromised patients present with encephalitis, chorioretinitis, pneumonitis, or systemic disease.
  c. Diagnosis
    i. Serology (IgG) to establish exposure.
    ii. Identify parasite in tissue.
    iii. CT or magnetic resonance imaging (MRI) of the brain for toxoplasmosis of the CNS.
     1. Multiple ring-enhancing lesions.
  d. Treatment
    i. Immunocompetent patient
     1. No treatment for lymphadenitis.
     2. Systemic disease treated with pyrimethamine, sulfadiazine, and folinic acid.
    ii. Immunocompromised patient
     1. Pyrimethamine, sulfadiazine, and folinic acid.
     2. Trimethoprim/sulfamethoxazole or dapsone plus pyrimethamine for prophylaxis.
      (a) Must be given for the lifetime of the patient.
    iii. Prevention
     1. Wash hands, fruits, and vegetables.

NOTES

2. Avoid contact with materials contaminated with cat feces.

SPIROCHETAL DISEASE

I. Lyme disease
   a. General
      i. Most common vector-borne disease in the United States.
      ii. Caused by a spirochete, *Borrelia burgdorferi.*
      iii. Transmitted by ticks of the *Ixodes* family.
      iv. Life cycle involves rodents (white-footed mouse) and larger mammals (deer).
   b. Clinical manifestations
      i. Three stages:
         1. First stage:
            (a) Acute onset of fever, rash, fatigue, headache, and lymphadenopathy.
            (b) Classic skin lesion is erythema chronicum migrans, which appears about 1 week after the tick bite, most commonly on the trunk, groin, thigh, or axilla.
            (c) The lesion is large. The outer border is red with an indurated center.
         2. Second stage:
            (a) Begins days to weeks after initial infection.
            (b) Due to hematogenous spread of the spirochete.
            (c) May have multiple erythema migrans lesions.
               (i) Lesions are usually annular, smaller, and without indurated centers.
               (ii) Can occur anywhere on the body except soles of feet and palms of hands.
            (d) May also present with facial nerve palsy, lymphocytic meningitis, arthritis, radiculopathy, or heart block.

Table 13-5 • Summary of Tapeworms

	Taenia solium	Taenia saginata	Diphyllobothrium latum
Disease	Pork tapeworm	Beef tapeworm	Fish tapeworm
Location	Mexico, South and Central America, Africa, Southeast Asia and India	Worldwide, but common in central Asia and eastern Africa	Europe, Canada, Alaska, and Japan
Intermediate host	Pig	Cow	Fish
Signs/Symptoms	Asymptomatic	Asymptomatic	Bloating, abdominal pain, and diarrhea
Labs	Eosinophilia	Eosinophilia	Eosinophilia and vitamin B12 deficiency
Diagnosis	Stool O & P	Stool O & P	Stool O & P
Treatment	Praziquantel or Niclosamide	Praziquantel or Niclosamide	Praziquantel or Niclosamide
Prevention	Adequate cooking (<65°C core temperature) of pork and pork products	Adequate cooking (>65°C core temperature) of beef and beef products. Meat inspection.	Adequate cooking or freezing (24–48 hours at −18°C) of fish.

NOTES

3. Third stage:
   (a) Occurs more than a year after initial infection.
   (d) Demonstrates chronic oligoarticular arthritis.
c. Diagnosis
   i. Based on history of tick bite in an endemic area, classic skin lesion, and other features of the disease.
   ii. Serologic testing is commonly used to confirm diagnosis in patients who do not present with clear history of the classic skin lesion.
      1. IgM antibodies appear 3–4 weeks after initial infection and peak at 6–8 weeks.
      2. IgG appear 6–8 weeks after initial infection and peak in 4–6 months.
      3. May have false-positive test in patients with autoimmune disorders.
   iii. Polymerase chain reaction (PCR) can be used to aid in the diagnosis of Lyme arthritis.
d. Treatment
   i. Without treatment patients may develop cardiac involvement, chronic arthritis, or neurologic disease.
   ii. Treatment is typically for 21–28 days total.
   iii. See Table 13-6 for treatment of Lyme disease.

Table 13-6 • Treatment of Lyme Disease

Early Localized Disease or Early Disseminated	Symptoms[a]	Arthritis, Early or Late
Doxycycline	Ceftriaxone	Doxycycline
Amoxicillin	Penicillin G	Amoxicillin
Cefuroxime axetil		Ceftriaxone
		Penicillin G

[a]Symptoms include meningitis, facial nerve palsy with abnormal CSF, severe neurologic or cardiac disease, and persistent or recurrent arthritis.

II. Rocky Mountain spotted fever
   a. General
      i. Generalized infection of the vascular endothelium, leading to widespread tissue injury.
      ii. Caused by an intracellular bacteria, *Rickettsia rickettsii*.
      iii. Transmitted by ticks in the *Dermacentor* family.
      iv. Disease noted in the western United States and the South Atlantic west central regions during the late spring and summer months.
   b. Clinical manifestations
      i. After a 2–14-day incubation period, presents as a nonspecific flu-like illness with fever (may exceed 39°C), severe headache, and myalgias.
      ii. May also note nausea, vomiting, abdominal pain, and diarrhea.
      iii. The rash appears on day 3 of the illness and is typically maculopapular and/or petechial. Appears first on the wrists or ankles. Appearance of the rash on the palms or soles occurs later, if at all.
   c. Diagnosis
      i. WBC count is normal but a left shift is present.
      ii. Thrombocytopenia is common.
      iii. Diagnosis is suggested by the typical rash and confirmed with retrospective serologic tests
   d. Treatment
      i. Treatment should be started in any patient where the diagnosis is suggested due to the rash, and before confirmation of the diagnosis.
      ii. Doxycycline is the drug of choice with chloramphenicol being used in pregnant women.
      iii. Mortality rate is 20% if untreated and 4% if treated.
      iv. Death occurs due to organ failure.
III. Syphilis
   a. General
      i. Caused by *Treponema pallidum*, a spirochete.
      ii. After inoculation through abraded skin or mucous membranes it attaches to the host cells and spreads in hours to regional lymph nodes.

NOTES

b. Clinical manifestations
   i. Primary
      1. Incubation period 2–6 weeks after exposure.
      2. Papule develops at site of infection and ulcerates into chancre.
      3. Chancre is a painless, indurated ulcer with well-defined borders and a clean base.
         (a) Chancre heals in 3–6 weeks without treatment.
   ii. Secondary
      1. Will develop in 60%–90% of patients with untreated primary syphilis.
      2. Occurs 4–10 weeks after chancre disappears.
      3. Systemic disease with generalized lymphadenopathy, fever, headache, sore throat, and arthralgias.
      4. Most common characteristic is the rash. Rash consists of macules and papules on the head, neck, trunk, and extremities, including the palms and soles.
   iii. Latent
      1. Defined as a patient having reactive serology in the absence of clinical signs or symptoms.
   iv. Tertiary
      1. Presentation may include cardiovascular disorders (aortic aneurysm, aortic insufficiency, and coronary stenosis), gummatous lesions (bones and skin), or CNS disorders (general paresis and tabes dorsalis).
   v. Neurosyphilis
      1. Can be noted at any time during the course of the disease.
      2. Meningitis may present with headache, nausea, vomiting, stiff neck, cranial nerve palsies, hearing loss, and tinnitus.
      3. Meningovascular meningitis can lead to hemiparesis, hemiplegia, aphasia, and seizures.
c. Diagnosis
   i. Primary syphilis diagnosed by noted treponemes on dark-field microscopic examination.

QUESTION

An 8-year-old patient presents with nocturnal peri-anal itching. Which of the following is the next best test to assist in the diagnosis of this patient?

A. Stool for ova and parasite
B. Fecal white blood cell count
C. Eosinophil count
D. Cellulose tape test

   ii. Serologic testing
      1. Treponemal
         (a) Fluorescent treponemal antibody absorption test (FTA-ABS)
         (b) Microhemagglutination assay-*Treponemal pallidum* (MHA-TP)
      2. Non-treponemal: detect anticardiolipin antibodies and are confirmatory tests.
         (a) Rapid plasma reagin (RPR)
         (b) Venereal Disease Research Laboratory test (VDRL)
   iii. Sensitivity of tests by stage:
      1. Primary
         (a) VDRL 75%–88%
         (b) RPR 75%–100%
         (c) FTA-ABS 70%–100%
      2. Secondary: diagnosed by a positive RPR and confirmatory test in a patient without signs or symptoms.
         (a) VDRL 100%
         (b) RPR 100%
         (c) FTA-ABS 100%
      3. Latent: diagnosed when syphilitic gumma, cardiovascular disease, or neurologic disease is noted.
         (a) VDRL 90%–100%
         (b) RPR 95%–100%
         (c) FTA-ABS 100%
      4. Neurosyphilis
         (a) Diagnosis made based on history and physical, serologic testing, and CSF examination.
         (b) A positive CSF VDRL is highly specific for neurosyphilis.

NOTES

ANSWER **D** EXPLANATION: *Perianal itching in young children could be due to pinworms. The scotch tape or cellulose tape test is indicated to make the diagnosis by revealing the presence of pinworms.*

correct ☐   incorrect ☐

---

d. Treatment
   i. All positive cases must be reported to the health department and the partner treated.
   ii. All patients with syphilis should be tested for HIV.
   iii. Treatment depends on the stage, but penicillin G is mainstay of therapy for all stages.
     1. Doxycycline or tetracycline is indicated in penicillin-allergic patients.

VIRAL DISEASE

I. Cytomegalovirus (CMV) infections
  a. General
   i. Member of the *Herpesviridae* family.
   ii. Can be acquired congenitally, perinatally, and via close contact or sexual transmission.
   iii. Leading cause of blindness in patients with AIDS.
  b. Clinical manifestations
   i. Immunocompetent patients seldom have any clinical manifestations of infection.
   ii. If symptoms do develop they are mononucleosis-like.
   iii. Congenital CMV infection:
     1. Typically asymptomatic at birth but may develop sensory nerve hearing loss and/or psychomotor mental retardation.
     2. While rare, symptomatic signs at birth may include hepatosplenomegaly, jaundice, anemia, thrombocytopenia, low birth weight, and microencephaly.
   iv. CMV infection in immunoincompetent patient:
     1. Infection may lead to chorioretinitis, gastroenteritis, and neurologic disorders.
     2. Reactivation of disease is common.

  c. Diagnosis
   i. Detection of CMV cytopathology: "owl eye" cells
   ii. Cell culture
   iii. Antibody detection
  d. Treatment
   i. Ganciclovir is used to treat CMV infection in children.
   ii. Ganciclovir or foscarnet is used in adults.
   iii. HIV-positive patients will need prophylactic treatment for CMV infections.
II. Epstein-Barr virus (EBV) infections
  a. General
   i. Member of the *Herpesviridae* family.
   ii. Cause of infectious mononucleosis and certain lymphoproliferative disease.
   iii. Transmission requires repeated close contact with infected secretions such as saliva.
  b. Clinical manifestations
   i. Infectious mononucleosis
     1. Fever, malaise, pharyngitis, lymphadenopathy, and splenomegaly.
     2. May persist for 1–2 weeks.
  c. Diagnosis
   i. Complete blood count reveals a lymphocytosis with many atypical lymphocytes (>10%).
   ii. Elevated liver function tests.
   iii. Presence of heterophile antibodies (positive Monospot).
   iv. Positive EBV-specific serology findings.
     1. See Table 13-7 for interpretation of EBV serology.
  d. Treatment
   i. Mainly supportive.
   ii. Corticosteroids can be used in severe disease or if CNS complications.
   iii. Complications
     1. Contact sports should be avoided to decrease the risk of splenic rupture.
     2. Laryngeal obstruction
     3. Aseptic meningitis
     4. Encephalitis
III. Erythema infectiosum
  a. General
   i. Also known as fifth disease.
   ii. Caused by the Parvovirus B19.

NOTES

    iii. Spread by respiratory transmission and is moderately infectious.

  b. Clinical manifestations

    i. Most cases are asymptomatic or subclinical.

    ii. Develops most often in children under age 10.

    iii. Starts with a nonspecific prodrome, then a nonspecific febrile illness with headache, coryza, and diarrhea. This is followed by a bright red "slapped-cheek" facial rash.

    iv. Later a maculopapular rash appears on the trunk and extremities.

    v. Adults infected with the virus are more likely to present with arthritis.

  c. Diagnosis

    i. Based on clinical findings or by presence of IgM antibodies.

  d. Treatment

    i. Usually a self-limited disease.

    ii. Complications

      1. Infection during pregnancy increases risk of miscarriage.

      2. Aplastic crisis can also develop in patients infected with the virus.

        (a) Treatment of the aplastic crisis includes IV immunoglobulin.

IV. Herpes simplex

  a. General

    i. Member of the *Herpesviridae* family.

    ii. Humans are the only natural reservoir.

QUESTION

Which of the following disorders presents with a chancre?

  A. Rocky mountain spotted fever

  B. Herpes simplex

  C. Lyme disease

  D. Syphilis

---

    iii. Direct contact with infected secretions is the major transmission mode.

    iv. Cause both acute and latent infection.

      1. Acute infection consists of development of multinucleated giant cells.

      2. Latent infection can be triggered by fever, trauma, and exposure to ultraviolet light.

  b. Clinical manifestations

    i. Herpes simplex virus-1 (HSV-1)

      1. Grouped or single vesicular lesions that become pustular and form single or multiple ulcers.

      2. Can involve any mucosal surface.

      3. Lesions are very painful and last for 5–10 days.

      4. May become latent within sensory nerve root ganglion.

      5. Recurrences are typically unilateral and last about 7 days.

Table 13-7 • Serology Results in Epstein-Barr Virus Infection

Antibody	Time of Appearance	Persistence	Percent of IM Patients with Antibody	Note
VCA-IgM	At clinical presentation	1–2 months	100	Best indicator of primary infection.
VCA-IgG	At clinical presentation	Lifelong	100	
EBNA	3–6 weeks after onset	Lifelong	100	Presence of EBNA plus VCA-IgG indicates past infection.

IM, infectious mononucleosis; VCA, viral capsid antigen; EBNA, Epstein-Barr nuclear antigen.

NOTES

ANSWER D EXPLANATION: *The initial presenting lesion of syphilis is called a chancre.*

correct ☐   incorrect ☐

6. Herpes whitlow is HSV infection involving the finger or nail area.
   ii. Herpes simplex virus-2 (HSV-2)
   1. Cause of genital herpes.
   2. Incubation period is 5 days from sexual contact to onset of lesions.
   3. Lesions are small erythematous papules that form into vesicles and then pustules.
   4. With primary disease the lesions are painful, multiple, and extensive.
      (a) May have systemic symptoms such as fever and myalgias.
   5. Recurrent disease is typically shorter in duration and typically localized to the genital region, without systemic symptoms.
      (a) Prodromal paresthesias may be noted 12–24 hours prior to the appearance of the lesions.
c. Diagnosis
   i. Can be made by cell culture, Tzanck smear, antigen detection, and PCR.
      1. Tzanck smear shows multinucleated giant cells.
      2. PCR is the test of choice for diagnosis of HSV encephalitis.
d. Treatment
   i. Use of acyclovir, valacyclovir, or famciclovir is indicated.
      1. IV acyclovir is needed in HSV encephalitis.
   ii. Prophylactic measures include avoidance of contact with HSV-positive secretions and daily acyclovir to suppress recurrences.
   iii. Because of high mortality and morbidity with neonatal HSV infection, Cesarean section should be used to prevent transmission to infant from actively infected mother.

V. Human immunodeficiency virus (HIV) infection
   a. General
      i. Due to infection with human immunodeficiency virus-1 (HIV-1)
         1. A lentivirus, which is a member of the retroviruses.
      ii. Uses reverse transcriptase to produce DNA copy from viral RNA, which is incorporated into the host nucleus to produce more viral RNA.
         1. Infects cells with a CD4 receptor (macrophages, T cells, and astrocytes).
      iii. Disease is noted worldwide and spread by parenteral or sexual routes.
   b. Clinical manifestations
      i. After infection, patient develops an acute retroviral syndrome with symptoms similar to mononucleosis, influenzae-like illness, or aseptic meningitis.
      ii. Patients are then asymptomatic until development of opportunistic infections, tumors, or wasting syndrome.
      iii. During this asymptomatic time frame patients' CD4 count declines and viral load increases, making them more susceptible to opportunistic infection.
      iv. Opportunistic infections
         1. See Table 13-8 for list of opportunistic infections seen in HIV.
   c. Diagnosis
      i. Antibodies to HIV can be detected within weeks to months after infection.
         1. Anti-HIV is typically detected by the enzyme-linked immunosorbent assay (ELISA) method within 3–6 months of infection.
      ii. Positive screening test is confirmed with the Western blot test.
         1. Detects antibodies in the core and envelope of HIV.
      iii. Staging of the illness is done with monitoring CD4 cell count and nucleic acid tests for HIV DNA or RNA with the PCR.
   d. Treatment
      i. Initial treatment, which should include at least three drugs, should begin before patient develops substantial immunocompromise.

NOTES

ii. When therapy changes, at least two drugs should be added or substituted to prevent resistance.

iii. During treatment viral load should be monitored to keep the level below the level of detection.

iv. Drugs
   1. See Table 13-9 for drugs, used in treatment of HIV, including side effects.

v. Prophylaxis treatment of opportunistic infections

Table 13-8 • Opportunistic Infections Noted in HIV

Bacterial	Protozoan	Fungal	Viruses	Malignancy
Mycobacterium tuberculosis	*Toxoplasma gondii*	*Candida* species	Varicella-zoster	Kaposi's sarcoma
Mycobacterium avium-intracellulare	*Cryptosporidium parvum*	*Cryptococcus neoformans*	Human papovavirus	Non-Hodgkin's lymphoma
	Isospora belli	*Pneumocystis carinii*		
	Microspora			

Table 13-9 • Drugs Used in the Treatment of HIV

Mechanism of Action	Generic Name	Trade Name	Abbreviation	Side Effects
Nucleoside reverse transcriptase inhibitors (NRTIs)	Zidovudine	Retrovir	AZT (ZDV)	Anemia, neutropenia, and myopathy
	Stavudine	Zerit	d4T	Peripheral neuropathy
	Didanosine	Videx	ddI	Pancreatitis and peripheral neuropathy
	Lamivudine	Epivir	3TC	Nausea, headache, and fatigue
	Zalcitabine	Hivid	ddC	Peripheral neuropathy and mouth sores
Nonnucleoside reverse transcriptase inhibitors (NNRTIs)	Nevirapine	Viramune	NVP	Hepatotoxicity, rash, and nausea
	Delavirdine	Rescriptor	DLV	Rash, headache, and elevated liver function tests.
Protease Inhibitors (PIs)	Saquinavir	Invirase	SQV	Lipodystrophy
	Ritonavir	Norvir	RTV	Inhibits P450 enzymes and elevates many drug levels
	Indinavir	Crixivan	IDV	Nephrolithiasis
	Nelfinavir	Viracept	NFV	Diarrhea

NOTES

ANSWER **D** EXPLANATION: *Infectious mononucleosis presents with fever, pharyngitis, and splenomegaly. Laboratory testing reveals the presence of heterophile antibodies (positive Monospot).*

correct ☐   incorrect ☐

    1. See Table 13-10 for treatment options of opportunistic infections seen in HIV.
  vi. Prevention
    1. Avoid high-risk partners and unprotected intercourse.
    2. Transmission to baby from mother can be reduced with the administration of a protease inhibitor.
VI. Human papillomavirus (HPV) infections
  a. General
    i. Member of the *Papovaviruses* family.
    ii. Cause warts and genital lesions.

    iii. Skin warts are common in children and young adults.
    iv. Genital warts are sexually transmitted and associated with cervical dysplasia and/or neoplasia.
  b. Clinical manifestations
    i. Skin warts
      1. Two types: flat and plantar
      2. Associated with HPV types 1-4
      3. Infect the keratinized surfaces, typically on the hands and feet.
      4. If given time will regress spontaneously.
    ii. Genital warts (*Condyloma acuminata*)
      1. Occur on the squamous epithelium of the external genitalia and perianal area.
      2. Associated with HPV types 6 and 11.
    iii. Cervical dysplasia
      1. HPV types 16 and 18 are associated with intraepithelial cervical dysplasia, neoplasia, and cancer.

Table 13-10 • Prophylaxis Treatment of Opportunistic Infections in HIV

Pathogen	Primary Prophylaxis	Alternative Primary	Secondary Prophylaxis	Alternative Secondary
Pneumocystis carinii	TMP/SMX			
Toxoplasma gondii	TMP/SMX		Pyrimethamine plus sulfadiazine plus folinic acid	Clindamycin plus pyrimethamine plus leucovorin
Mycobacterium tuberculosis (INH-sensitive)	INH	Rifabutin plus pyrazinamide		
Mycobacterium tuberculosis (INH-resistant)	Rifampin plus pyrazinamide	Rifabutin plus pyrazinamide		
Mycobacterium avium complex	Azithromycin or clarithromycin	Azithromycin or clarithromycin plus rifabutin	Clarithromycin plus ethambutol	Azithromycin plus ethambutol
Cytomegalovirus retinitis			Ganciclovir plus foscarnet	Cidofovir
Cryptococcus neoformans			Fluconazole	Itraconazole
Histoplasma capsulatum			Itraconazole	

NOTES

c. Diagnosis
   i. Confirm by biopsy with the appearance of hyperplasia of prickle cells and production of excess keratin.
   ii. DNA probes for HPV.
      (a) Suggested by the presence of koilocytotic squamous epithelial cells on smear.
d. Treatment
   i. Spontaneous disappearance occurs, but may take years.
   ii. Methods of removal include electrocautery, cryotherapy, and chemical (podophyllin or salicylic acid).
   iii. Injection with interferon may also be helpful.
   iv. Best prevention is avoidance of infected tissue.

VII. Influenzae
  a. General
    i. Two types of viruses:
      1. Influenzae A: the cause of epidemic or pandemic influenzae.
        (a) Characterized by envelope glycoproteins known as hemagglutinin (H) and neuraminidase (N).
        (b) Highly infectious and increased rates of disease are noted in institutional settings.
      2. Influenzae B: milder illness.
        (a) Increased incidence in schools and military camps.
  b. Clinical manifestations
    i. Symptoms begin abruptly.
    ii. After a 2–4-day incubation period, present with high fever, headache, photophobia, myalgia, pharyngitis, nonproductive cough, and malaise.
    iii. Physical examination findings are nonspecific.
    iv. Symptoms resolve over 2–5 days.
  c. Diagnosis
    i. Viral culture and antigen detection are available.
  d. Treatment
    i. Symptomatic therapy with fluids, rest, and acetaminophen.
    ii. Three classes of agents used in treatment.

QUESTION

Which of the following malignancies has been linked to the human papillomavirus?

  A. Oral
  B. Esophageal
  C. Cervical
  D. Rectal

---

      1. Tricyclic amines
        (a) Effective in preventing influenzae A in institutional settings.
        (b) CNS side effects include insomnia, anxiety, confusion, and, rarely, seizures.
      2. Nucleoside analog
        (a) Active against both influenzae A and B.
      3. Neuraminidase inhibitors
        (a) Shorten duration of disease if given within the first 48 hours of symptoms.
    iii. Immunization
      1. Best strategy for prevention.
      2. Recommended for those at increased risk for complications or those with increased potential to transmit the disease.
    iv. Complications
      1. Pneumonia
      2. Reye syndrome: secondary to use of aspirin in treatment.
      3. Acute myositis and rhabdomyolysis
      4. *S. aureus* superinfection
      5. Myocarditis and pericarditis
      6. Encephalitis, transverse myelitis, or Guillain-Barré syndrome.

VIII. Mumps
  a. General
    i. Mumps virus is a paramyxovirus.
    ii. Spread via respiratory droplets with humans as the only reservoir.
    iii. Incubation period is 12–25 days.
    iv. Patient infectious from 2 days before to 9 days after the development of parotid swelling.

NOTES

ANSWER C EXPLANATION: *cervical cancer has been linked to exposure and infection with human papillomavirus*

correct ❏   incorrect ❏

b. Clinical manifestations
  i. Rarely have a prodromal period, but may develop fever, myalgias, and headache.
  ii. Parotid pain and swelling are the hallmarks of the disease.
c. Diagnosis
  i. Based on physical findings and culture or serology results.
d. Treatment
  i. Control of symptoms with analgesics and fluids.
  ii. Vaccine given at age 12–15 months with a second dose at age 4–5 years of age.
e. Complications
  i. Orchitis
  ii. Meningoencephalitis
  iii. Deafness
  iv. Arthritis
  v. Pancreatitis
IX. Rabies
  a. General
    i. Virus is a bullet-shaped virus of the rhabdovirus group.
    ii. Acute fatal viral illness of the CNS.
    iii. Transmitted by infected secretions between mammals.
    iv. Human exposure to the disease is through infected dogs, cats, skunks, foxes, wolves, raccoons, bats, and mongooses.
    v. Pathogenesis
      1. Virus enters epidermis through a bite.
      2. Virus replicates in the striated muscle at the site of inoculation.
      3. Enters peripheral nerve and spreads up the nerve to the CNS.
      4. Replicates in the gray matter and then passes centrifugally along autonomic nerves to other tissues.

  b. Clinical manifestations
    i. Begins as a nonspecific illness with fever, headache, malaise, nausea, and vomiting.
    ii. Onset of encephalitis noted with excess motor activity and agitation.
    iii. Hallucinations, combativeness, muscle spasms, meningeal irritation, seizures, and focal paralysis are noted.
    iv. Increased salivation noted due to autonomic nervous system involvement.
    v. Double vision, facial palsies, and difficulty swallowing noted due to brain stem and cranial nerve dysfunction.
    vi. Hydrophobia also noted.
    vii. With onset of symptoms the survival time is 4 days.
  c. Diagnosis
    i. Demonstration of the virus in brain tissue at autopsy.
    ii. Classic finding is Negri bodies.
  d. Treatment
    i. Prevention of disease is the key. Done through immunization of animals.
    ii. Preexposure: prophylaxis immunization.
    iii. Postexposure treatment:
      1. Wound care
      2. Observation of animal for development of signs of rabies.
      3. Treat with vaccine and rabies immune globulin (RIG) if animal suspected to be rabid.
        (a) RIG should be injected into the wound site if possible. If not, then give IM.
X. Roseola
  a. General
    i. Caused by human herpesviruses 6 and 7.
    ii. Occurs in infancy after an incubation period of 10 days.
  b. Clinical manifestations
    i. Present with high fever for 1–4 days.
    ii. During febrile period patient is listless and may have cough, diarrhea, or lymphadenopathy.
    iii. Fever resolves, followed by a maculopapular rash on the face or trunk and rapidly spreads over rest of the body.
    iv. Rash lasts for 2–5 days.

NOTES

c. Diagnosis
    i. Based on clinical findings.
d. Treatment
    i. Symptomatic treatment only.
    ii. Complications include seizures and rare cases of encephalitis.

XI. Rubella
  a. General
    i. Due to a Rubivirus in the Togaviridae family.
    ii. Transmitted via respiratory droplets.
  b. Clinical manifestations
    i. Begins with a sore throat, conjunctivitis, and a low-grade fever.
    ii. On day 2 or 3 the fine macular rash appears on the face and moves downward.
    iii. Fever disappears within 24 hours of the onset of the rash.
    iv. Petechial lesions (Forchheimer's spots) are occasionally noted on the soft palate.
    v. Posterior cervical and occipital lymphadenopathy can be noted.
  c. Diagnosis
    i. Clinical features seldom permit diagnosis.
    ii. IgM antibodies can be detected to confirm diagnosis.
  d. Treatment
    i. There is no specific treatment.
    ii. First dose of immunization given at between 12–15 months of age and the second dose given at age 4–6 years.
    iii. Immunization status must be checked in all pregnant women.
    iv. Complications
      1. Congenital rubella
        (a) Can cause a variety of transient, permanent, and developmental problems.
        (b) The severity of the illness is related to time during gestation fetus was infected.
        (c) Manifestations include low birth weight, hepatosplenomegaly, meningoencephalitis, mental retardation, and congenital anomalies.
      2. Thrombocytopenia purpura
      3. Encephalitis

QUESTION

Which of the following HIV medications has pancreatitis and peripheral neuropathy as common side effects?

    A. Indinavir (Crixivan)
    B. Nevirapine (Viramune)
    C. Didanosine (Videx)
    D. Zidovudine (Retrovir)

XII. Rubeola (Measles)
  a. General
    i. A paramyxovirus that is highly contagious.
    ii. Transmitted by droplets, by person-to-person contact, or airborne spread.
  b. Clinical manifestations
    i. Begins with a fever, irritability, malaise, conjunctivitis, and evidence of a respiratory infection.
    ii. Koplik's spots appear within several days as small, raised white or blue-gray lesions on an erythematous base on the buccal mucosa opposite the upper molar.
    iii. On day 3 or 4 the nonpruritic maculopapular rash begins, starting at the hairline and descending to the trunk and extremities.
      1. See Color Plate 19.
    iv. Fever resolves as the rash appears.
  c. Diagnosis
    i. Based on clinical grounds.
    ii. IgM antibodies can be detected to confirm diagnosis.
  d. Treatment
    i. No specific treatment.
    ii. Large doses of vitamin A have been reported to reduce the severity of the disease.
    iii. Immunization
      1. First dose given at between 12–15 months of age and the second dose given at age 4–6 years.
    iv. Complications
      1. Usually a self-limited disease. Resolving in 7–10 days.

NOTES

ANSWER C EXPLANATION: *The nucleoside reverse transcriptase, didanosine (Videx), has pancreatitis and peripheral neuropathy as common side effects.*

correct ☐   incorrect ☐

2. Complications include pneumonia, bacterial superinfections, otitis media, abnormal liver function tests, post-measles encephalitis, and subacute sclerosing encephalitis.

XIII. Varicella-zoster virus infections
  a. General
    i. Causes chickenpox.
  b. Clinical manifestations
    i. Lesions start as erythematous macules, which become vesicles, then pustules, which crust over.
    ii. The hallmark to diagnose chickenpox is the presence of lesions in various stages.
      1. In smallpox all lesions must be at the same stage of development at a given time.
      2. See Color Plate 20.
    iii. Lesions can be noted on mucous membranes.
    iv. The rash is very pruritic.
  c. Diagnosis
    i. Based on clinical presentation.

  d. Treatment
    i. Treatment is symptomatic.
    ii. Vaccine is given at 12–18 months.
    iii. Can use acyclovir in immunocompromised patients.
    iv. Neonates with perinatal varicella-zoster should be treated with varicella-zoster immune globulin to decrease mortality.
    v. Complications
      1. Herpes zoster (shingles)
        (a) Due to reactivation of latent varicella-zoster virus.
      2. Varicella encephalitis
      3. Cerebellar ataxia
      4. Pneumonia
      5. Bacterial superinfection with group A beta-hemolytic *Streptococcus* or *S. aureus*.

XIV. Other
  a. Herpangina
    i. Caused by coxsackie A virus.
    ii. Note 1–4 mm vesicles on uvula and soft palate.
    iii. Present with fever and sore throat.
    iv. Recover in 1 week.
  b. Hand-foot-and-mouth disease
    i. Caused by coxsackie A16.
    ii. Note small vesicles in anterior part of the mouth and on palms and soles.
    iii. Present with fever and sore throat.
    iv. Recover in 1 week.

XV. See Table 13-11 for summary of viral disease infections.

NOTES

Table 13-11 • Viral Disease Infections

Condition	Agent	Incubation Period (days)	Prodrome	Rash	Complications
Chickenpox	Varicella-zoster	10–21	Rare in children, may present with headache, myalgia, and malaise.	Pruritic, vesicles that crust over starting on the face or trunk and spread to the rest of the body.	Pneumonia, secondary bacterial infections, and encephalitis.
Erythema infectiosum	Parvovirus	12–18	None	Slapped cheeks.	Arthritis and hemolytic anemia
Measles	Paramyxovirus	9–14	Cough, coryza, conjunctivitis, and fever.	Confluent, erythematous rash starting at the head and moving caudally.	Meningoencephalitis, pneumonia, otitis media, and laryngotracheitis.
Mumps	Paramyxovirus	12–25	Rare, can have fever, myalgia, and headache.	None	Orchitis, deafness
Roseola	Human herpes virus 6	10–14	Fever	Maculopapular rash on the face or trunk with spread over rest of body.	Febrile seizures
Rubella	Togavirus	14–21	Rare, but may have cough, coryza, and lymphadenopathy.	Erythematous, maculopapular rash starting on the face and then moving peripherally.	Encephalitis and thrombocytopenia

NOTES

Question 1

Which of the following physical examination findings is typically noted in patients with diphtheria?

A. Papular rash on the trunk
B. Supraclavicular nodes
C. Pharyngeal pseudomembrane
D. Splenomegaly

Question 2

A 3-year-old presents with nocturnal anal itching. Which of the following is the best test to aid in the diagnosis of this patient?

A. Stool for ova and parasite
B. Fecal white blood cell count
C. Eosinophil count
D. Cellulose tape test

Question 3

A 25-year-old patient with AIDS presents with fever, non-productive cough, and worsening shortness of breath. On chest x-ray diffuse bilateral interstitial infiltrates are noted. Which of the following is the most likely diagnosis?

A. Aspergillus pneumonia
B. Pneumococcal pneumonia
C. Tuberculosis
D. Pneumocystic pneumonia

Question 4

A 4 year-old presents with a four day history of fever, irritability, and cough. On examination small, irregular, grayish-white lesions on the upper buccal mucosa and a maculopapular rash is noted in the hairline. What is the next best step in the management of this patient?

A. Large dose Vitamin C
B. Prophylactic antibiotics
C. Antipyretics and analgesics
D. Active immunization

Question 5

A 20-year-old female presents with vaginal itching and thick discharge. On physical examination the vaginal mucosa is inflamed and patches of white material are noted on the vaginal walls. Which of the following is the best treatment option for this patient?

A. Nystatin
B. Metronidazole
C. Clindamycin
D. Acyclovir

Question 6

The first dose of measles, mumps, and rubella (MMR) vaccine is typically given at what age?

A. Birth
B. 2 months
C. 12 months
D. 24 months

NOTES

Question 7

A 40-year-old patient who returned from Japan 4 months ago presents with abdominal pain and diarrhea. Stool cultures are negative. Ova and parasite study reveal bile stained eggs and proglottids. Which of the following is the most likely infectious agent?

    A. Taenia solium

    B. Ascaris lumbricoides

    C. Necator americanus

    D. Diphyllobothrium latum

Answer 1

ANSWER **C** EXPLANATION: *Diphtheria presents with fever, malaise, and sore throat. On physical examination a grayish pseudomembrane that bleeds easily on attempted removal is noted.*

Topic: Diphtheria

correct ☐   incorrect ☐

Answer 2

ANSWER **D** EXPLANATION: *Pinworms, or Enterobius vermicularis, presents with severe perianal itching. Diagnosis is made by observing ovoid eggs under the microscope with the cellophane tape test.*

Topic: Pinworm

correct ☐   incorrect ☐

Answer 3

ANSWER **D** EXPLANATION: *Pneumocystic pneumonia is most commonly noted in AIDS patients and presents with fever, non-productive cough, and dyspnea. Chest x-ray may be normal or reveal diffuse bilateral interstitial infiltrates.*

Topic: Pneumocystis

correct ☐   incorrect ☐

Answer 4

ANSWER **C** EXPLANATION: *Rubeola (measles) presents with fever, irritability, malaise, and cough. Within days small, raised white or blue gray lesions appear on a red base in the buccal mucosa, opposite the upper molars, called Koplik's spots. Later the maculopapular rash appears on the hairline and then the trunk.*

Topic: Rubeola

correct ☐   incorrect ☐

Answer 5

ANSWER **A** EXPLANATION: *Candida infection of the vagina presents with an inflamed vaginal mucosa and white vaginal discharge. Treatment consists of antifungal agents, such as nystatin.*

Topic: Candidiasis

correct ☐   incorrect ☐

NOTES

Answer 6

ANSWER C EXPLANATION: *Measles, mumps, and rubella (MMR) vaccine is first given at age 12-15 months and repeated at age 4-6 years.*

Topic: Measles/Mumps/Rubella

correct ☐   **incorrect** ☐

Answer 7

ANSWER D EXPLANATION: *The tapeworm, Diphyllobothrium latum (Fish tapeworm), is more commonly noted in Asia and Japan and due to consumption of raw seafood/fish. Diagnosis is made by noting bile stained eggs and proglottids on examination of the stool.*

Topic: Tapeworms

correct ☐   **incorrect** ☐

NOTES

Appendix 1
Pediatric Milestones

Table A1-1 • Language Screening in Pediatrics		
Age (Years)	Speech Production	Command Following
1	1–3 words	1-step commands
2	2–3 word phrases	2-step commands
3	Routine sentence use	
4	Routine sentence use and give and take with conversation	
5	Complex sentences	

Table A1-2 • Developmental Milestones		
Age	Gross Motor	Visual Motor
1 month	Raises head slightly from prone Lifts chin up	Tight grasp, follow to midline
2 months	Lifts chest off table	Follows objects past midline
3 months	Supports self on forearms in prone, holds head up steadily	Follows in a circular pattern
6 months	Sits well unsupported	Reaches with either hand, grasp
9 months	Creeps and crawls Pulls to stand	Use pincer grasp, holds bottle, finger feeds
12 months	Walks alone	Throws objects, lets go of objects
18 months	Runs, throws toy without falling	Turns 2–3 pages, fills spoon and feeds self
24 months	Walks up and down stairs without assistance	Turns page one at a time, removes clothes
36 months	Pedals tricycle, alternates feet when going up stairs	Partially dresses and undresses, draws a circle
4 years	Hops, skips, alternates feet when going down stairs	Buttons clothes, catches ball
5 years	Skips, jumps over low objects	Ties shoes, spreads with knife

Appendix 2
Common Signs in Medicine

Sign	Clinical Indication	Description
Babinski	Pyramidal tract involvement	Extension of great toe and abduction of other toes with plantar stimulation.
Barlow	Congenital hip dislocation	Click of femoral head with bringing hip into mid-abduction with posterior and lateral pressure while infant supine and hips flexed 90 degrees.
Battle	Base of skull fracture	Postauricular ecchymosis
Biot	Increased intracranial pressure	Abnormal breathing with periods of apnea and periods of several breaths of similar volumes.
Brudzinski	Meningitis	With passive flexion of the leg on one side, movement occurs in the opposite leg.
Bulge	Knee joint effusion	Bulge in the hollow medial hollow to the patella after milking the knee and pressing the knee behind the lateral margin of the patella.
Chadwick	Pregnancy	Bluish discoloration of the cervix and vagina.
Chvostek	Tetany	Spasm of the orbicular oculi or oris with tapping of facial nerve.
Courvoisier	Pancreatic cancer	Palpable gallbladder in a jaundiced patient.
Cullen	Ruptured ectopic pregnancy Hemorrhagic pancreatitis	Periumbilical darkening of skin from blood.
Drawer	Cruciate ligament injury	Forward or backward sliding of the tibia under applied stress.
Gower	Muscular dystrophy	Use of limb muscles to assume an upright sitting position.
Grey Turner	Hemorrhagic pancreatitis	Local areas of discoloration in the region of the loins.
Hegar	Early pregnancy	Softening and compressibility of the lower segment of the uterus
Homans	Deep venous thrombosis	Pain in calf with dorsiflexion of the ankle, with the knee bent.
Impingement	Rotator cuff tendinitis	Pain with provocative physical examination maneuvers.
Kernig	Meningitis	Incomplete extension of the leg on the thigh when patient supine and the thigh flexed to a right angle with the axis of the trunk.
Lasègue	Lumbar nerve irritation Sciatic nerve irritation	Pain or spasms in the posterior thigh with hip flexed and knee extended, and ankle dorsiflexed, while patient supine.
Lhermitte	Multiple sclerosis Cervical spinal cord injury	Sudden electric-like shocks extending down spine when flexing the neck.

Sign	Clinical Indication	Description
McBurney	Appendicitis	Tenderness at site two-thirds of the distance between umbilicus and anterior superior iliac spine.
Murphy	Acute cholecystitis	Pain on palpation in right upper quadrant with inspiration.
Obturator	Appendicitis	Pain in right hypogastric region with flexion of right leg at the hip with the knee bent and internally rotated.
Ortolani	Congenital hip dysplasia	Snapping with relocation of a dislocated femoral hip.
Phalen	Carpal tunnel syndrome	Pain with wrist flexion.
Psoas	Appendicitis	Pain with flexion of leg against resistance.
Romberg	Cerebellar dysfunction	Unsteadiness with closing of eyes in patient standing with feet approximated.
Rovsing	Appendicitis	Pain at McBurney's point with pressure over descending colon.
Russell	Bulimia	Abrasions and scars on back of hands and fingers due to self-induced vomiting.
Snellen	Graves disease	Bruit heard on auscultation over the eye.
String	Pyloric stenosis	Narrowed pyloric canal on abdominal X-ray.
Tinel	Carpal tunnel syndrome	Sensation of tingling with percussion over medial nerve.
Trendelenburg	Congenital hip dislocation Hip abductor weakness	Sagging of pelvis on the side opposite the affected side during single leg stance on the affected side.
Trousseau	Tetany	Carpopedal spasm when upper arm is compressed.
Westermark	Pulmonary embolism	Decreased lung markings from oligemia.
Wrist	Marfan syndrome	Overlapping of thumb and fifth finger when the wrist is gripped with the opposite hand.

Appendix 3
Common Dermatomes

Dermatome	Location
C3	Front and back of neck
C6	Thumb
C8	Ring and little finger
T4	Nipples
T10	Umbilicus
S1	Heel
S5	Perianal
L1	Inguinal
L3	Knee
L5	Anterior ankle and foot

Appendix 4
Cranial Nerves and Function

Number	Nerve	Function
I	Olfactory	Sense of smell
II	Optic	Visual acuity
III	Oculomotor	Pupillary constriction Elevation of upper eyelid Extraocular movements
IV	Trochlear	Downward, inward eye movement
V	Abducens	Lateral deviation of the eye
VI	Trigeminal	Motor: Temporal and masseter muscles Lateral movement of the jaw Sensory: Facial, three divisions: • Ophthalmic • Maxillary • Mandibular
VII	Facial	Motor: Muscles of the face Sensory: Taste anterior two-thirds of tongue
VIII	Auditory	Hearing and balance
IX	Glossopharyngeal	Sensory: Posterior tongue, including taste Motor: Pharynx
X	Vagus	Motor: Palate, pharynx, and larynx Sensory: Pharynx and larynx
XI	Spinal accessory	Motor to sternomastoid and upper trapezius
XII	Hypoglossal	Motor to tongue

Appendix 5
Apgar Scoring[a]

	Sign	0	1	2
A	Activity (Muscle tone)	Absent	Arms/legs flexed	Active movement
P	Pulse (bpm)	Absent	<100	>100
G	Grimace (Irritability)	No response	Grimace	Coughs, pulls away
A	Appearance (Skin color)	Pale all over	Pink, except extremities	Pink all over
R	Respirations	Absent	Slow	Good, crying

[a]Measure at 1 minute and 5 minutes after birth.
Scores:
7–10 Normal
4–7 Possible resuscitation
≤3 Immediate resuscitation needed

Appendix 6
Poisoning Antidotes

Poison	Antidote
Acetaminophen	N-acetylcysteine
Arsenic	Dimercaptosuccinic acid
Atropine	Physostigmine
Carbon monoxide	Oxygen
Cyanide	Amyl nitrite
Ethylene glycol	Ethyl alcohol
Gold	Dimercaptosuccinic acid
Iron	Deferoxamine
Lead	Calcium disodium edetate
Mercury	Dimercaptosuccinic acid
Methyl alcohol	Ethyl alcohol
Nitrites	Methylene blue
Opiates	Naloxone
Organophosphates	Pralidoxime

Appendix 7
Secondary Prevention of Common Cancers in Average-Risk Patients

Cancer Location	Method of Detection	Onset of Screening (Years)	Frequency of Screening
Skin	Cancer related check-up		Routine
Oral	Cancer related check-up		Routine
Thyroid	Cancer related check-up		Routine
Lymph node	Cancer related check-up		Routine
Breast	Mammogram Breast exam	40 years of age 20 years of age	Every 1–2 years Monthly
Cervix	Pap smear	21 years of age or within 3 years of onset of sexual activity.	Yearly
Ovarian	CA-125	Postmenopause	
Prostate	Digital rectal exam PSA	50 years of age 50 years of age	Yearly Yearly
Testicular	Self-testicular exam Cancer-related check-up	18 years of age	Monthly Routine
Colon	Fecal occult blood Sigmoidoscopy and digital rectal exam	50 years of age 50 years of age	Yearly Every 5 years

Appendix 8
Normal Laboratory Values

Hematology and Coagulation	
Test	**Normal Range**
Antithrombin III	22–39 mg/dL
Bleeding time	2–10 min
CBC	
White blood cell count	$5.0–10.5 \times 10^3/\mu L$
Red blood cell count	$4.5–5.5 \times 10^6/mm^3$
Hemoglobin	Female 12–14 g/dL
	Male 14–16 g/dL
Hematocrit	Female 36–42%
	Male 42–48%
MCV	80–100 fl
MCH	26–34 pg/cell
MCHC	31–36 g/dL
Platelet count	$150–350 \times 10^9/L$
Differential	
Neutrophils	40–70%
Bands	1–10%
Lymphocytes	25–45%
Monocytes	4–10%
Eosinophils	0–8%
Basophils	0–2%
D-Dimer	<0.5 mg/L
Eosinophil count	40–500/μL
Erythrocyte sedimentation rate	0–20 mm/hr
Ferritin	30–300 ng/mL
Fibrinogen degradation products	<2.5 mg/L
Fibrinogen	150–400 mg/dL
Folate	3.0–17.0 ng/mL
Haptoglobin	15–200 mg/dL
Hemoglobin electrophoresis	
Hemoglobin A	95–98%
Hemoglobin A_2	1.5–3.5%
Hemoglobin F	0–2%
Other	Absent
Iron	30–160 μg/dL

Test	Normal Range
Iron binding capacity	225–430 μg/dL
Partial thromboplastin time	22–35 sec
Prothrombin time	11–13 sec
Reticulocyte count	0.5–1.5 %
Sickle cell test	Negative
Thrombin time	16–25 sec
Transferrin	190–375 mg/dL
Vitamin B12	125–250 pg/mL

Immunology

Test	Normal Range
Anti-ds DNA	Negative at 1:10
Antinuclear antibody	Negative at 1:40
C-reactive protein	0.08–3.0 mg/L
Immunoglobulins 　IgA 　IgE 　IgG 　IgM	 60–310 mg/dL 10–180 IU/mL 615–1300 mg/dL 55–330 mg/dL
Rheumatoid factor	<30 IU/mL
Serum protein electrophoresis 　Albumin 　Globulin 　Alpha 1 　Alpha 2 　Gamma	 3.5–5.5 g/dL 2.0–3.5 g/dL 0.2–0.4 g/dL 0.5–0.9 g/dL 0.7–1.7 g/dL

Toxicology

Test	Therapeutic Range	Toxic Range
Acetaminophen	10–30 μg/mL	>200 μg/mL
Digoxin	0.8–2.0 ng/mL	>2.5 ng/mL
Ethanol	—	>20 mg/dL
Lithium	0.6–1.3 mEq/L	>2 mEq/L
Phenobarbital	10–40 μg/mL	>65 μg/mL
Phenytoin	10–20 μg/mL	>20 μg/mL
Salicylates	150–300 μg/mL	>300 μg/mL
Theophylline	8–20 μg/mL	>20 μg/mL

Lipid Classification	
Test	**Interpretation**
LDL cholesterol	
<100	Optimal
100–129	Above normal
130–159	Borderline high
160–189	High
190	Very high
Total cholesterol	
<200	Desirable
200–239	Borderline high
240	High
HDL cholesterol	
<40	Low
60	High

Chemistry	
Test	**Normal Range**
Acetoacetate	<1 mg/dL
Adrenocorticotropin (ACTH)	6.0–76.0 pg/mL
Albumin	3.5–5.5 g/dL
Aldosterone	2–9 ng/dL
Alkaline phosphatase	30–120 U/L
Alpha-1-antitrypsin	85–213 mg/dL
Alpha-fetoprotein	<15 ng/mL
ALT	0–40 U/L
Ammonia	10–80 µg/dL
Amylase	60–180 U/L
Angiotensin-converting enzyme	<40 U/L
Anion gap	7–16 mmol/L
Arterial blood gases	
pH	7.38–7.44
pCO_2	35–45 mmHg
pO_2	80–100 mmHg
Bicarbonate	21–30 mEq/L
Oxygen saturation	>95%
AST	0–40 U/L
Beta-human chorionic gonadotropin	<5 mIU/mL
Beta-hydroxybutyrate	<3 mg/dL

Test	Normal Range
Bilirubin	
Total	0.3–1.0 mg/dL
Direct	0.1–0.3 mg/dL
Indirect	0.2–0.7 mg/dL
Blood urea nitrogen	5–20 mg/dL
Brain natriuretic peptide (BNP)	<167 pg/mL
Calcium, ionized	1.1–1.4 mmol/L
Calcium	8.5–10.5 mg/dL
Carbon dioxide	21–30 mEq/L
Carcinoembryonic antigen (CEA)	0.0–3.4 ng/mL
Ceruloplasmin	27–37 ng/dL
Chloride	98–106 mEq/L
Cortisol	5–25 µg/dL
C-peptide	0.5–2.0 ng/mL
Creatine kinase, total (CK)	40–200 U/L
CK-MB	0–7 ng/mL
Creatinine	0.5–1.5 mg/dL
Creatinine clearance (Cl_{cr})	90–140 mL/min/1.73 m^2 BSA
Ferritin	15–200 ng/mL
Follicle-stimulating hormone (FSH)	
Female	
Follicular phase	3.0–20.0 U/L
Ovulatory phase	9.0–26.0 U/L
Luteal phase	1.0–12.0 U/L
Postmenopausal	18.0–153.0 U/L
Male	1.0–12.0 U/L
Gamma glutamyltransferase	5–95 U/L
Gastrin	<100 pg/mL
Glucose	65–110 mg/dL
Growth hormone	0.5–17.0 ng/mL
Hemoglobin A$_1$C	3.8–6.4%
Insulin	6–35 µU/mL
Iron	30–160 µg/dL
Iron binding capacity	225–430 µg/dL
Percent saturation	20–45%
Ketone (acetone)	Negative

Test	Normal Range
Lactate dehydrogenase	100–190 U/L
Lactate	5–15 mg/dL
Lead	
Children	<25 µg/mL
Adult	<40 µg/mL
Lipase	0–160 U/L
Luteinizing hormone (LH)	
Female	
Follicular phase	2.0–15.0 I/L
Ovulatory phase	22.0–105.0 U/L
Luteal phase	0.6–19.0 U/L
Postmenopausal	16.0–64.0 U/L
Male	2.0–12.0 U/L
Magnesium	1.8–3.0 mg/dL
Osmolality	
Plasma	285–295 mOsmol/kg
Urine	300–900 mOsmol/kg
Parathyroid hormone	10–60 pg/mL
Phosphorus	3.0–4.5 mg/dL
Potassium	3.5–5.5 mEq/L
Progesterone	
Female	
Follicular phase	<1.0 ng/mL
Mid-luteal	3–20 ng/mL
Male	<1.0 ng/mL
Prolactin	
Female	2.0–26 ng/mL
Male	1.6–23 ng/mL
Prostate-specific antigen (PSA)	
Female	<0.5 ng/mL
Male <40 yr	0.0–2.0 ng/mL
Male >40 yr	0.0–4.0 ng/mL
Sodium	135–145 mEq/L
Testosterone	
Female	5–85 ng/dL
Male	270–1050 ng/dL
Thyroid stimulating hormone	0.5–4.5 µU/mL
Thyroxine (T_4)	4.5–10.5 µg/dL
Triiodothyronine (T_3)	60–180 ng/dL
Thyroxine, free (FT_4)	0.8–2.7 ng/dL

Test	Normal Range
Total protein	5.5–8.0 g/dL
Transferrin	230–390 mg/dL
Triglycerides	<160 mg/dL
Troponin I	0.0–0.4 ng/mL
Uric acid	1.5–7.0 mg/dL

Test Taking Strategies

THE EXAMINATION

The PANCE and PANRE are developed by the National Commission on the Certification of Physician Assistants (NCCPA). The exam questions are developed by committees comprised of physician assistants and physicians. The committee members are selected based on the area of expertise, geographic location, and test writing skills.

Each test item goes through multiple levels of review before being placed on the exam for pre-testing. Every NCCPA exam contains questions that are scored and others being pre-tested. The examinee has no way of knowing which item is being scored and which are being pre-tested. The examinee should treat each question as if it is being scored.

A number of different versions of the exam are used during each examination block. When the exam is scored, candidates are given one point for every correct answer and zero points for incorrect answers to produce the raw exam score. This is why you should answer each question; there is no penalty for guessing. After the raw score has been calculated by two different computer systems the raw score is used to calculate the examinees proficiency measure. The proficiency measure is based on item difficulty and the number of correct responses. This process assures that all proficiency measures are calculated as if each student took the same exam.

This proficiency measure is then converted to a scaled score so that results can be compared over time and between different groups of examinees. Scores are scaled so that the average score is 500 with a standard deviation of 100. Most scores are in the range of 200 to 800.

The PANCE and PANRE examinations have the following breakdown of tasks, which make up the corresponding percent of the total examination questions:

Task	Percent of Exam
History taking and performing physical examination	16%
Using laboratory and diagnostic studies	14%
Formulating most likely diagnosis	18%
Health maintenance	10%
Clinical intervention	14%
Pharmaceutical therapeutics	18%
Applying basic science concepts	10%

Each of the task areas are defined by the NCCPA. The history taking and performing physical examination area assesses the test takers knowledge in the areas of pertinent historical information, signs, symptoms, and physical examination findings associated with medical conditions, risk factors for selected medical conditions, and physical examination techniques.

The using laboratory and diagnostic studies area assesses the test takers knowledge in the areas of indications for initial and subsequent diagnostic and laboratory studies, relevance of common screening tests, diagnostic studies and procedural risk factors, and the selecting and interpreting appropriate diagnostic and laboratory studies.

The formulating the most likely diagnosis area assesses the test takers knowledge in the areas of the significance of history, physical examination findings, and diagnostic and laboratory studies as they relate to formulating a diagnosis.

The health maintenance area assesses the test takers knowledge in the areas of epidemiology of selected medical conditions, early detection and prevention of

NOTES

selected medical conditions, patient education, prevention of communicable diseases, immunizations, human sexuality, and barriers to care.

The clinical intervention area assesses the test takers knowledge in the areas of management and treatment of selected medical conditions, follow-up and monitoring of therapeutic regimens, indications, contraindications, complications, risks, and benefits of selected procedures, end-of-life issues, and the risks and benefits of alternative medicine.

The pharmaceutical therapeutics area assesses the test takers knowledge in the areas of mechanisms of action, indications for use, contraindications, side effects, adverse reactions, drug interactions, drug toxicity, and selecting appropriate pharmacologic therapy for selected medical conditions.

The applying of basic science concepts area assesses the test takers knowledge in the areas of human anatomy, physiology, pathophysiology, microbiology, and biochemistry.

The approximate percentage of questions based on each organ system is noted below.

Organ System	Percent of Exam
Cardiovascular	16%
Pulmonary	12%
Gastrointestinal/Nutritional	10%
Musculoskeletal	10%
Eyes, ears, Nose, and Throat	9%
Reproductive	8%
Endocrine	6%
Genitourinary	6%
Neurologic system	6%
Psychiatry/Behavioral	6%
Dermatologic	5%
Hematologic	3%
Infectious disease	3%

See the NCCPA web site (*www.nccpa.net*) for complete details on task areas and organ system information related to the exam.

Testing Taking Strategies

You have been preparing for this exam since the start of PA school or through all the years of clinical practice. Now is the time to focus on the exam.

BEFORE THE EXAM

- Take a refresher course that offers sample testing. See the AAPA web site (*www.aapa.org*) for a list of current board review courses.
- Set up a schedule to study for the exam.
- It is better to study 1-2 hours per day for one month prior to the exam, than to try and study 12 hours per day just a few days prior to the exam.
- See below for sample 31-day and 15-day studying schedule.
- Practice as many sample questions as possible before the exam.
  - Questions must match the types seen on the exam.
- Design your review schedule to follow the organ systems as noted above.
- If time is limited, review and study for the systems that make up the largest part of the exam.
- Remember that the exam is primary care focused.
- Review the NCCPA web site for sample questions and to familiarize yourself with the exam format.
- Remember to register for the exam on time, make sure you know the location of the testing center, and arrive at the testing center at least 30 minutes prior to your exam time.
- Review the exam policies and procedures on the NCCPA web site.

DAY OF THE EXAM

- Get plenty of rest the night before.
- Eat before the exam, but not a large meal since it may make you sleepy.
- Dress in layers so that you can adjust to the temperature in the room.
- Remember your admission card and identification.

NOTES

- No personal belongings are allowed in the testing room.
- Test anxiety strategies
- Being well prepared is the best way to reduce anxiety.
- Space out your studying.

Maintain a positive attitude

- Write down important facts, formulas, facts etc, on the laminated noteboard supplied by the testing center prior to starting the exam.
- Do not worry about how fast others are completing the exam. They may not even be taking the PANCE or PANRE examinations.

- The PANCE exam is a six-hour exam consisting of 360 multiple-choice questions.
- The PANRE exam is a five-hour exam consisting of 300 multiple-choice questions.

DURING THE EXAM

- Read directions carefully and complete computer tutorial.
- Pace yourself to avoid rushing at the end of the exam.
- Answer all items. Mark the questions you are not sure of to review once you have completed the exam.

Table 1-31 • Day Sample Study Schedule

Day 1	Day 2	Day 3	Day 4	Day 5	Day 6	Day 7
Take sample test	Cardiovascular review-2 hours	Cardiovascular review-2 hours	Cardiovascular review-2 hours	Cardiovascular review-2 hours	EKG review-2 hours	Pulmonary review-2hours
Day 8	**Day 9**	**Day 10**	**Day 11**	**Day 12**	**Day 13**	**Day 14**
Pulmonary review-2 hours	Pulmonary - review- 2 hours	Pulmonary- review- 2 hours	Gastrointestinal review-2.5 hours	Gastrointestinal review-2.5 hours	Musculoskeletal review-2.5 hours	Musculoskeletal review-2.5 hours
Day 15	**Day 16**	**Day 17**	**Day 18**	**Day 19**	**Day 20**	**Day 21**
Take day off.	Eyes, ears, nose, and throat review-2 hours	Eyes, ears, nose, and throat review-2hours	Reproductive review-2 hours	Reproductive review-2 hours	Endocrine review-2 hours	Genitourinary review-2 hours
Day 22	**Day 23**	**Day 24**	**Day 25**	**Day 26**	**Day 27**	**Day 28**
Genitourinary review-2 hours	Take day off.	Neurology review- 2 hours	Neurology review- 2 hours	Psychiatry review-2 hours	Psychiatry review-2 hours	Dermatology review-2 hours
Day 29	**Day 30**	**Day 31**				
Hematology review-2 hours	Infectious disease review-2 hours	Take sample test				

NOTES

- Do not change answers unless you are sure you marked the answer wrong.
- Remember the exam is professionally written and the test writers are not out to trick you.
- Multiple choice question strategies
- Read the question carefully and try to answer it before looking at the choices.

- Read all the choices before answering the question.
- Answer all questions; there is no penalty for guessing.

AFTER THE EXAM

Relax and celebrate.

Table 2. 15-Day Sample Study Schedule

Day 1	Day 2	Day 3	Day 4	Day 5	Day 6	Day 7
Take sample test	Cardiology review-4 hours	Pulmonary review-3 hours	Gastrointestinal review-3 hours	Musculoskeletal review-3 hours	Eyes, ears, nose and throat review-3 hours	Reproductive review-3.5 hours
Day 8	**Day 9**	**Day 10**	**Day 11**	**Day 12**	**Day 13**	**Day 14**
Endocrine review-2 hours	Genitourinary review-3 hours	Neurology review-2.5 hours	Psychiatry review-2.5 hours	Dermatology review-2.5 hours	Hematology review-2 hours	Infectious disease review-2.5 hours
Day 15						
Take sample test						

NOTES

Subject index